Frontiers in Natural Product Chemistry

(Volume 11)

Edited by

Shazia Anjum
Institute of Chemistry
The Islamia University of Bahawalpur
Pakistan

Frontiers in Natural Product Chemistry

(Volume 11)

Editor: Shazia Anjum

ISSN (Online): 2212-3997

ISSN (Print): 1574-0897

ISBN (Online): 978-981-5136-59-3

ISBN (Print): 978-981-5136-60-9

ISBN (Paperback): 978-981-5136-61-6

First published in 2023.

need for a court order if at any point you breach any terms of this License Agreement. In no event will any delay or failure by Bentham Science Publishers in enforcing your compliance with this License Agreement constitute a waiver of any of its rights.

3. You acknowledge that you have read this License Agreement, and agree to be bound by its terms and conditions. To the extent that any other terms and conditions presented on any website of Bentham Science Publishers conflict with, or are inconsistent with, the terms and conditions set out in this License Agreement, you acknowledge that the terms and conditions set out in this License Agreement shall prevail.

Bentham Science Publishers Pte. Ltd.
80 Robinson Road #02-00
Singapore 068898
Singapore
Email: subscriptions@benthamscience.net

BENTHAM SCIENCE

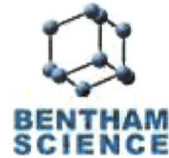

CONTENTS

PREFACE

The 11ᵗʰ volume of **Frontiers in Natural Product Chemistry** maintains the tradition of publishing updated knowledge on the subject. Leading scientists contributed 05 extensive book chapters in this volume including advanced methods of isolation, syntheses, computational studies and SARs. Each chapter bears a uniqueness that will definitely attract readers' and postgraduate students' attention.

For instance, in Chapter 01, Kumar *et al.* discussed the medicinal importance of Turmeric (*Curcuma Longa*)- a blessed plant and its phytochemicals that have diverse medicinal properties.

While Öneri and Çolak reviewed some novel natural compounds for hepatocellular carcinoma treatment. The authors have discussed the effect of these natural compounds on the genetic hallmarks of various signaling pathways and important cellular metabolism molecules of hepatocellular carcinoma.

Shivakumar *et al.* in Chapter 03, explained the prevention of overexploited herbs for balancing a sustainable ecosystem. It has been emphasized that in the Ayurvedic system of medicine, there is an in-depth biochemical classification of herbs, based on which substitutes can be deduced. Moreover, ancient texts also describe alternate herbs for some key ingredients.

Microbial control is an ever-increasing economic burden that is disturbing human beings and as well as animals. Radhakrishnan and Benny, in Chapter 04, discussed the over-smartness of bacteria by forming some biofilms as safety walls for their existence. Therefore, the multi-drug resistance of bacterial biofilm has constantly challenged the existing anti-bacterial drugs. This chapter deals with a few methods by which biofilm inhibition can be achieved by making use of various synthetic and natural compounds.

The updated review on quercetin chemistry, its structural modifications, SARs and therapeutic applications by Banday *et al.* can be found in Chapter 05. Quercetin is a naturally occurring flavone with tremendous medicinal potential and it has a wider scope in medicines as evidenced from this chapter.

It is hoped that this volume will be thought-provoking and trigger further research in the quest for new and novel natural therapies. I am indebted for the great efforts of the entire editorial team, especially Mr. Mahmood Alam (Director Publications) and Ms. Asma Ahmed (Editorial Manager Publications) at Bentham Science Publishers.

Shazia Anjum
Dean, Faculty of Chemical & Biological Science
The Islamia University of Bahawalpur
Pakistan

List of Contributors

Arun Shivakumar	Dubai Science Park, Al Barsha, Himalaya Global Research Center FZ LLC, Dubai, UAE
Atul Namdeorao Jadhav	Himalaya Wellness Company, Bengaluru, Research and Development Cente, Karnataka, India
Ashok Bast Krishnaiah	Himalaya Wellness Company, Bengaluru, Research and Development Cente, Karnataka, India
Anjitha Theres Benny	Department of Chemistry, School of Advanced Science, VIT, Vellore, Tamil Nadu-632014, India
Archana	Department of Morphology and Physiology, Karaganda Medical University, Karaganda-100008, Kazakhstan
Çağrı ÖNER	Medical Faculty, Department of Medical Biology and Genetics, Maltepe University, İstanbul, Turkey
Emine ÇOLAK	Medical Faculty, Department of Medical Biology, Eskişehir Osmangazi University, Eskişehir, Turkey
Ethiraj Kannatt Radhakrishnan	Department of Chemistry, School of Advanced Science, VIT, Vellore, Tamil Nadu-632014, India
Mudasir Maqbool	Pharmacy Practice Division, Department of Pharmaceutical Sciences, University of Kashmir, Hazratbal, Srinagar, 190006, Kashmir, India
Nazia Banday	Pharmacognosy and Phytochemistry Lab, Department of Pharmaceutical Sciences, University of Kashmir, Hazratbal, Srinagar-190006, Kashmir, India
Nyira Shafi	Pharmacology Division, Department of Pharmaceutical Science, University of Kashmir, Hazratbal, Srinagar, 190006, Kashmir, India
Punit Kumar	Department of Biological Sciences & Bioengineering, Indian Institute of Technology Kanpur, Uttar Pradesh-208016, India
Prince Ahad Mir	Khalsa College of Pharmacy, G.T. Road, Amritsar-143002 Punjab, India
Rangesh Paramesh	Manal Family Office Holdings Ltd, Dubai International Financial Centre, Dubai, UAE
Rafia Jan	Defence Research and Development Organization (DRDO), Hospital, Khonmoh, Srinagar, 190001, Jammu & Kashmir, India
Rooh Mohi-ud-din	Pharmacognosy and Phytochemistry Lab, Department of Pharmaceutical Sciences, University of Kashmir, Hazratbal, Srinagar-190006, Kashmir, India Sher-I-Kashmir Institute of Medical Sciences, Soura, Srinagar, Jammu, and Kashmir, India
Reyaz Hassan Mir	Pharmaceutical Chemistry Division, Chandigarh College of Pharmacy, Landran, Punjab-140301, India Pharmaceutical Chemistry Division, Department of Pharmaceutical Sciences, University of Kashmir, Srinagar-190006, Kashmir, India
Sujata	Department of Electronics and Communication Engineering, Kashi Institute of Technology Varanasi, Uttar Pradesh-221307, India

CHAPTER 1

Medicinal Importance of Turmeric (*Curcuma Longa*) and its Natural Products

Punit Kumar[3,*], Sujata[1] and Archana[2]

[1] *Department of Biological Sciences & Bioengineering, Indian Institute of Technology Kanpur, Uttar Pradesh-208016, India*

[2] *Department of Electronics and Communication Engineering, Kashi Institute of Technology Varanasi, Uttar Pradesh-221307, India*

[3] *Department of Morphology and Physiology, Karaganda Medical University, Karaganda-100008, Kazakhstan*

Abstract: It is believed that natural products exhibiting medicinal benefits do not cause systemic side effects or they cause acceptable side effects. Due to the increase in research output and increased awareness about the importance of natural products, nowadays, a large fraction of the population is now shifting their orientation towards the use of natural products in daily use. Turmeric (*Curcuma longa*) is one such blessing for all of us. It is one of the most important and abundant spices used in Asian food. It is cultivated around the world and originated in India, Indonesia, and Southeast Asia. Turmeric powder has a bitter, sharp taste and is yellow. It is used to provide color and flavor to various food products such as; butter, mustard, cheese, *etc.* Turmeric belongs to the Zingiberaceae family. It is one of the most commonly used medicinal herbs in India and China and is used for the treatment of jaundice and liver problems. Turmeric is known to have a wide range of pharmacological properties such as anti-microbial, anti-protozoal, anti-malarial, anti-venom, anti-proliferative, anti-aging, anti-inflammatory, anti-tumor, *etc.* It is identified that the yellow color of the turmeric is due to the presence of Curcumin which is the most important and potent bioactive compound of turmeric. Curcumin is a curcuminoid that is extracted from the rhizomes of *Curcuma Longa*. Curcumin possesses remarkable medicinal properties and can also be used in cosmetic products. Curcumin has powerful anti-inflammatory and antioxidant properties. It helps to treat various diseases, some of them are; hay fever, depression, Alzheimer's, treat cholesterol, itching, and osteoarthritis. It is involved in maintaining the functioning of the brain and reduces the risk of brain and heart diseases. Investigators are focusing to find out the therapeutic role of curcumin in asthma, diabetes, cancer, indigestion, and many other disorders. In this chapter, we will discuss the natural compounds present in turmeric and their medicinal importance.

* **Corresponding author Punit Kumar:** Department of Morphology and Physiology, Karaganda Medical University, Karaganda-100008, Kazakhstan; E-mail: punitdariyapur@gmail.com

Shazia Anjum (Ed.)

Keywords: Anti-inflammatory Activities, Anticancer Activities, Antioxidant Activities, Cardioprotective Protective Properties, *Curcuma longa*, Curcumin, Curcuminoids, Medicinal Herbs, Natural Products, Turmeric.

INTRODUCTION

Natural products are the type of compounds that are produced by living organisms (microbes, animals, plants, *etc.*). These compounds comprise all chemical compounds or substances found in nature and are called natural products if they are produced by a living organism [1]. Natural products may be classified according to their chemical property, biological function, biosynthetic pathway, or source. The estimated number of known natural products around the world is about 326,000 [2]. Natural products may be extracted from the cells, tissues, and secretions of microorganisms, plants, and animals. A crude (unfractionated) extract from any one of these sources will contain a range of structurally diverse and often novel chemical compounds [3].

The natural product can be categorized as a compound that is produced by living organisms and includes the types of biotic materials (*e.g.* wood, silk), bio-based materials (*e.g.* bioplastics, cornstarch), bodily fluids (*e.g.* milk, plant exudates), and other natural materials (*e.g.* soil, coal) [4]. According to Albrecht Kossel's original proposal, natural products are divided into two classes; primary and secondary metabolites [5]. Primary metabolites have an important internal function in the survival of the organism that produces them. The secondary metabolites in contrast have an external function that significantly affects other organisms. Second metabolites are not essential for survival but increase biological competition in their environment. Because of their ability to alter biochemical pathways and signal transduction, some secondary metabolites have beneficial therapeutic properties. The most common classes of secondary metabolites include alkaloids, phenylpropanoids, polyketides, and terpenoids [6]. Although traditional medicines and other biological materials are considered an excellent source of novel compounds, the extraction, and isolation of these compounds can be slow and expensive. Because natural products are usually secondary metabolites with complex chemical properties, their total/semisynthesis is not always commercially viable. In these cases, attempts may be made to design simpler analogs with the same power and safety as the one that combines the essence/structure of the natural product [7]. There is a list of uses of natural compounds in various industries such as medicines, pharmaceuticals, cosmetics, food preservation, food safety, *etc.* Shen *et al.* (2021) reported the antifungal activity of Loquat leaves extract against citrus postharvest pathogens and provided a complete overview of the activity of anti-*Penicillium digitatum* activity. The antifungal activity of this extract against *P. digitatum* was said to be caused by abnormal cell membranes and disruption of energy metabolism [8]. Jiménez-Gómez *et al.* (2021) explored another potential method to increase crop production: the replacement of chemical fertilizers with biofertilizers (including plant-root-associated beneficial bacteria). They describe their work, which assesses the use of *B. halotolerans* SCCPVE07 and *R. laguerreae* PEPV40 strains as efficient biofertilizers for escarole crops. Natural products have been used since ancient times to enhance food attributes [9]. Plants are added to foodstuff for their aromatic features, but also for preserving and coloring purposes. On the other hand, plants have also been playing an important role in fighting health issues, mostly due to their richness in secondary metabolites. Natural products have been used in the cosmetic industry to avoid side effects with traditional preparations for herbal beauty such as *Emblica officinalis* (Amla), *Acacica concinna* (Shikakai), and *Callicarpa macrophylla* (Priyangu) have been used strongly in skincare and hair care. Moreover, Indian women are still using natural products such as *Pterocarpus santalinus* L. and *Curcuma longa* (skincare), *Lawsonia inermis* L. (hair color), and natural oils such as coconut, olive, shea butter, jojoba, and essential oils in perfumes for their bodies [10].

Natural products may be extracted from the cells, tissues, and secretions of microorganisms, plants, and animals. Crude (unfractionated) extract from any one of these sources will contain a range of structurally diverse and often novel chemical compounds. Chemical diversity in nature is based on biological diversity, so researchers travel around the world to obtain samples to analyze and evaluate in drug discovery or bioassays. This effort to search for natural products is known as bioprospecting [11]. Examples of biological sources along with their natural products are described below Table **1**.

Table 1. Medicinal uses of different natural products and their sources.

Source	Strain	Natural Compound	Medicinal Use	Ref.
Bacterium	*Streptomyces griseus*	Streptomycin	Antibiotic agent	[12]
-	*Paenibacillus polymyxa*	Polymyxins	Antibiotic agent	[13]
-	*Amycolatopsis rifamycinica*	Rifamycins	Used to cure tuberculosis and leprosy	[14]
-	*Clostridium botulinum*	Botulinum toxin	Used cosmetically to help reduce facial wrinkles	[15]
-	*Streptomyces verticillus*	Bleomycin	Used for the treatment of several cancers including Hodgkin's lymphoma, head and neck cancer, and testicular cancer	[16]
Archaea	*Pyrococcus furiosus*	Lactase enzyme	breakdown lactose, a disaccharide sugar found in milk	[17]

(Table 1) cont.....

Source	Strain	Natural Compound	Medicinal Use	Ref.
Fungi	*Penicillium chrysogenum*	Penicillins	Antibacterial drug	[18]
-	*Cephalosporium acremonium*	Cephalosporins	Antibacterial drug	[19]
-	*Penicillium griseofulvum*	Griseofulvin	Antifungal drug	[20]
-	*Aspergillus terreus*	Lovastatin	Lower cholesterol	[21]
-	*Claviceps spp.*	Ergometrine	Acts as vasoconstrictor	[22]
-	*Tolypocladium inflatum*	Cyclosporine	Used to suppress immune response during organ transplant	[23]
Plants	*Taxus brevifolia*	Paclitaxel	Anticancer agent	[24]
-	*Catharanthus roseus*	Vinblastine	Anticancer agent	[25]
-	*Artemisia annua*	Artemisinin	Antimalarial agent	[26]
-	*Papaver somniferum*	Morphine	Opioid analgesic drug	[27]
-	*Galanthus spp.*	Galantamine	Used in Alzheimer's disease drugs	[28]
-	*Zingiber officinale*	Gingerols, shogaols, and paradols	Treat diarrhea, colic infections, nausea, arthritis	[29]
-	*Curcuma longa*	Curcuminoids, sesquiterpenoids, and turmerones	Indigestion, ulcerative colitis, osteoarthritis, atherosclerosis in some animals	[30]
-	*Mentha arvensis*	4-Hydroxy benzoic, caffeic, p-coumaric, chlorogenic, and rosmarinic acids	Treat stomach ache and other digestive disorders, chest pain, teeth whitening, diuretic	[31]
-	*Agaricus bisporus*	Lectins, beta-glucans, ergosterol, ergothioneine	Cholesterol regulation, some species possess antifungal, antibacterial, antiviral, or antimicrobial properties as a defense mechanism	[32]
-	*Azadirachta indica*	6-desacetylnimbinene, nimbandiol, nimbolide, ascorbic acid, n-hexacosanol	Treat various skin disorders (*i.e.* leprosy, skin ulcers, chickenpox, acne), pest repellant	[33]
-	*Ocimum sanctum*	Oleanolic acid, Ursolic acid, Rosmarinic acid, Eugenol, Carvacrol, Linalool, and β-caryophyllene	Used to clear the bronchial tube, treatment for fever and the common cold, coughs, sore throat, respiratory disorder, kidney stones, heart disorder, diarrhea, stress	[34]
Animals	*Leiurus quinquestriatus*	Chlorotoxin	Anticancer agent	[35]
-	*Bothrops jararaca*	Teprotide	Antihypertensive agent	[36]

(Table 1) cont.....

Source	Strain	Natural Compound	Medicinal Use	Ref.
-	*Conus magus*	ω-conotoxin	Used to relieve severe and chronic pain	[37]
-	*Ecteinascidia turbinata*	ecteinascidin 743	Used to treat cancer	[38]

The discipline of pharmacognosy, which is the study of natural products with biological activity, provides the tools to identify select, and process natural products destined for different uses. Usually, a natural extract has some form of biological activity that can be detected and attributed to a single compound or a set of related compounds produced by the organism. These active compounds can be used in the medical field directly as they are, or they may be synthetically modified to enhance biological properties or reduce side effects [39].

The World Health Organization conducted a study between 1999 and 2009, and a list of over 21 000 plants was prepared that are used for medicinal purposes all over the world [40]. This effort was made for the proper identification of safe plants, as it is estimated that plant-based traditional medicines are used by 60% of the world's population [41]. In addition to efforts to establish formal, DNA-based identification of such plants for wider use [42], collections of medicinal plant species, associated with their therapeutic activities and physicochemical properties are being established around the world. This is particularly the case in Asia and Africa, where traditional medicines remain an important part of everyday life for cultural, traditional, and economic reasons [43]. The Indian Traditional System of Medicine is one of the oldest systems of medical practice in the world and has played an essential role in providing healthcare services to human civilization, right from its inception. India has the exclusive distinction of its own recognized traditional medicine; Ayurveda, Yoga, Unani, Siddha, and Homoeopathy (AYUSH) [44]. These systems are based on definite medical philosophies and represent a way of achieving a healthy lifestyle with conventional and established ideas on the prevention of diseases and the promotion of health. The basic treatment approach of all these systems is holistic and the pharmacological modalities are based on natural products of plants and herbs [45]. In India, around 25,000 effective plant-based formulations are used in traditional and folk medicine. It is estimated that more than 7800 manufacturing units are involved in the production of natural health products and traditional plant-based formulations in India, which requires more than 2000 tons of medicinal plant raw material annually [46]. More than 1500 herbals are sold as dietary supplements or ethnic traditional medicines [47]. Some of them are Triphala Churna, Cinnamon, Brahmi, Cumin, Turmeric, Licorice root, Gotu Kola, Giloy, Cardamom, Manjistha, Aloe vera, Neem, Lavender, Chamomile, Rosemary Guduchi, Ginger, and Hibiscus, *etc.*

TURMERIC (*CURCUMA LONGA*)

Turmeric is commonly used in Chinese and Indian (Ayurvedic) medicine system; possess curcumin. It is also called Curcuma. It is a perennial plant that grows 3 to 5 feet high in the tropical regions of Southern Asia. The rhizome, the root of Curcuma is used in medicinal and food preparations. Curcumin is the main active component of this herb and exhibits antioxidant properties. Turmeric is especially useful for the treatment of skin disorders, such as acne, when administered orally. It can also be used to treat liver and stomach disorders, skin discoloration, constipation, and haemorrhoids [48, 49]. Significant improvement in morning stiffness, walking time and joint swelling has been observed as anti-arthritic effects after regular Curcuma consumption by Rheumatoid arthritis patients [50].

General Study: Habitat, Classification & Uses

Turmeric is a spice, and is used in folk medicine since ancient times, has received interest from both the medical/and scientific community, and it is considered the potent source of the polyphenolic compound known as curcumin. Turmeric is a rhizomatous herbaceous perennial plant (*Curcuma longa*) of the ginger family *i.e.* Zingiberaceae [51]. It is native to tropical South Asia. The medicinal properties of turmeric have been known for thousands of years; however, the ability to determine the exact mechanism(s) of action and to determine the bioactive components have only recently been investigated [52].

About 133 species of turmeric (*Curcuma*) have been identified worldwide. It is commonly found in Cambodia, China, India, Nepal, Indonesia, Madagascar, Malaysia, Philippines and Viet Nam [52]. Most of them have common local names and are used for various drug formulations. Turmeric needs temperature between 20 °C and 30 °C to grow and significant annual rainfall to thrive [50]. The individual plant attains 1 m height and has long oblong leaves. Plants are harvested annually for their rhizomes and bred from some of these rhizomes the following season. The rhizome, from turmeric, is tuberous, with rough and segmented skin. Rhizomes mature under foliage at ground level. They are golden brown with a dull orange interior. The main rhizome is pointed or tapered at the distal end and 2.5–7.0 cm long and approximately 2.5 cm in diameter, with small branched tubers. Turmeric rhizome, when dried, can be ground into a yellow powder, with a bitter, slightly acrid but sweet taste [52].

Curcuma is being recognized and used across the world in different ways for a large number of health benefits (Fig. **1**). There are many notable examples of consumption of turmeric in the world such as; in India, turmeric has been used in curries, and in spices as an important ingredient of cooked food products; in China, in Malaysia, it is used as antiseptic material; it is used as a colorant; in

Thailand, it is used in the preparation of cosmetics; in Japan, it is used in the preparation of tea; in Korea, it is mixed in drinks; in Pakistan, it is used as an anti-inflammatory agent; and in the United States, it is used in mustard sauce, cheese, butter, and chips, as a preservative and a coloring agent, in addition to capsules and powder forms.

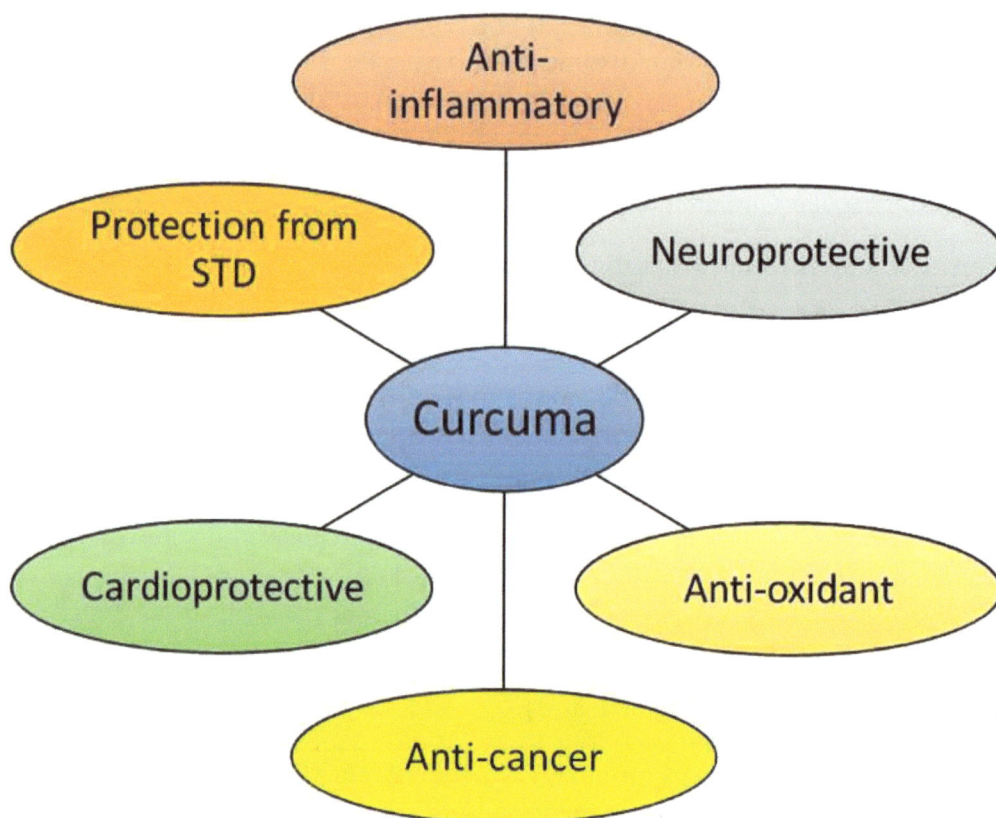

Fig. (1). Schematic illustration of Curcumin biological activities.

Curcuma longa possesses different medicinal properties such as antioxidant, anti-inflammatory [53], antimutagenic, antimicrobial [54, 55], and anticancer properties [56, 57], and due to these properties, it has been traditionally used as a medical herb in many Asian countries. A composition comprising ethanol, curcumin and a dissolved whole tumeric powder for the preparation of an alcoholic curcumin and turmeric liquid pharmaceutical composition for treating proliferative and other clinical disorders in a human patient enhanced bioavailability vis-a-vis a comparable dosage of curcumin in dry powder form [58].

Medicinal Uses of Turmeric

Neuroprotective Effects

The pathogenesis of neurodegenerative diseases includes toxic biochemical reactions including inflammation, change of mitochondrial activity and ubiquitin/proteasome system, glutamatergic toxicity, activation of pathways for apoptosis, an increase of iron and nitric oxide, and the effect on the homeostasis of antioxidants/oxidation [59]. It is suggested that major neurodegenerative diseases for example Alzheimer's, and Parkinson's; are the result of multiple factor involvement along with the combination of genetic and environmental factors. Research groups have worked on the use of rhizomes of *C. longa* for the treatment of neurogenerative diseases. The mechanism of neuroprotective properties against experimental cerebral ischemia by Curcuma oil that is isolated from the rhizomes of *C. longa* is well elaborated [60]. It is well known that calcium ions are a common component of signal transduction pathways. It has been observed that turmeric oil inhibits the increases in intracellular calcium ion concentrations and reduces high levels of nitric oxide (NO) produced by nitric oxide synthase (NOS) isoforms responsible for neuroinflammation [60]. Turmeric oil has also been found to reduce ROS production and inhibit elevated levels of the Bax protein, an early sign of cell death. Thus, turmeric oil exhibits major action in the semi-pubic region of the infarct, which is protected by the regulation of apoptosis. Sahoo *et al.* (2008) studied the role of curcumin (CUR) in oxidative stress parameters, antioxidant defense enzymes, and oxidative levels (GSSG) and reduced glutathione (GSH) in the testis of mice with l-thyroxine (T4)-induced hyperthyroidism in rats [61]. CUR was primarily effective in protecting the testes from T4-induced oxidative stress by restoring antioxidant enzymes [61]. Therefore, this suggests that *C. longa* extract can be used as a potential therapeutic agent for neurodegenerative diseases [61, 62]. Hyperhomo cysteinemia is one of the pathological causes of neurodegenerative diseases, and Ataie *et al.* (2010) studied the effect of turmeric as a prophylactic agent to prevent oxidative stress in homocysteinemia [59]. Chronic administration of turmeric significantly improved memory recognition ability in older male mice on novel object recognition and passive avoidance tasks through positive interaction of the neuronal nitric oxide synthase (nNOS)/nitric oxide (NO) pathway [63]. Wang *et al.* (2017) also described the role of *C. longa* extract in the treatment of Parkinson's disease [64].

Anticancer Activity

Extensive preclinical studies evaluating the anticancer effects of curcumin can be found in the literature, with increasing interest in the relevant mechanisms of action. Curcuminoids are assumed as excellent antioxidant polyphenols with radiomodulatory properties, radioprotective for noncancerous cells, and radiosensitizing the cancer cells [65]. Semsri *et al.* (2011) reported that turmeric in its pure form affects Wilms tumor protein 1 (WT1) promoter binding, WT1 mRNA reduction, and protein levels in K562 cells, which is due to the antiproliferative effect of turmeric [66]. Jiang *et al.* (2012) studied and identified the anticancer nature of curcuminoids of *C. longa* in HeLa cells [67]. Anticancer activity of the rhizomes of turmeric was evaluated *in vitro* using tissue culture methods and *in vivo* in mice using Dalton's lymphoma cells grown as ascites form. Turmeric extract inhibited cell growth in Chinese Hamster Ovary (CHO) cells at a concentration of 0.4 mg/ml and was cytotoxic to lymphocytes and Dalton's lymphoma cells at the same concentration. The active constituent was found to be 'curcumin' which showed cytotoxicity to lymphocytes and Dalton's lymphoma cells at a concentration of 4 µg/ml [68]. Turmeric treatment also attenuated TNFα-mediated lipolysis by downregulating extracellular signal kinase 1/2 (ERK1/2) phosphorylation and reversing the downregulation of perilipin protein in TNFα-stimulated adipocytes. The anti-lipolytic effect may be cell-based, reducing plasma-free fatty acids and improving insulin sensitivity [69]. Crude extract in combination with cisplatin augmented the decrease in the viability of cancer cells compared with single compound treatment in A549 lung cancer cells. The total extract of *Curcuma longa* could be regarded as being more effective against lung cancer cells *in vitro* than its separated compounds [70]. The combination of turmeric and paridis rhizome saponins also demonstrated good anticancer properties. This combination product significantly inhibited the tumor growth rate by inhibiting the levels of metabolites such as amino acids, lipids, and carbohydrates in the tumor tissue [71].

Antioxidant Activity

A list of *in vitro* and *in vitro* tests shows the antioxidant activity of curcuminoids. Jayaprakash *et al.* (2006) studied the antioxidant capacity of curcuminoids in an *in vitro* model system using various methods such as phosphomolybdenum and linoic acid peroxidation methods [72]. The antioxidant mechanism of turmeric was demonstrated through density functional theory, along with five other mechanisms: H atom transfer from neutral curcumin (HAT), H atom transfer from deprotonated curcumin (HAT-D), radical adduct formation (RAF), single electron transfer (SET), and sequential electron transfer with proton loss (SPLET). The chemical interaction between curcumin and DPPH actually proceeds only by the SPLET mechanism, while the chemical reaction with -OCH3 and other alkoxy radicals are regulated by the HAT mechanism. The role of the GAT mechanism in the overall reaction with curcumin and -OCH3 was found to be more than 95% irrespective of the solvent and the polarity of the reacting curcumin isomer. The antioxidant activity of curcumin has been experimentally confirmed and phenolic groups in turmeric are found involved in this activity [73]. Curcuminoids may be used to improve oxidative damage in patients with beta-thalassemia/Hb disease. Naik *et al.* (2011) demonstrated the protective effect of turmeric against experimentally induced clinical conditions such as inflammation, cardiotoxicity, and hepatotoxicity in animal models by analyzing the level of serum marker enzymes and antioxidants in target tissues [74]. Curcumin may be a useful adjunct to medication, along with standard medications for diseases caused by oxidative stress. Turmeric treatment also suppresses the formation of edema and cotton granulomas caused by carrageenan and albumin. Turmeric also tends to inhibit iron-catalyzed lipid peroxidation in liver homogenates, the removal of spontaneously formed nitric oxide from nitroprusside, and heat-induced hemolysis of rat red blood cells. The anti-inflammatory, hepatoprotective and cardioprotective effects of curcuminoids may be related to their antioxidant activity both *in vitro* and *in vivo* [75].

Cardioprotective Effects

Curcuminoids have been shown to have therapeutic effects on diabetes-associated cardiovascular complications, myocardial infarction, and cardiac hypertrophy. Cardioprotective effects are associated with interactions with cytokine receptors, ECM receptors, and local spikes [76]. Curcumin is also useful in the treatment of idiopathic pulmonary arterial hypertension [77]. Turmeric extract works through a variety of therapeutic mechanisms, depending on the type of cardiovascular disease. As with aortic aneurysms, this helps reduce the diameter of the aorta, increasing its structural integrity. In atherosclerosis, curcuminoids help reduce cholesterol accumulation, white blood cell adhesion, and migration, along with a decrease in foam cells and oxidized LDL levels. Curcumin normalizes calcium levels in heart enlargement and heart failure. These conditions also reduce cardiomyocyte growth, apoptosis, and cardiac fibrosis. Turmeric extract has been shown to normalize lipid disorders in cardiovascular complications with a reduction in cardiac fibrosis and an increase in vasodilatory function. In myocardial infarction, curcumin increases the fractional shortening of the left ventricle with a decrease in the level of myocardial cell death, perivascular fibrosis, and cardiac remodeling. Turmeric extract has also been found to help with stroke. In stroke, it reduces apoptosis and increases endothelial and mitochondrial function [78]. While all extracts of turmeric have proven useful as a treatment for cardiovascular disease, of all extracts, curcumin has been extensively studied for its mechanism of action.

Anti-inflammatory Activity

Inflammation is the root cause of a list of diseases therefore preventing inflammation in any diseased condition is the first step toward the cure of that disease.

Ca^{2+}/calmodulin-dependent protein kinase II, extracellular signal-regulated kinase ½-NF-E2- related factor-2 cascade as a novel anti-inflammatory pathway mediating bisdemethoxycurcumin (BDMC) signaling to heme oxygenase-1 expression in macrophages. The biological relevance of the signaling pathway to the anti-inflammatory nature of BDMC was studied by *in vitro* inflammation model caused by blocking the Ca^{2+} release from IP3 channels or inhibition of calmodulin-dependent protein kinase II or extracellular signal-regulated kinase ½. Kim *et al.*, (2010) studied the anti-inflammatory BDMC signaling pathway leading to the expression of heme oxygenase-1 and it was mediated *via* a rapid increase in the level of intracellular (Ca^{2+}), which subsequently influenced the activity of calmodulin/calmodulin-dependent protein kinase II, extracellular signal-regulated kinase ½, and NF-E2- related factor-2 [79].

Cooney *et al.* (2016) reported the ability of curcuminoid to reduce colon infection inside the Mdr1a−/− mouse model of human inflammatory bowel disease. This study was conducted using transcriptomics and proteomics methods. Colon mRNA transcript tiers were analyzed by microarrays, and colon protein expression was analyzed through 2D gel electrophoresis. Including this, liquid chromatography-mass spectrometry (LC-MS) based protein identification and the colonic histological damage rating were also additionally determined [80]. The anti-inflammatory properties of curcuminoids have been demonstrated by multiple molecular pathways along with increased xenobiotic metabolism, reduced immune reaction, reduced neutrophil migration, and barrier remodeling [80-82].

Therapeutic Agent for Sexually Transmitted Infections/Diseases (STD)

Sexually transmitted infections and unplanned pregnancies present a high risk to the reproductive fitness of females. Thus there is an urgent need for female-controlled vaginal products for sickness prevention and contraception. Patel *et al.* (2015) reported the development of advanced poloxamer-based thermosensitive contraceptive vaginal *in situ* hydrogels of curcuminoids. Biodegradable hydrogels impregnated with Poloxamers and HPMC K4M may be used to develop dosage for women-friendly, non-hormonal, long-performing, and biocompatible intravaginal contraceptives [83]. During the development of hydrogel, dosage optimization was performed by the use of a three-factor, three-level of Box-Behnken Design (BBD). The optimized composition was found to have

Poloxamer 188 (3.83%), Poloxamer 407 (19.96%), and HPMC K4M (0.91%). Moreover, the dosage form may use a spermicide inside a condom. Turmeric extracts represented many beneficial effects like the management of polycystic ovary syndrome (PCOS) situations, ovulation, and improved fertility. Curcuminoids restored the hormone and lipid profile, antioxidant and glycemic level in addition to ovarian morphology in Letrozole-induced PCOS animals. Curcuminoids may be a promising drug for treating scientific and pathological abnormalities in PCOS situations [84]. Turmeric also showed an improvement in the male reproductive system. Akinyemi *et al.* (2015) investigated the preventive outcomes of turmeric rhizomes on some biomarkers of male reproductive features in l-NAME-induced hypertensive rats. Dietary supplementation with turmeric rhizome was related to the recovery of systolic blood pressure, level of testosterone, sperm motility, and development of antioxidant status within the epididymis and testes of l-NAME-triggered hypertensive rats [85].

Hepatoprotective Effect

Turmeric extracts are significantly studied for their hepatoprotective outcomes. Choudhury *et al.* (2016) reported that curcumin injection (8.98 µM) decreased the NADH oxidase level, increased the Glutathione reductase (GR), Glutathione S - transferase (GST) levels, and succinate dehydrogenase activity in Swiss albino rats with CCl4-induced hepatotoxicity [86]. For similar hepatotoxicity, curcumin (200 mg/kg) in Sprague-Dawley rats improved the level of hepatic glutathione level and reduced the lipid peroxidase level and activities of aspartate aminotransferase (AST), and alanine transaminase (ALT) [87]. So, curcumin may be a promising agent to prevent oxidative stress-related liver disease, by using decreasing ALT, AST, and alkaline phosphatase degrees, increasing GST, GR, Glutathione Peroxidase (GPx), Superoxide Dismutase (SOD), and catalase (CAT), and reducing nitric oxide (NO) in addition to inhibiting reactive oxygen species (ROS) production [88]. Furthermore, Badria *et al.* (2015) reported curcumin-associated increased antioxidant levels (CAT, SOD, glutathione, and ascorbic acid) in the liver of chronic iron-overloaded male rats [88]. Curcumin also showed hepatoprotective properties for hepatoxicity caused by streptozotocin and paracetamol in mice [89]. Afrin *et al.* (2015) found that curcumin reduced the level of mitogen-activated protein kinases (MAPK), IL-1ß, TNFa, and apoptosis signal-regulating kinase 1 (ASK1) in liver tissues in Sprague Dawley rats with streptozotocin-induced diabetes [90]. In the study conducted on non-alcoholic steatohepatitis triggered by a high-fat diet, and low-dose streptozotocin, Afrin *et al.* (2017) demonstrated that curcumin treatment decreased lipogenesis, oxidatively stressed, infection, attenuated fibrosis, and HMGB1-NF-kB signaling [91]. In the case of paracetamol-triggered hepatotoxicity, curcumin managed mitochondrial disorder by removing free radicals, increasing the expression of antioxidant enzymes, and controlling transient receptor potential melastatin 2 (TRPM2) channels, and NF-kB [92, 93]. Including this, curcumin was also found effective in liver fibrosis and cirrhosis [94, 95].

Other Medicinal Uses

Curcuminoids and oil showed a zone of inhibition against all tested strains of bacteria *i.e. Bacillus subtilis, Bacillus macerans, Bacillus licheniformis* and *Azotobacter*. Among all the bacterial strains, *B. subtilis* was the most sensitive to turmeric extracts of curcuminoids and oil. The MIC value for different strains and varieties ranged from 3.0 to 20.6 mm in diameter [96]. Also, curcumin showed significant antibacterial activity with MIC values between 5 and 50 µg/mL against 65 clinical isolates of *Helicobacter pylori*. An *in vivo* study of *H. pylori*-infected C57BL/6 mice administered with curcumin, exhibited immense therapeutic potential and pronounced eradication effect against *H. pylori* infection associated with restoration of gastric damage [97]. *Curcuma longa* possesses powerful antifungal activity also. The study of addition of turmeric powder in plant tissue culture showed that turmeric at 0.8 and 1.0 g/L had appreciable inhibitory activity against fungal contaminations [98]. The crude methanol extract of *C. longa* has an inhibitory effect against some clinical isolates of dermatophytes. It was demonstrated that 18-month-old and freshly distilled oil isolated from the rhizome of *C. longa* showed the most potent antifungal effect against 29 clinical isolates of dermatophytes with MIC values of 7.2 and 7.8 mg/mL, respectively [99]. The strong antifungal activity of *C. longa* rhizome and its low side effects were the main reasons to investigate its probable synergistic effect with existing fungicides. Curcumin has been defined as the most active component in *C. longa* and has considerable gastroprotective and antiulcerogenic effect. The antiulcer activity of curcumin was displayed by attenuating the different ulcerative effectors including gastric acid hypersecretion, total peroxides, myeloperoxiase activity, IL-6, and apoptotic incidence, along with its inhibitory activity for pepsin [100]. Surprisingly, curcumin showed immense therapeutic potential against *H. pylori* infection, as it was highly effective in the eradication of *H. pylori* from infected mice as well as in the restoration of *H. pylori*-induced gastric damage. Curcumin does this by preventing the growth of *H. pylori* cagA + strain to control H. pylori-mediated ulcer, suggesting its antiulcer potential [97]. The powdered rhizome of CA exhibited wound-healing activity in rabbits. Studies also showed significant wound healing activity in excision wound models, conducted to assess the wound healing activity of topical application of CA rhizome extracts and its cream formulations [101].

CURCUMINOIDS

Curcuminoids (polyphenols) are the main components of turmeric. *C. longa* consists of a list of curcuminoids, among all the most active ones is curcumin. These curcuminoids contribute aromatic and coloring properties to turmeric. Curcumin, a yellow polyphenolic pigment that has been used for centuries for culinary and food coloring purposes, along with as an ingredient for various medicinal preparations, is widely used in Ayurveda and Chinese medicine [82].

Curcuminoid content in turmeric is also influenced by the origin, and soil conditions where it is cultivated. The approximate amount of curcuminoids varies between 2%-9%. The main curcuminoids of turmeric are of three following types (Fig. **2**).

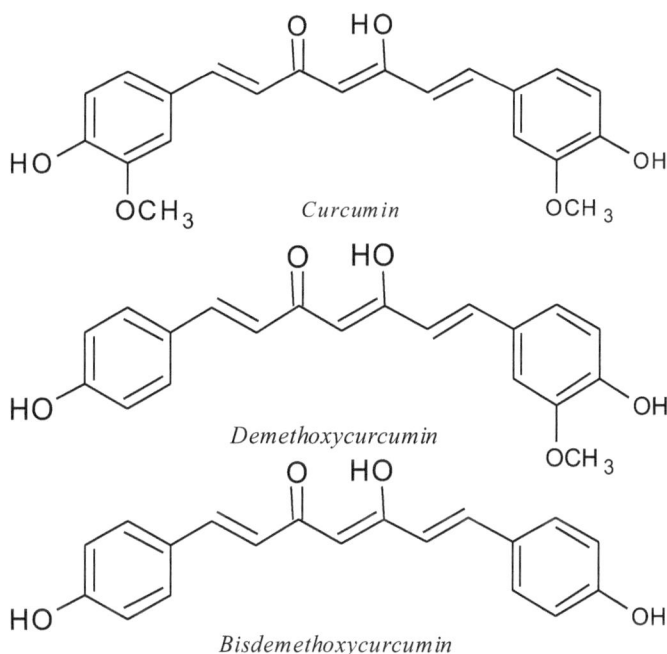

Fig. (2). Chemical structure of curcumin [82].

1. Curcumin (CUR)
2. Desmethoxycurcumin (DMC)
3. Bisdemethoxycurcumin (BDMC)

Out of these curcuminoids, curcumin is the major component, and including this cyclic curcumin is also a type of curcuminoid but it is a minor component [49].

CURCUMIN

Curcumin is the most prevalent of these curcuminoids. Curcumin (1,7-bis(-hydroxy-3-methoxyphenyl)-1,6-heptadiene-3,5-dione), also called diferuloyl methane. It is one of the main polyphenols found in the rhizome of *Curcuma longa* (turmeric) and others *Curcuma* spp [102].

Due to its medicinal activities, curcumin has received the attention of researchers. Curcumin was first isolated in 1815, but not in its purest form [103]. The purified crystalline form was reported in 1870 by Dauble [104]. After the discovery of the purified form, extensive research was done to determine the structure and molecules present in curcumin. Polish scientists in 1910 proposed the structure of curcumin for the first time [105]. Basically, curcumin is a diferuloylmethane with a generalized chemical formula $C12H20O6$. It is purified in crystalline form having yellow-orange color. It has a molecular weight of 368.39 g/mol and a melting temperature of 183°C. Its chemical properties include keto-enol tautomerism. However, the predominant keto form exists in neutral and acidic solutions, while the predominant enol form exists in solid-state and alkaline solutions and it is also considered a stable enol form [106]. Based on chemical modifications curcumin is of three types known as curcumin I, II, and III. Chemically, they are referred to as 1,7-bis(4-hydroxy-3-methoxyphenyl--1,6-heptadiene-3,5-dione, demethoxycurcumin, 1-(4-hydroxy-3-methoxyphe-yl)-7-(4-hydroxyphenyl)-1,6-heptadiene-3,5-dione, bisdemethoxycurcumin, 1,7-bis(4-hydroxyphenyl)-1,6-heptadiene-3,5-dione for curcumin I, II and III respectively [107].

Curcumin incorporates a seven carbon-linker and three major functional groups: an α,β-unsaturated β-diketone moiety and an aromatic O-methoxy-phenolic group [108]. The aromatic ring systems, which are phenols, are connected by two α,β-unsaturated carbonyl groups [105]. It is a diketone tautomer, existing in enolic form in organic solvents and in keto form in water [109]. The diketones form stable enols and are readily deprotonated to form enolates; the α,β-unsaturated carbonyl group is a good Michael acceptor and undergoes nucleophilic addition [108]. Because of its hydrophobic nature, curcumin is poorly soluble in water. However, it is easily soluble in organic solvents [108]. Curcumin is used as a complexometric indicator for boron. It reacts with boric acid to form a red-colored compound, rosocyanine [109].

This polyphenolic compound is worldwide known as the 'wonder drug of life' [110]. Turmeric is being used as a therapeutic agent since ancient times. Its crude form *i.e.*, whole turmeric, is the source of all types of curcuminoids. Still, its use in medicinal clinics is rare due to its low bioavailability. On the other hand, curcumin seems to offer a promising potential for therapeutic development in its pure form, with stable metabolism and low toxicity [111]. Therefore, the isolation of curcumin from the rhizome is of great advantage. Research has been reported in recent years on the isolation of curcumin. Its pure form is extensively used as a therapeutic agent for the treatment of various diseases and hence, health promotion.

Isolation and Analysis of Curcumin

Solvent extraction followed by chromatography is one of the most commonly used methods for curcumin isolation [51]. As curcumin is insoluble in water therefore different research groups have used a combination of different organic solvents (polar and non-polar) for its isolation (Fig. **3**). Out of the organic solvents, ethanol is preferred and including these chlorinated solvents are considered efficient. Soxhlet, ultrasonic, and microwave extraction methods are the general methods used for extraction (Fig. **3**). Including this, pulse ultrasonic and microwave-assisted extraction methods are also being conducted. A high temperature of about 60-80°C is also considered for improved extraction. Bagchi (2012) used a mixture of ethanol and acetone as a solvent to isolate curcumin from turmeric powder [112]. Anderson *et al.* (2000) have used dichloromethane as an organic solvent for curcumin extraction from ground turmeric. They magnetically stirred the whole turmeric in dichloromethane and heated it for one hour. Followed by the suction filter of the mixture and finally, the filtrate was concentrated in a vacuum filter attached to the hot water bath, maintained at 50°C. The resulting deep orangish-yellow oil residue was titrated with hexane and the resulting solid material was collected. Thin layer chromatography (TLC) based analysis (3% methanol and 97% dichloromethane) showed the presence of all three types of curcumin [113]. Kang's method for curcumin extraction is also extensively used for its isolation, on the basis of ethanolic extract preparation [114]. The method given by Pothitirat *et al.* (2006) had also been extensively used for the isolation of curcumin [115]. Chromatography and electrophoresis methods are commonly used for further purification and analysis of curcumin. These methods are column chromatography, high-performance liquid chromatography (HPLC) using a C-18 column, Liquid chromatography-coupled mass spectrometry, High-performance-thin layer chromatography, and Microemulsion electrokinetic chromatography, Capillary electrophoresis, and Ultraperformance liquid chromatography (UPLC) coupled with tandem mass spectrometry.

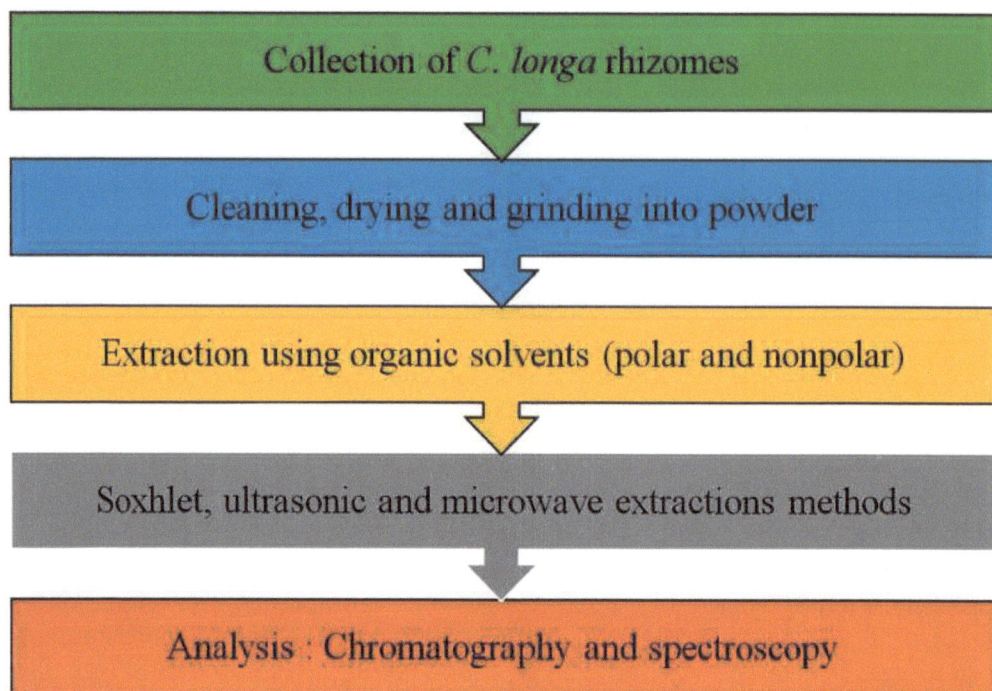

Fig. (3). Schematic representation of the scheme for isolation and analysis of curcuminoids from *C. longa*.

Health Benefits of Curcumin

Curcumin is mainly used in dairy products, beverages, cereals, mustard, food concentrates, pickles, sausages, confectionery, meat, and bakery products [116, 117]. As an additive, it is stable during thermal treatment and it is inert to react with other ingredients [118]. Curcumin and its derivatives are well studied for their biological effect on health promotion and disease prevention [119].

Curcumin helps in the management of oxidative and inflammatory conditions, metabolic syndrome, arthritis, anxiety, and hyperlipidemia. The hydrophobic nature of curcumin after oral administration triggers a poor absorption rate by the gastrointestinal (GI) tract. Including this, rapid metabolism, and rapid elimination also lead to poor bioavailability. Thus consuming curcumin may not contribute to the associated health benefits. Several components can improve the bioavailability of curcumin. For example, piperine (a major active component of black pepper) combined with curcumin, has increased the bioavailability by 2000%.

Curcumin is considered a chain-breaking antioxidant, and because of its lipophilic nature, it acts as a peroxyl radicals scavenger [120]. Its chemical structure is said to be responsible for the antioxidant properties due to the bonds like carbon-

carbon double bonds, B-diketo group, and phenyl rings with hydroxyl, and methoxy groups [120-122]. Techniques like laser flash photolysis and pulse radiolysis have been used to elucidate the mechanism of action of curcumin's antioxidant activity [123, 124].

A list of anti-inflammatory actions of curcumin is also reported in the literature. It was shown that curcumin can:

I. Control pro-inflammatory transcription factors (NF-kB and AP-1);
II. Reduce the proinflammatory cytokines TNFa, IL-1b, IL-2, IL-6, IL-8, MIP-1a, MCP-1, CRP, and PGE2;
III. Down-regulate enzymes such as 5- lipoxygenase and COX-2 and -5;
IV. Control the mitogen-activated protein kinases (MAPK) and pathways involved in nitric oxide synthase (NOS) enzymes synthesis [81, 124-128].

It is well-known that oxidative stress triggers chronic inflammation, therefore, a relationship between the antioxidant and anti-inflammatory activity of curcumin becomes clear. Its anti-inflammatory activity only results in its neuroprotective effect as neuroinflammation leads to neuronal metabolism changes that finally result in neuronal degradation. Neuronal degradation results in disorders such as Parkinson's disease (PD), Alzheimer's disease (AD), major depression, and epilepsy. Therefore, curcumin has shown neuroprotective effects through different mechanisms, including antioxidant, anti-inflammatory, and anti-proliferative, along with modulating several molecular targets [82].

Curcumin has been shown to prevent carcinogenesis by affecting angiogenesis and cancer cell growth (Fig. **4**). It also suppresses cancer cell metastasis and induces cancer cell apoptosis through a p53-dependent pathway [129]. Curcumin has been found to have antiangiogenic activity by regulating the angiogenic stimulators, such as VEGF and basic fibroblast growth factor. Curcumin is reported to downregulate the expression of VEGF *via* NF-kB and AP-1 regulation and decrease the expression of IL-8 [130, 131]. Curcumin has been suggested as highly effective against Ras-overexpressed cancer conditions. In a study conducted by Cao *et al.* (2015), it was demonstrated that curcumin controlled the proliferation of AGS gastric cancer cells by downregulating the Ras proteins and upregulating ERK [132].

Studies also support the activity of curcumin in favor of the prevention of cardiovascular disease (Fig. **5**). Curcumin mainly shows protective effects on atherosclerosis, cardiac hypertrophy, heart failure, aortic aneurysm, stroke, myocardial infarction, and diabetic cardiovascular complications [133]. Yao *et al.* (2016) found that curcumin reduces angiotensin II type 1 receptor (AT1R) expression, thus preventing cardiovascular diseases [134]. Cao *et al.* (2018) studied that curcumin may reduce the risk of chronic heart failure by increasing the ASK1, JNK, p38, and MAPK [135].

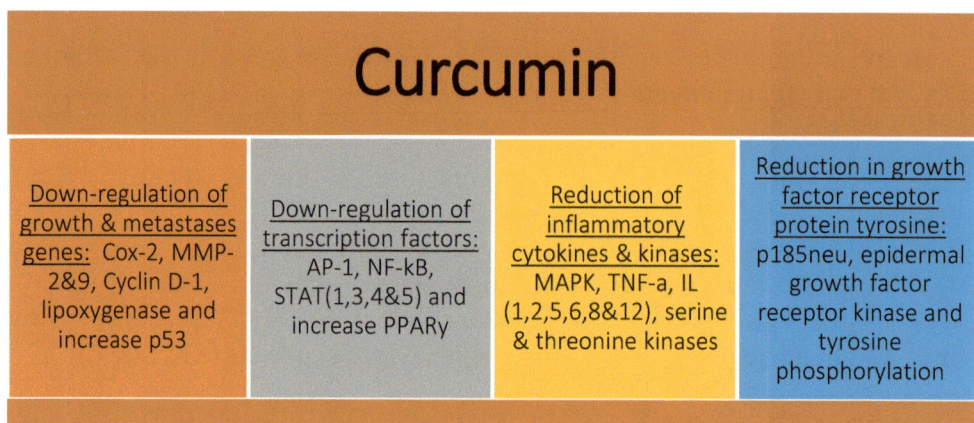

Fig. (4). Curcumin molecular targets in cancer cells (Adapted from Sharifi-Rad *et al.,* 2020) [82].

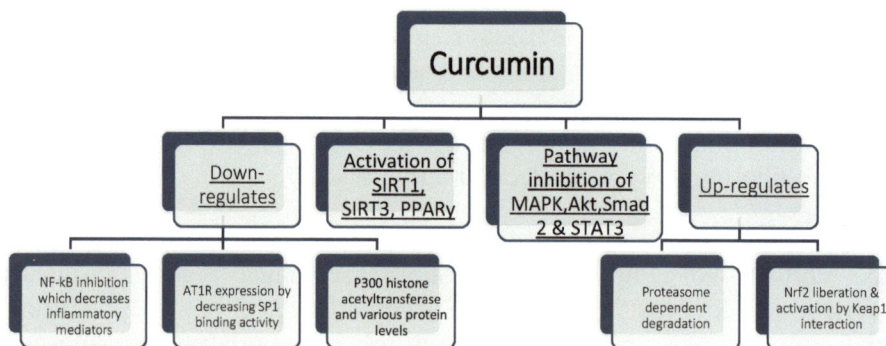

Fig. (5). Mode of action of curcumin as a therapeutic agent for cardiovascular diseases (adapted from Li *et al.,* 2019) [78].

Availability of Curcumin

Curcumin is available in several forms including capsules, tablets, ointments, energy drinks, soaps, and cosmetics. Even, US Food and Drug Administration (FDA) has recognized curcuminoids as "Generally Recognized As Safe" (GRAS) [52]. Moreover, clinical trials conducted with doses between 4000 and 8000 mg/day showed good tolerability and safety profiles [136] and of doses up to 12,000 mg/day of 95% concentration of three curcuminoids: curcumin, bisdemethoxycurcumin, and desmethoxycurcumin [137].

Clinical Investigation of Curcumin as an Anticancer Product

Clinical trials have been studied for many diseases and these clinical trials are increased in a progressive manner, remarkable disproportionalities have been reported with respect to biological effects assessment. Clinical trials have been conducted to evaluate the therapeutic effects of curcumin effect on cancer, eye, skin, urogenital, gastrointestinal, central nervous system, inflammation, cardiovascular, respiratory, and metabolic disorders [138].

Many preclinical studies have represented the anticancer properties of curcumin. Phase I/II clinical studies conducted with patients with pancreatic cancer using oral administration of curcumin alone or in combination with Gem revealed the improvement in survival time/rate and quality of life without exhibiting major collective toxicity. Though it was found that absorption is limited during oral administration of curcumin, and for clinical study, Theracurmin has been developed [139]. Curcuminoids were reported to exhibit anticancer activity for pancreatic cancer by inducing caspase-3 activity in pancreatic ductal adenocarcinoma cells and stimulating the activity of natural killer cells [140]. Further studies revealed that curcuminoids inhibited cell proliferation *via* induction of ROS, and regulation of NF-κB, specificity protein (SP), and antiapoptotic genes [140].

In colorectal cancer, curcumin resulted in a reduction in glutathione S-transferase activity, reduction in prostaglandin E2, reduction in the size of polyps with any significant toxicity, and improved body weight [141-143]. In multiple myeloma, curcumin caused a reduction in Paraproteins, NF–κB, pSTAT3, and COX-2 [144, 145]. Clinical trials of curcumin on inflammatory bowel disease revealed a reduction in symptoms and inflammatory indices in patients with proctitis [146]. Analysis of the anti-inflammatory study revealed a reduction in postoperative inflammation [147]. In case of the antiobesity study, turmeric exhibited anti-diabetic effects and showed activities like appetite stimulant and laxative. Curcuminoids caused a reduction in inflammatory markers, and oxidative stress [148].

CONCLUSION

Turmeric has been used since ancient times as an essential food ingredient for coloring, and as spices. Including this, turmeric also exhibits many medicinal properties and it is also used as a therapeutic product in folk medicine. The chemical analysis of turmeric extract revealed the presence of polyphenol curcuminoids that contribute medicinal properties like antioxidant, anticancer, anti-inflammatory, *etc.* Though clinical trials demonstrated the medicinal benefits of Curcumin, clinical studies are to be regularly established for its use as a medicine.

CONSENT FOR PUBLICATION

Not applicable.

CONFLICT OF INTEREST

The author declares no conflict of interest, financial or otherwise.

ACKNOWLEDGEMENTS

Declared none.

REFERENCES

[1]   Gunnar, S.; Bohlin, L. Drugs of Natural Origin, A Textbook of Pharmacognosy.; Swedish Pharmaceutical society: Stockholm, 1999.

[2]   Banerjee, P.; Erehman, J.; Gohlke, B.O.; Wilhelm, T.; Preissner, R.; Dunkel, M. Super Natural II—a database of natural products. *Nucleic Acids Res.,* **2015**, *43*(D1), D935-D939.
        [http://dx.doi.org/10.1093/nar/gku886] [PMID: 25300487]

[3]   Cushnie, T.P.T.; Cushnie, B.; Echeverría, J.; Fowsantear, W.; Thammawat, S.; Dodgson, J.L.A.; Law, S.; Clow, S.M. Bioprospecting for antibacterial drugs: a multidisciplinary perspective on natural product source material, bioassay selection and avoidable pitfalls. *Pharm. Res.,* **2020**, *37*(7), 125.
        [http://dx.doi.org/10.1007/s11095-020-02849-1] [PMID: 32529587]

[4]   Bhat, S.V.; Nagasampagi, B.A.; Sivakumar, M. *Chemistry of Natural Products*; Springer: Berlin, **2005**.

[5]   Kossel, A. About the chemical composition of the cell. *Du Bois-Reymond's Archives/Arch Anat Physiol Physiol Dept,* **1891**, *278*, 181-6.

[6]   Hanson, J.R. *Natural products: the secondary metabolites*; Royal Society of Chemistry, **2003**.

[7]   Maier, M.E. Design and synthesis of analogues of natural products. *Org. Biomol. Chem.,* **2015**, *13*(19), 5302-5343.
        [http://dx.doi.org/10.1039/C5OB00169B] [PMID: 25829247]

[8]   Shen, Y.; Chen, C.; Cai, N.; Yang, R.; Chen, J.; Kahramanoğlu, İ.; Okatan, V.; Rengasamy, K.R.; Wan, C The antifungal activity of loquat (*Eriobotrya japonica* Lindl.) leaves extract against *Penicillium digitatum. Front. Nutr.,* **2021**, 8.
        [http://dx.doi.org/10.3389/fnut.2021.663584]

[9]   Jiménez-Gómez, A.; García-Estévez, I.; Escribano-Bailón, M.T.; García-Fraile, P.; Rivas, R. Bacterial fertilizers based on *Rhizobium laguerreae* and *Bacillus halotolerans* enhance Cichorium endivia L. phenolic compound and mineral contents and plant development. *Foods,* **2021**, *10*(2), 424.
        [http://dx.doi.org/10.3390/foods10020424] [PMID: 33671987]

[10]   Desam, N.R.; Al-Rajab, A.J. The Importance of Natural Products in Cosmetics. *Bioactive Natural Products for Pharmaceutical Applications*; Pal, D.; Nayak, A.K., Eds.; Springer: Cham, **2021**, pp. 643-685.
        [http://dx.doi.org/10.1007/978-3-030-54027-2_19]

[11]   Strobel, G.; Daisy, B. Bioprospecting for microbial endophytes and their natural products. *Microbiol. Mol. Biol. Rev.,* **2003**, *67*(4), 491-502.

[http://dx.doi.org/10.1128/MMBR.67.4.491-502.2003] [PMID: 14665674]

[12]   Westhoff, S.; Otto, S.B.; Swinkels, A.; Bode, B.; Wezel, G.P.; Rozen, D.E. Spatial structure increases the benefits of antibiotic production in *Streptomyces*. *Evolution,* **2020**, *74*(1), 179-187.
[http://dx.doi.org/10.1111/evo.13817] [PMID: 31393002]

[13]   He, Z.; Kisla, D.; Zhang, L.; Yuan, C.; Green-Church, K.B.; Yousef, A.E. Isolation and identification of a Paenibacillus polymyxa strain that coproduces a novel lantibiotic and polymyxin. *Appl. Environ. Microbiol.,* **2007**, *73*(1), 168-178.
[http://dx.doi.org/10.1128/AEM.02023-06] [PMID: 17071789]

[14]   Singh, P.; Kumari, R.; Mukherjee, U.; Saxena, A.; Sood, U.; Lal, R. Draft genome sequence of rifamycin derivatives producing Amycolatopsis mediterranei strain DSM 46096/S955. *Genome Announc.,* **2014**, *2*(4), e00837-14.
[http://dx.doi.org/10.1128/genomeA.00837-14] [PMID: 25125653]

[15]   Sakaguchi, G. Clostridium botulinum toxins. *Pharmacol. Ther.,* **1982**, *19*(2), 165-194.
[http://dx.doi.org/10.1016/0163-7258(82)90061-4] [PMID: 6763707]

[16]   Sánchez, C.; Du, L.; Edwards, D.J.; Toney, M.D.; Shen, B. Cloning and characterization of a phosphopantetheinyl transferase from Streptomyces verticillus ATCC15003, the producer of the hybrid peptide–polyketide antitumor drug bleomycin. *Chem. Biol.,* **2001**, *8*(7), 725-738.
[http://dx.doi.org/10.1016/S1074-5521(01)00047-3] [PMID: 11451672]

[17]   Li, B.; Wang, Z.; Li, S.; Donelan, W.; Wang, X.; Cui, T.; Tang, D. Preparation of lactose-free pasteurized milk with a recombinant thermostable β-glucosidase from *Pyrococcus furiosus. BMC Biotechnol.,* **2013**, *13*(1), 73.
[http://dx.doi.org/10.1186/1472-6750-13-73] [PMID: 24053641]

[18]   Barreiro, C.; Martín, J.F.; García-Estrada, C. Proteomics shows new faces for the old penicillin producer *Penicillium chrysogenum. J. Biomed. Biotechnol.,* **2012**, *2012*, 1-15.
[http://dx.doi.org/10.1155/2012/105109] [PMID: 22318718]

[19]   Demain, A.L.; Zhang, J. Cephalosporin C production by Cephalosporium acremonium: the methionine story. *Crit. Rev. Biotechnol.,* **1998**, *18*(4), 283-294.
[http://dx.doi.org/10.1080/0738-859891224176] [PMID: 9887506]

[20]   Zhang, D.; Zhao, L.; Wang, L.; Fang, X.; Zhao, J.; Wang, X.; Li, L.; Liu, H.; Wei, Y.; You, X.; Cen, S.; Yu, L. Griseofulvin derivative and indole alkaloids from *Penicillium griseofulvum* CPCC 400528. *J. Nat. Prod.,* **2017**, *80*(2), 371-376.
[http://dx.doi.org/10.1021/acs.jnatprod.6b00829] [PMID: 28117586]

[21]   Hajjaj, H.; Niederberger, P.; Duboc, P. Lovastatin biosynthesis by Aspergillus terreus in a chemically defined medium. *Appl. Environ. Microbiol.,* **2001**, *67*(6), 2596-2602.
[http://dx.doi.org/10.1128/AEM.67.6.2596-2602.2001] [PMID: 11375168]

[22]   Hafner, M.; Sulyok, M.; Schuhmacher, R.; Crews, C.; Krska, R. Stability and epimerisation behaviour of ergot alkaloids in various solvents. *World Mycotoxin J.,* **2008**, *1*(1), 67-78.
[http://dx.doi.org/10.3920/WMJ2008.x008]

[23]   Ramana Murthy, M.V.; Mohan, E.V.S.; Sadhukhan, A.K. Cyclosporin-A production by Tolypocladium inflatum using solid state fermentation. *Process Biochem.,* **1999**, *34*(3), 269-280.
[http://dx.doi.org/10.1016/S0032-9592(98)00095-8]

[24]   Wani, M.C.; Taylor, H.L.; Wall, M.E.; Coggon, P.; McPhail, A.T. Plant antitumor agents. VI. Isolation and structure of taxol, a novel antileukemic and antitumor agent from *Taxus brevifolia. J. Am. Chem. Soc.,* **1971**, *93*(9), 2325-2327.
[http://dx.doi.org/10.1021/ja00738a045] [PMID: 5553076]

[25]   Kumar, A.; Patil, D.; Rajamohanan, P.R.; Ahmad, A. Isolation, purification and characterization of vinblastine and vincristine from endophytic fungus Fusarium oxysporum isolated from *Catharanthus roseus. PLoS One,* **2013**, *8*(9), e71805.

[http://dx.doi.org/10.1371/journal.pone.0071805] [PMID: 24066024]

[26] Delabays, N.; Simonnet, X.; Gaudin, M. The genetics of artemisinin content in Artemisia annua L. and the breeding of high yielding cultivars. *Curr. Med. Chem.*, **2001**, *8*(15), 1795-1801.
       [http://dx.doi.org/10.2174/0929867013371635] [PMID: 11772351]

[27] Miller, R.J.; Jolles, C.; Rapoport, H. Morphine metabolism and normorphine in Papaver somniferum. *Phytochemistry*, **1973**, *12*(3), 597-603.
       [http://dx.doi.org/10.1016/S0031-9422(00)84450-7]

[28] Santos, G.S.; Sinoti, S.B.P.; de Almeida, F.T.C.; Silveira, D.; Simeoni, L.A.; Gomes-Copeland, K.K.P. Use of galantamine in the treatment of Alzheimer's disease and strategies to optimize its biosynthesis using the *in vitro* culture technique. *Plant Cell Tissue Organ Cult.*, **2020**, *143*(1), 13-29. [PCTOC].
       [http://dx.doi.org/10.1007/s11240-020-01911-5]

[29] Shahrajabian, M.H.; Sun, W.; Cheng, Q. Clinical aspects and health benefits of ginger (*Zingiber officinale*) in both traditional Chinese medicine and modern industry. *Acta Agric. Scand. B Soil Plant Sci.*, **2019**, *69*(6), 546-556.
       [http://dx.doi.org/10.1080/09064710.2019.1606930]

[30] Nishiyama, T.; Mae, T.; Kishida, H.; Tsukagawa, M.; Mimaki, Y.; Kuroda, M.; Sashida, Y.; Takahashi, K.; Kawada, T.; Nakagawa, K.; Kitahara, M. Curcuminoids and sesquiterpenoids in turmeric (Curcuma longa L.) suppress an increase in blood glucose level in type 2 diabetic KK-Ay mice. *J. Agric. Food Chem.*, **2005**, *53*(4), 959-963.
       [http://dx.doi.org/10.1021/jf0483873] [PMID: 15713005]

[31] Sharangi, A.B.; Bhutia, P.H.; Raj, A.C.; Sreenivas, M. *Underexploited spice crops: present status, agrotechnology, and future research directions,* 1st ed; Apple Academic Press: New York, **2018**.
       [http://dx.doi.org/10.1201/9781351136464]

[32] Rathore, H.; Prasad, S.; Sharma, S. Mushroom nutraceuticals for improved nutrition and better human health: A review. *PharmaNutrition*, **2017**, *5*(2), 35-46.
       [http://dx.doi.org/10.1016/j.phanu.2017.02.001]

[33] Rahmani, A.; Almatroudi, A.; Alrumaihi, F.; Khan, A. Pharmacological and therapeutic potential of neem (*Azadirachta indica*). *Pharmacogn. Rev.*, **2018**, *12*(24), 250.
       [http://dx.doi.org/10.4103/phrev.phrev_8_18]

[34] Panchal, P.; Parvez, N. Phytochemical analysis of medicinal herb (*Ocimum sanctum*). *Int. J. Nanomater. Nanotechnol. Nanomedicine.*, **2019**, *5*(2), 008-11.
       [http://dx.doi.org/10.17352/2455-3492.000029]

[35] Ojeda, P.G.; Wang, C.K.; Craik, D.J. Chlorotoxin: Structure, activity, and potential uses in cancer therapy. *Biopolymers*, **2016**, *106*(1), 25-36.
       [http://dx.doi.org/10.1002/bip.22748] [PMID: 26418522]

[36] Alekseenko, L.P.; Orekhovich, V.N. Human erythrocyte prolyl endopeptidase II hydrolysing teprotid, an inhibitor of peptidyl peptidase from snake venom. *Biull. Eksp. Biol. Med.*, **1985**, *99*(3), 308-311.
       [PMID: 2985149]

[37] Monje, V.D.; Haack, J.A.; Naisbitt, S.R.; Miljanich, G.; Ramachandran, J.; Nasdasdi, L.; Olivera, B.M.; Hillyard, D.R.; Gray, W.R. A new Conus peptide ligand for Ca channel subtypes. *Neuropharmacology*, **1993**, *32*(11), 1141-1149.
       [http://dx.doi.org/10.1016/0028-3908(93)90008-Q] [PMID: 8107968]

[38] Kerr, R.G.; Miranda, N.F. Biosynthetic studies of ecteinascidins in the marine tunicate Ecteinascidia turbinata. *J. Nat. Prod.*, **1995**, *58*(10), 1618-1621.
       [http://dx.doi.org/10.1021/np50124a025]

[39] Sarker, S. Pharmacognosy in modern pharmacy curricula. *Pharmacogn. Mag.*, **2012**, *8*(30), 91-92.
       [http://dx.doi.org/10.4103/0973-1296.96545] [PMID: 22701278]

[40] World Health Organization. WHO monographs on selected medicinal plants. *Geneva*, **2009**; 4.

[41]   Polur, H.; Joshi, T.; Workman, C.T.; Lavekar, G.; Kouskoumvekaki, I. Back to the roots: prediction of biologically active natural products from ayurveda traditional medicine. *Mol. Inform.,* **2011**, *30*(2-3), 181-187.
[http://dx.doi.org/10.1002/minf.201000163] [PMID: 27466772]

[42]   Palhares, R. M.; Gonçalves Drummond, M.; dos Santos Alves Figueiredo Brasil, B.; Pereira Cosenza, G. Medicinal plants recommended by the world health organization: DNA barcode identification associated with chemical analyses guarantees their quality. *PloS one.,* **2015**, *15*(10)(5), e0127866.
[http://dx.doi.org/10.1371/journal.pone.0127866]

[43]   Sorokina, M.; Steinbeck, C. Review on natural products databases: Where to find data in 2020. *J. Cheminform.,* **2020**, *12*(1), 20.
[http://dx.doi.org/10.1186/s13321-020-00424-9] [PMID: 33431011]

[44]   Adhikari, P.P.; Paul, S.B. History of Indian traditional medicine: A medical inheritance. *Asian J. Pharm. Clin. Res.,* **2018**, *11*(1), 421.
[http://dx.doi.org/10.22159/ajpcr.2018.v11i1.21893]

[45]   Ahmad, S.; Zahiruddin, S.; Parveen, B.; Basist, P.; Parveen, A.; Gaurav, ; Parveen, R.; Ahmad, M. Indian medicinal plants and formulations and their potential against COVID-19–Preclinical and clinical research. *Front. Pharmacol.,* **2021**, *11*, 578970.
[http://dx.doi.org/10.3389/fphar.2020.578970] [PMID: 33737875]

[46]   Pandey, M.M.; Rastogi, S.; Rawat, A.K. Indian herbal drug for general healthcare: An overview. *Internet J. Altern. Med.,* **2008**, *6*(1), 3.
[http://dx.doi.org/10.5580/1c51]

[47]   Patwardhan, B.; Warude, D.; Pushpangadan, P.; Bhatt, N. Ayurveda and traditional Chinese medicine: a comparative overview. *Evid. Based Complement. Alternat. Med.,* **2005**, *2*(4), 465-473.
[http://dx.doi.org/10.1093/ecam/neh140] [PMID: 16322803]

[48]   Nguyen, V.B. Turmeric for treating skin disorders. U.S. Patent No. US5897865A, 1997.

[49]   Suman, K. Use of turmeric in wound healing. U.S. Patent No. US5401504A, 1993.

[50]   Dcodhar, S.D.; Sethi, R.; Srimal, R.C. Preliminary study on antirheumatic activity of curcumin (diferuloyl methane). *Indian J. Med. Res.,* **2013**, *138*(1).

[51]   Priyadarsini, K. The chemistry of curcumin: from extraction to therapeutic agent. *Molecules,* **2014**, *19*(12), 20091-20112.
[http://dx.doi.org/10.3390/molecules191220091] [PMID: 25470276]

[52]   Gupta, S.C.; Patchva, S.; Aggarwal, B.B. Therapeutic roles of curcumin: lessons learned from clinical trials. *AAPS J.,* **2013**, *15*(1), 195-218.
[http://dx.doi.org/10.1208/s12248-012-9432-8] [PMID: 23143785]

[53]   Lestari, M.L.A.D.; Indrayanto, G. Curcumin. *Profiles Drug Subst. Excip. Relat. Methodol.,* **2014**, *39*, 113-204.
[http://dx.doi.org/10.1016/B978-0-12-800173-8.00003-9] [PMID: 24794906]

[54]   Mahady, G.B.; Pendland, S.L.; Yun, G.; Lu, Z.Z. Turmeric (Curcuma longa) and curcumin inhibit the growth of *Helicobacter pylori*, a group 1 carcinogen. *Anticancer Res.,* **2002**, *22*(6C), 4179-4181.
[PMID: 12553052]

[55]   Reddy, R.C.; Vatsala, P.G.; Keshamouni, V.G.; Padmanaban, G.; Rangarajan, P.N. Curcumin for malaria therapy. *Biochem. Biophys. Res. Commun.,* **2005**, *326*(2), 472-474.
[http://dx.doi.org/10.1016/j.bbrc.2004.11.051] [PMID: 15582601]

[56]   Vera-Ramirez, L.; Pérez-Lopez, P.; Varela-Lopez, A.; Ramirez-Tortosa, M.C.; Battino, M.; Quiles, J.L. Curcumin and liver disease. *Biofactors,* **2013**, *39*(1), 88-100.
[http://dx.doi.org/10.1002/biof.1057] [PMID: 23303639]

[57]   Wright, L.; Frye, J.; Gorti, B.; Timmermann, B.; Funk, J. Bioactivity of turmeric-derived

curcuminoids and related metabolites in breast cancer. *Curr. Pharm. Des.,* **2013**, *19*(34), 6218-6225.
[http://dx.doi.org/10.2174/1381612811319340013] [PMID: 23448448]

[58] Rabinovich, M.; Rabinovich, A. Turmeric compositions and methods for the preparation thereof. French Patent no. WO2008096343A1, 2008.

[59] Ataie, A.; Sabetkasaei, M.; Haghparast, A.; Moghaddam, A.H.; Kazeminejad, B. Neuroprotective effects of the polyphenolic antioxidant agent, Curcumin, against homocysteine-induced cognitive impairment and oxidative stress in the rat. *Pharmacol. Biochem. Behav.,* **2010**, *96*(4), 378-385.
[http://dx.doi.org/10.1016/j.pbb.2010.06.009] [PMID: 20619287]

[60] Dohare, P.; Varma, S.; Ray, M. Curcuma oil modulates the nitric oxide system response to cerebral ischemia/reperfusion injury. *Nitric Oxide,* **2008**, *19*(1), 1-11.
[http://dx.doi.org/10.1016/j.niox.2008.04.020] [PMID: 18485279]

[61] Sahoo, D.K.; Roy, A.; Chainy, G.B.N. Protective effects of vitamin E and curcumin on l-thyroxin--induced rat testicular oxidative stress. *Chem. Biol. Interact.,* **2008**, *176*(2-3), 121-128.
[http://dx.doi.org/10.1016/j.cbi.2008.07.009] [PMID: 18723006]

[62] Zhang, L.J.; Wu, C.F.; Meng, X.L.; Yuan, D.; Cai, X.D.; Wang, Q.L.; Yang, J.Y. Comparison of inhibitory potency of three different curcuminoid pigments on nitric oxide and tumor necrosis factor production of rat primary microglia induced by lipopolysaccharide. *Neurosci. Lett.,* **2008**, *447*(1), 48-53.
[http://dx.doi.org/10.1016/j.neulet.2008.09.067] [PMID: 18838107]

[63] Yu, S.Y.; Zhang, M.; Luo, J.; Zhang, L.; Shao, Y.; Li, G. Curcumin ameliorates memory deficits *via* neuronal nitric oxide synthase in aged mice. *Prog. Neuropsychopharmacol. Biol. Psychiatry,* **2013**, *45*, 47-53.
[http://dx.doi.org/10.1016/j.pnpbp.2013.05.001] [PMID: 23665290]

[64] Wang, X.S.; Zhang, Z.R.; Zhang, M.M.; Sun, M.X.; Wang, W.W.; Xie, C.L. Neuroprotective properties of curcumin in toxin-base animal models of Parkinson's disease: a systematic experiment literatures review. *BMC Complement. Altern. Med.,* **2017**, *17*(1), 412.
[http://dx.doi.org/10.1186/s12906-017-1922-x] [PMID: 28818104]

[65] Lopez-Jornet, P.; Gómez-García, F.; García Carrillo, N.; Valle-Rodríguez, E.; Xerafin, A.; Vicente-Ortega, V. Radioprotective effects of lycopene and curcumin during local irradiation of parotid glands in Sprague Dawley rats. *Br. J. Oral Maxillofac. Surg.,* **2016**, *54*(3), 275-279.
[http://dx.doi.org/10.1016/j.bjoms.2016.01.013] [PMID: 26830066]

[66] Semsri, S.; Krig, S.R.; Kotelawala, L.; Sweeney, C.A.; Anuchapreeda, S. Inhibitory mechanism of pure curcumin on *Wilms' tumor 1* (*WT1*) gene expression through the PKCα signaling pathway in leukemic K562 cells. *FEBS Lett.,* **2011**, *585*(14), 2235-2242.
[http://dx.doi.org/10.1016/j.febslet.2011.05.043] [PMID: 21658388]

[67] Jiang, J.L.; Jin, X.L.; Zhang, H.; Su, X.; Qiao, B.; Yuan, Y.J. Identification of antitumor constituents in curcuminoids from *Curcuma longa* L. based on the composition–activity relationship. *J. Pharm. Biomed. Anal.,* **2012**, *70*, 664-670.
[http://dx.doi.org/10.1016/j.jpba.2012.05.011] [PMID: 22682511]

[68] Kuttan, R.; Bhanumathy, P.; Nirmala, K.; George, M.C. Potential anticancer activity of turmeric (Curcuma longa). *Cancer Lett.,* **1985**, *29*(2), 197-202.
[http://dx.doi.org/10.1016/0304-3835(85)90159-4] [PMID: 4075289]

[69] Xie, X.; Kong, P.R.; Wu, J.; Li, Y.; Li, Y. Curcumin attenuates lipolysis stimulated by tumor necrosis factor-α or isoproterenol in 3T3-L1 adipocytes. *Phytomedicine,* **2012**, *20*(1), 3-8.
[http://dx.doi.org/10.1016/j.phymed.2012.09.003] [PMID: 23083815]

[70] Kukula-Koch, W.; Grabarska, A.; Łuszczki, J.; Czernicka, L.; Nowosadzka, E.; Gumbarewicz, E.; Jarząb, A.; Audo, G.; Upadhyay, S.; Główniak, K.; Stepulak, A. Superior anticancer activity is demonstrated by total extract of *Curcuma longa* L. as opposed to individual curcuminoids separated by centrifugal partition chromatography. *Phytother. Res.,* **2018**, *32*(5), 933-942.

[http://dx.doi.org/10.1002/ptr.6035] [PMID: 29368356]

[71]   Man, S.; Chai, H.; Qiu, P.; Liu, Z.; Fan, W.; Wang, J.; Gao, W. Turmeric enhancing anti-tumor effect of Rhizoma paridis saponins by influencing their metabolic profiling in tumors of H22 hepatocarcinoma mice. *Pathol. Res. Pract.,* **2015**, *211*(12), 948-954.
[http://dx.doi.org/10.1016/j.prp.2015.09.011] [PMID: 26471217]

[72]   Jayaprakasha, G.K.; Jaganmohan Rao, L.; Sakariah, K.K. Antioxidant activities of curcumin, demethoxycurcumin and bisdemethoxycurcumin. *Food Chem.,* **2006**, *98*(4), 720-724.
[http://dx.doi.org/10.1016/j.foodchem.2005.06.037]

[73]   Galano, A.; Álvarez-Diduk, R.; Ramírez-Silva, M.T.; Alarcón-Ángeles, G.; Rojas-Hernández, A. Role of the reacting free radicals on the antioxidant mechanism of curcumin. *Chem. Phys.,* **2009**, *363*(1-3), 13-23.
[http://dx.doi.org/10.1016/j.chemphys.2009.07.003]

[74]   Naik, S.R.; Thakare, V.N.; Patil, S.R. Protective effect of curcumin on experimentally induced inflammation, hepatotoxicity and cardiotoxicity in rats: Evidence of its antioxidant property. *Exp. Toxicol. Pathol.,* **2011**, *63*(5), 419-431.
[http://dx.doi.org/10.1016/j.etp.2010.03.001] [PMID: 20363603]

[75]   Amalraj, A.; Pius, A.; Gopi, S.; Gopi, S. Biological activities of curcuminoids, other biomolecules from turmeric and their derivatives – A review. *J. Tradit. Complement. Med.,* **2017**, *7*(2), 205-233.
[http://dx.doi.org/10.1016/j.jtcme.2016.05.005] [PMID: 28417091]

[76]   Hong, D.; Zeng, X.; Xu, W.; Ma, J.; Tong, Y.; Chen, Y. Altered profiles of gene expression in curcumin-treated rats with experimentally induced myocardial infarction. *Pharmacol. Res.,* **2010**, *61*(2), 142-148.
[http://dx.doi.org/10.1016/j.phrs.2009.08.009] [PMID: 19747544]

[77]   Bronte, E.; Coppola, G.; Di Miceli, R.; Sucato, V.; Russo, A.; Novo, S. Role of curcumin in idiopathic pulmonary arterial hypertension treatment: A new therapeutic possibility. *Med. Hypotheses,* **2013**, *81*(5), 923-926.
[http://dx.doi.org/10.1016/j.mehy.2013.08.016] [PMID: 24054817]

[78]   Li, L.; Su, Z.; Zou, Z.; Tan, H.; Cai, D.; Su, L.; Gu, Z. Ser46 phosphorylation of p53 is an essential event in prolyl-isomerase Pin1-mediated p53-independent apoptosis in response to heat stress. *Cell Death Dis.,* **2019**, *10*(2), 96.
[http://dx.doi.org/10.1038/s41419-019-1316-8] [PMID: 30718466]

[79]   Kim, A.N.; Jeon, W.K.; Lee, J.J.; Kim, B.C. Up-regulation of heme oxygenase-1 expression through CaMKII-ERK1/2-Nrf2 signaling mediates the anti-inflammatory effect of bisdemethoxycurcumin in LPS-stimulated macrophages. *Free Radic. Biol. Med.,* **2010**, *49*(3), 323-331.
[http://dx.doi.org/10.1016/j.freeradbiomed.2010.04.015] [PMID: 20430097]

[80]   Cooney, J.M.; Barnett, M.P.G.; Dommels, Y.E.M.; Brewster, D.; Butts, C.A.; McNabb, W.C.; Laing, W.A.; Roy, N.C. A combined omics approach to evaluate the effects of dietary curcumin on colon inflammation in the Mdr1a−/− mouse model of inflammatory bowel disease. *J. Nutr. Biochem.,* **2016**, *27*, 181-192.
[http://dx.doi.org/10.1016/j.jnutbio.2015.08.030] [PMID: 26437580]

[81]   He, Y.; Yue, Y.; Zheng, X.; Zhang, K.; Chen, S.; Du, Z. Curcumin, inflammation, and chronic diseases: how are they linked? *Molecules,* **2015**, *20*(5), 9183-9213.
[http://dx.doi.org/10.3390/molecules20059183] [PMID: 26007179]

[82]   Sharifi-Rad, J.; Rayess, Y.E.; Rizk, A.A.; Sadaka, C.; Zgheib, R.; Zam, W.; Sestito, S.; Rapposelli, S.; Neffe-Skocińska, K.; Zielińska, D.; Salehi, B.; Setzer, W.N.; Dosoky, N.S.; Taheri, Y.; El Beyrouthy, M.; Martorell, M.; Ostrander, E.A.; Suleria, H.A.R.; Cho, W.C.; Maroyi, A.; Martins, N. Turmeric and its major compound curcumin on health: bioactive effects and safety profiles for food, pharmaceutical, biotechnological and medicinal applications. *Front. Pharmacol.,* **2020**, *11*, 01021.
[http://dx.doi.org/10.3389/fphar.2020.01021] [PMID: 33041781]

[83]   Patel, N.; Thakkar, V.; Moradiya, P.; Gandhi, T.; Gohel, M. Optimization of curcumin loaded vaginal in-situ hydrogel by box-behnken statistical design for contraception. *J. Drug Deliv. Sci. Technol.,* **2015**, *29*, 55-69.
[http://dx.doi.org/10.1016/j.jddst.2015.06.002]

[84]   Reddy, P.S.; Begum, N.; Mutha, S.; Bakshi, V. Beneficial effect of Curcumin in Letrozole induced polycystic ovary syndrome. *Asian Pac. J. Reprod.,* **2016**, *5*(2), 116-122.
[http://dx.doi.org/10.1016/j.apjr.2016.01.006]

[85]   Akinyemi, A.J.; Adedara, I.A.; Thome, G.R.; Morsch, V.M.; Rovani, M.T.; Mujica, L.K.S.; Duarte, T.; Duarte, M.; Oboh, G.; Schetinger, M.R.C. Dietary supplementation of ginger and turmeric improves reproductive function in hypertensive male rats. *Toxicol. Rep.,* **2015**, *2*, 1357-1366.
[http://dx.doi.org/10.1016/j.toxrep.2015.10.001] [PMID: 28962478]

[86]   Choudhury, S.T.; Das, N.; Ghosh, S.; Ghosh, D.; Chakraborty, S.; Ali, N. Vesicular (liposomal and nanoparticulated) delivery of curcumin: a comparative study on carbon tetrachloride-mediated oxidative hepatocellular damage in rat model. *Int. J. Nanomedicine,* **2016**, *11*, 2179-2193.
[PMID: 27274242]

[87]   Lee, H.Y.; Kim, S.W.; Lee, G.H.; Choi, M.K.; Jung, H.W.; Kim, Y.J.; Kwon, H.J.; Chae, H.J. Turmeric extract and its active compound, curcumin, protect against chronic CCl4-induced liver damage by enhancing antioxidation. *BMC Complement. Altern. Med.,* **2016**, *16*(1), 316.
[http://dx.doi.org/10.1186/s12906-016-1307-6] [PMID: 27561811]

[88]   Badria, F.A.; Ibrahim, A.S.; Badria, A.F.; Elmarakby, A.A. Curcumin Attenuates Iron Accumulation and Oxidative Stress in the Liver and Spleen of Chronic Iron-Overloaded Rats. *PLoS One,* **2015**, *10*(7), e0134156.
[http://dx.doi.org/10.1371/journal.pone.0134156] [PMID: 26230491]

[89]   Farzaei, M.; Zobeiri, M.; Parvizi, F.; El-Senduny, F.; Marmouzi, I.; Coy-Barrera, E.; Naseri, R.; Nabavi, S.; Rahimi, R.; Abdollahi, M. Curcumin in liver diseases: a systematic review of the cellular mechanisms of oxidative stress and clinical perspective. *Nutrients,* **2018**, *10*(7), 855.
[http://dx.doi.org/10.3390/nu10070855] [PMID: 29966389]

[90]   Afrin, R.; Arumugam, S.; Soetikno, V.; Thandavarayan, R.A.; Pitchaimani, V.; Karuppagounder, V.; Sreedhar, R.; Harima, M.; Suzuki, H.; Miyashita, S.; Nomoto, M.; Suzuki, K.; Watanabe, K. Curcumin ameliorates streptozotocin-induced liver damage through modulation of endoplasmic reticulum stress-mediated apoptosis in diabetic rats. *Free Radic. Res.,* **2015**, *49*(3), 279-289.
[http://dx.doi.org/10.3109/10715762.2014.999674] [PMID: 25536420]

[91]   Afrin, R.; Arumugam, S.; Rahman, A.; Wahed, M.I.I.; Karuppagounder, V.; Harima, M.; Suzuki, H.; Miyashita, S.; Suzuki, K.; Yoneyama, H.; Ueno, K.; Watanabe, K. Curcumin ameliorates liver damage and progression of NASH in NASH-HCC mouse model possibly by modulating HMGB1-NF-κB translocation. *Int. Immunopharmacol.,* **2017**, *44*, 174-182.
[http://dx.doi.org/10.1016/j.intimp.2017.01.016] [PMID: 28110063]

[92]   Granados-Castro, L.F.; Rodríguez-Rangel, D.S.; Fernández-Rojas, B.; León-Contreras, J.C.; Hernández-Pando, R.; Medina-Campos, O.N.; Eugenio-Pérez, D.; Pinzón, E.; Pedraza-Chaverri, J. Curcumin prevents paracetamol-induced liver mitochondrial alterations. *J. Pharm. Pharmacol.,* **2016**, *68*(2), 245-256.
[http://dx.doi.org/10.1111/jphp.12501] [PMID: 26773315]

[93]   Kheradpezhouh, E.; Barritt, G.J.; Rychkov, G.Y. Curcumin inhibits activation of TRPM2 channels in rat hepatocytes. *Redox Biol.,* **2016**, *7*, 1-7.
[http://dx.doi.org/10.1016/j.redox.2015.11.001] [PMID: 26609559]

[94]   Chen, N.; Geng, Q.; Zheng, J.; He, S.; Huo, X.; Sun, X. Suppression of the TGF-β/Smad signaling pathway and inhibition of hepatic stellate cell proliferation play a role in the hepatoprotective effects of curcumin against alcohol-induced hepatic fibrosis. *Int. J. Mol. Med.,* **2014**, *34*(4), 1110-1116.
[http://dx.doi.org/10.3892/ijmm.2014.1867] [PMID: 25069637]

[95]   Zhong, W.; Qian, K.; Xiong, J.; Ma, K.; Wang, A.; Zou, Y. Curcumin alleviates lipopolysaccharide induced sepsis and liver failure by suppression of oxidative stress-related inflammation *via* PI3K/AKT and NF-κB related signaling. *Biomed. Pharmacother.,* **2016**, *83*, 302-313.
[http://dx.doi.org/10.1016/j.biopha.2016.06.036] [PMID: 27393927]

[96]   Naz, S.; Jabeen, S.; Ilyas, S.; Manzoor, F.; Aslam, F.; Ali, A. Antibacterial activity of *Curcuma longa* varieties against different strains of bacteria. *Pak. J. Bot.,* **2010**, *42*(1), 455-462.

[97]   De, R.; Kundu, P.; Swarnakar, S.; Ramamurthy, T.; Chowdhury, A.; Nair, G.B.; Mukhopadhyay, A.K. Antimicrobial activity of curcumin against *Helicobacter pylori* isolates from India and during infections in mice. *Antimicrob. Agents Chemother.,* **2009**, *53*(4), 1592-1597.
[http://dx.doi.org/10.1128/AAC.01242-08] [PMID: 19204190]

[98]   Upendra, R.S.; Khandelwal, P.; Reddy, A.H.M. Turmeric powder (Curcuma longa Linn.) as an antifungal agent in plant tissue culture studies. *Int. J. Eng. Sci.,* **2011**, *3*(11), 7899-7904.

[99]   Wuthi-udomlert, M.; Grisanapan, W.; Luanratana, O.; Caichompoo, W. Antifungal activity of *Curcuma longa* grown in Thailand. *Southeast Asian J. Trop. Med. Public Health,* **2000**, *31*(1) Suppl. 1, 178-182.
[PMID: 11414453]

[100] Mei, X.; Xu, D.; Wang, S.; Xu, S. Pharmacological researches of curcumin solid dispersions on experimental gastric ulcer. *Zhongguo Zhongyao Zazhi,* **2009**, *34*(22), 2920-2923.
[PMID: 20209961]

[101] Kumar, A.; Chomwal, R.; Kumar, P.; Renu, S. Antiinflammatory and wound healing activity of Curcuma aromatica salisb extract and its formulation. *J. Chem. Pharm. Res.,* **2009**, *1*(1), 304-310.

[102] Aggarwal, B.B.; Kumar, A.; Bharti, A.C. Anticancer potential of curcumin: preclinical and clinical studies. *Anticancer Res.,* **2003**, *23*(1A), 363-398.
[PMID: 12680238]

[103] Vogel, A.; Pelletier, J. Examen chimique de la racine de Curcuma. *J. Pharm. (Cairo),* **1815**, *1*, 289-300.

[104] Daube, F.W. *About curcumin the dye of turmeric root,* **1870**.

[105] Miłobędzka, J.; Kostanecki, S.; Lampe, V. Zur kenntnis des curcumins. *Ber. Dtsch. Chem. Ges.,* **1910**, *43*(2), 2163-2170.
[http://dx.doi.org/10.1002/cber.191004302168]

[106] Anand, P.; Kunnumakkara, A.B.; Newman, R.A.; Aggarwal, B.B. Bioavailability of curcumin: problems and promises. *Mol. Pharm.,* **2007**, *4*(6), 807-818.
[http://dx.doi.org/10.1021/mp700113r] [PMID: 17999464]

[107] Buckingham, J., Ed. *Dictionary of natural products*; CRC Press, **1993**.

[108] Farooqui, T.; Farooqui, A.A. *Curcumin: Historical Background, Chemistry, Pharmacological Action, and Potential Therapeutic Value*; Curcumin for Neurological and Psychiatric Disorders, **2019**, pp. 23-44.

[109] Manolova, Y.; Deneva, V.; Antonov, L.; Drakalska, E.; Momekova, D.; Lambov, N. The effect of the water on the curcumin tautomerism: A quantitative approach. *Spectrochim. Acta A Mol. Biomol. Spectrosc.,* **2014**, *132*, 815-820.
[http://dx.doi.org/10.1016/j.saa.2014.05.096] [PMID: 24973669]

[110] Gera, M.; Sharma, N.; Ghosh, M.; Huynh, D.L.; Lee, S.J.; Min, T.; Kwon, T.; Jeong, D.K. Nanoformulations of curcumin: an emerging paradigm for improved remedial application. *Oncotarget,* **2017**, *8*(39), 66680-66698.
[http://dx.doi.org/10.18632/oncotarget.19164] [PMID: 29029547]

[111] Parsamanesh, N.; Moossavi, M.; Bahrami, A.; Butler, A.E.; Sahebkar, A. Therapeutic potential of curcumin in diabetic complications. *Pharmacol. Res.,* **2018**, *136*, 181-193.

[http://dx.doi.org/10.1016/j.phrs.2018.09.012] [PMID: 30219581]

[112] Bagchi, A. Extraction of Curcumin. *IOSR J. Environ. Sci. Toxicol. Food Technol.,* **2012**, *1*(3), 01-16.
[http://dx.doi.org/10.9790/2402-0130116]

[113] Anderson, A.M.; Mitchell, M.S.; Mohan, R.S. Isolation of curcumin from turmeric. *J. Chem. Educ.,* **2000**, *77*(3), 359.
[http://dx.doi.org/10.1021/ed077p359]

[114] Kang, H.W. Antioxidant activity of ethanol and water extracts from lentil (Lens culinaris). *J. Food Nutr. Res.,* **2015**, *3*(10), 667-669.
[http://dx.doi.org/10.12691/jfnr-3-10-8]

[115] Pothitirat, W.; Gritsanapan, W. Variation of bioactive components in *Curcuma longa* in Thailand. *Curr. Sci.,* **2006**, 1397-1400.

[116] Chaitanya Lakshmi, G. Food coloring: the natural way. *Res. J. Chem. Sci.,* **2014**, *2231*(8), 606X.

[117] Solymosi, K.; Latruffe, N.; Morant-Manceau, A.; Schoefs, B. Food colour additives of natural origin.*Colour Additives For Foods And Beverages*; Scotter, M.J., Ed.; Woodhead Publishing: Cambridge, **2015**, pp. 3-34.
[http://dx.doi.org/10.1016/B978-1-78242-011-8.00001-5]

[118] Stankovic, I. *Curcumin: chemical and technical assessment (CTA)*; JECFA: Rome, **2004**, p. 8.

[119] Xu, X.Y.; Meng, X.; Li, S.; Gan, R.Y.; Li, Y.; Li, H.B. Bioactivity, health benefits, and related molecular mechanisms of curcumin: Current progress, challenges, and perspectives. *Nutrients,* **2018**, *10*(10), 1553.
[http://dx.doi.org/10.3390/nu10101553] [PMID: 30347782]

[120] Priyadarsini, K.I.; Maity, D.K.; Naik, G.H.; Kumar, M.S.; Unnikrishnan, M.K.; Satav, J.G.; Mohan, H. Role of phenolic O-H and methylene hydrogen on the free radical reactions and antioxidant activity of curcumin. *Free Radic. Biol. Med.,* **2003**, *35*(5), 475-484.
[http://dx.doi.org/10.1016/S0891-5849(03)00325-3] [PMID: 12927597]

[121] Wright, J.S. Predicting the antioxidant activity of curcumin and curcuminoids. *J. Mol. Struct. THEOCHEM,* **2002**, *591*(1-3), 207-217.
[http://dx.doi.org/10.1016/S0166-1280(02)00242-7]

[122] Padmaja, S.; Raju, T.N. Antioxidant effect of curcumin in selenium induced cataract of Wistar rats. *Indian J. Exp. Biol.,* **2004**, *42*(6), 601-603.
[PMID: 15260112]

[123] Jovanovic, S.V.; Steenken, S.; Boone, C.W.; Simic, M.G. H-atom transfer is a preferred antioxidant mechanism of curcumin. *J. Am. Chem. Soc.,* **1999**, *121*(41), 9677-9681.
[http://dx.doi.org/10.1021/ja991446m]

[124] Aggarwal, B.B.; Sung, B. Pharmacological basis for the role of curcumin in chronic diseases: An age-old spice with modern targets. *Trends Pharmacol. Sci.,* **2009**, *30*(2), 85-94.
[http://dx.doi.org/10.1016/j.tips.2008.11.002] [PMID: 19110321]

[125] Meng, B.; Li, J.; Cao, H. Antioxidant and antiinflammatory activities of curcumin on diabetes mellitus and its complications. *Curr. Pharm. Des.,* **2013**, *19*(11), 2101-2113.
[PMID: 23116316]

[126] Panahi, Y.; Rahimnia, A.R.; Sharafi, M.; Alishiri, G.; Saburi, A.; Sahebkar, A. Curcuminoid treatment for knee osteoarthritis: A randomized double-blind placebo-controlled trial. *Phytother. Res.,* **2014**, *28*(11), 1625-1631.
[http://dx.doi.org/10.1002/ptr.5174] [PMID: 24853120]

[127] Panahi, Y.; Saadat, A.; Beiraghdar, F.; Sahebkar, A. Adjuvant therapy with bioavailability-boosted curcuminoids suppresses systemic inflammation and improves quality of life in patients with solid tumors: A randomized double-blind placebo-controlled trial. *Phytother. Res.,* **2014**, *28*(10), 1461-

1467.
[http://dx.doi.org/10.1002/ptr.5149] [PMID: 24648302]

[128]   Machova Urdzikova, L.; Karova, K.; Ruzicka, J.; Kloudova, A.; Shannon, C.; Dubisova, J.; Murali, R.; Kubinova, S.; Sykova, E.; Jhanwar-Uniyal, M.; Jendelova, P. The anti-inflammatory compound curcumin enhances locomotor and sensory recovery after spinal cord injury in rats by immunomodulation. *Int. J. Mol. Sci.,* **2015,** *17*(1), 49.
[http://dx.doi.org/10.3390/ijms17010049] [PMID: 26729105]

[129]   Kandoth, C.; McLellan, M.D.; Vandin, F.; Ye, K.; Niu, B.; Lu, C.; Xie, M.; Zhang, Q.; McMichael, J.F.; Wyczalkowski, M.A.; Leiserson, M.D.M.; Miller, C.A.; Welch, J.S.; Walter, M.J.; Wendl, M.C.; Ley, T.J.; Wilson, R.K.; Raphael, B.J.; Ding, L. Mutational landscape and significance across 12 major cancer types. *Nature,* **2013,** *502*(7471), 333-339.
[http://dx.doi.org/10.1038/nature12634] [PMID: 24132290]

[130]   Atsumi, T.; Kakiuchi, N.; Mikage, M. DNA sequencing analysis of ITS and 28S rRNA of Poria cocos. *Biol. Pharm. Bull.,* **2007,** *30*(8), 1472-1476.
[http://dx.doi.org/10.1248/bpb.30.1472] [PMID: 17666806]

[131]   Astinfeshan, M.; Rasmi, Y.; Kheradmand, F.; Karimipour, M.; Rahbarghazi, R.; Aramwit, P.; Nasirzadeh, M.; Daeihassani, B.; Shirpoor, A.; Gholinejad, Z.; Saboory, E. Curcumin inhibits angiogenesis in endothelial cells using downregulation of the PI3K/Akt signaling pathway. *Food Biosci.,* **2019,** *29*, 86-93.
[http://dx.doi.org/10.1016/j.fbio.2019.04.005]

[132]   Cao, A.L.; Tang, Q.F.; Zhou, W.C.; Qiu, Y.Y.; Hu, S.J.; Yin, P.H. Ras/ERK signaling pathway is involved in curcumin-induced cell cycle arrest and apoptosis in human gastric carcinoma AGS cells. *J. Asian Nat. Prod. Res.,* **2015,** *17*(1), 56-63.
[http://dx.doi.org/10.1080/10286020.2014.951923] [PMID: 25492214]

[133]   Salehi, B.; Del Prado-Audelo, M.L.; Cortés, H.; Leyva-Gómez, G.; Stojanović-Radić, Z.; Singh, Y.D.; Patra, J.K.; Das, G.; Martins, N.; Martorell, M.; Sharifi-Rad, M.; Cho, W.C.; Sharifi-Rad, J. Therapeutic applications of curcumin nanomedicine formulations in cardiovascular diseases. *J. Clin. Med.,* **2020,** *9*(3), 746.
[http://dx.doi.org/10.3390/jcm9030746] [PMID: 32164244]

[134]   Yao, Y.; Wang, W.; Li, M.; Ren, H.; Chen, C.; Wang, J.; Wang, W.E.; Yang, J.; Zeng, C. Curcumin exerts its anti-hypertensive effect by down-regulating the AT1 receptor in vascular smooth muscle cells. *Sci. Rep.,* **2016,** *6*(1), 25579.
[http://dx.doi.org/10.1038/srep25579] [PMID: 27146402]

[135]   Cao, Q.; Zhang, J.; Gao, L.; Zhang, Y.; Dai, M.; Bao, M. Dickkopf-3 upregulation mediates the cardioprotective effects of curcumin on chronic heart failure. *Mol. Med. Rep.,* **2018,** *17*(5), 7249-7257.
[http://dx.doi.org/10.3892/mmr.2018.8783] [PMID: 29568962]

[136]   Basnet, P.; Skalko-Basnet, N. Curcumin: an anti-inflammatory molecule from a curry spice on the path to cancer treatment. *Molecules,* **2011,** *16*(6), 4567-4598.
[http://dx.doi.org/10.3390/molecules16064567] [PMID: 21642934]

[137]   Lao, C.D.; Ruffin, M.T., IV; Normolle, D.; Heath, D.D.; Murray, S.I.; Bailey, J.M.; Boggs, M.E.; Crowell, J.; Rock, C.L.; Brenner, D.E. Dose escalation of a curcuminoid formulation. *BMC Complement. Altern. Med.,* **2006,** *6*(1), 10.
[http://dx.doi.org/10.1186/1472-6882-6-10] [PMID: 16545122]

[138]   Salehi, B.; Stojanović-Radić, Z.; Matejić, J.; Sharifi-Rad, M.; Anil Kumar, N.V.; Martins, N.; Sharifi-Rad, J. The therapeutic potential of curcumin: A review of clinical trials. *Eur. J. Med. Chem.,* **2019,** *163*, 527-545.
[http://dx.doi.org/10.1016/j.ejmech.2018.12.016] [PMID: 30553144]

[139]   Kanai, M. Therapeutic applications of curcumin for patients with pancreatic cancer. *World J. Gastroenterol.,* **2014,** *20*(28), 9384-9391.

[PMID: 25071333]

[140] Halder, R.C.; Almasi, A.; Sagong, B.; Leung, J.; Jewett, A.; Fiala, M. Curcuminoids and Ï‰-3 fatty acids with anti-oxidants potentiate cytotoxicity of natural killer cells against pancreatic ductal adenocarcinoma cells and inhibit interferon Î³ production. *Front. Physiol.,* **2015,** *6,* 129.
[http://dx.doi.org/10.3389/fphys.2015.00129] [PMID: 26052286]

[141] Sharma, R.A.; McLelland, H.R.; Hill, K.A.; Ireson, C.R.; Euden, S.A.; Manson, M.M.; Pirmohamed, M.; Marnett, L.J.; Gescher, A.J.; Steward, W.P. Pharmacodynamic and pharmacokinetic study of oral Curcuma extract in patients with colorectal cancer. *Clin. Cancer Res.,* **2001,** *7*(7), 1894-1900.
[PMID: 11448902]

[142] Pan, M.H.; Huang, T.M.; Lin, J.K. Biotransformation of curcumin through reduction and glucuronidation in mice. *Drug Metab. Dispos.,* **1999,** *27*(4), 486-494.
[PMID: 10101144]

[143] Cruz-Correa, M.; Shoskes, D.A.; Sanchez, P.; Zhao, R.; Hylind, L.M.; Wexner, S.D.; Giardiello, F.M. Combination treatment with curcumin and quercetin of adenomas in familial adenomatous polyposis. *Clin. Gastroenterol. Hepatol.,* **2006,** *4*(8), 1035-1038.
[http://dx.doi.org/10.1016/j.cgh.2006.03.020] [PMID: 16757216]

[144] Vadhan-Raj, S.; Weber, D.M.; Wang, M.; Giralt, S.A.; Thomas, S.K.; Alexanian, R.; Zhou, X.; Patel, P.; Bueso-Ramos, C.E.; Newman, R.A.; Aggarwal, B.B. Curcumin Downregulates NF-kB and related genes in patients with multiple myeloma: Results of a Phase I/II Study. *Blood,* **2007,** *110*(11), 1177.
[http://dx.doi.org/10.1182/blood.V110.11.1177.1177]

[145] Golombick, T.; Diamond, T.H.; Badmaev, V.; Manoharan, A.; Ramakrishna, R. The potential role of curcumin in patients with monoclonal gammopathy of undefined significance--its effect on paraproteinemia and the urinary N-telopeptide of type I collagen bone turnover marker. *Clin. Cancer Res.,* **2009,** *15*(18), 5917-5922.
[http://dx.doi.org/10.1158/1078-0432.CCR-08-2217] [PMID: 19737963]

[146] Holt, P.R.; Katz, S.; Kirshoff, R. Curcumin therapy in inflammatory bowel disease: A pilot study. *Dig. Dis. Sci.,* **2005,** *50*(11), 2191-2193.
[http://dx.doi.org/10.1007/s10620-005-3032-8] [PMID: 16240238]

[147] Satoskar, R.R.; Shah, S.J.; Shenoy, S.G. Evaluation of anti-inflammatory property of curcumin (diferuloyl methane) in patients with postoperative inflammation. *Int. J. Clin. Pharmacol. Ther. Toxicol.,* **1986,** *24*(12), 651-654.
[PMID: 3546166]

[148] Usharani, P.; Mateen, A.A.; Naidu, M.U.R.; Raju, Y.S.N.; Chandra, N. Effect of NCB-02, atorvastatin and placebo on endothelial function, oxidative stress and inflammatory markers in patients with type 2 diabetes mellitus: A randomized, parallel-group, placebo-controlled, 8-week study. *Drugs R D.,* **2008,** *9*(4), 243-250.
[http://dx.doi.org/10.2165/00126839-200809040-00004] [PMID: 18588355]

CHAPTER 2

Novel Natural Compounds for Hepatocellular Carcinoma Treatment

Çağrı ÖNER[1,*] and **Emine ÇOLAK**[2]

[1] *Maltepe University, Medical Faculty, Department of Medical Biology and Genetics, İstanbul, Turkey*

[2] *Eskişehir Osmangazi University, Medical Faculty, Department of Medical Biology, Eskişehir, Turkey*

Abstract: Due to the increase in cancer cases nowadays, an increase in studies related to treatment has been observed. Although many natural or synthetic compounds have been described as therapeutic today, the effects of these treatments are seen in both healthy and cancer cells. In order to reduce these undesirable effects seen in chemotherapy and radiotherapy, alternative treatments that have less effect on healthy cells or alternative attitudes that will allow the minimum use of therapeutics in these treatments continue to be investigated. In particular, such studies focus on natural compounds with phenolic properties. This chapter focuses on the relationship between coumarin derivatives, curcumin, *Olea europaea* leaf extract, and *Cynara scolymus* leaf extract with hepatocellular carcinoma. Furthermore, the effect of these natural compounds on the genetic hallmarks of various signalling pathways and important cellular metabolism molecules of hepatocellular carcinoma are discussed.

Keywords: Coumarin, Curcumin, *Cynara scolymus*, Hepatocellular Carcinoma, *Olea europaea*.

INTRODUCTION

Hepatocellular carcinoma (HCC) is the most occurring cancer type and cause of cancer-related death worldwide. HCC is seen more in males than females, and its development is also related to the age of individuals. There are some risk factors/diseases which might cause hepatocellular carcinoma to occur. The main diseases that cause hepatocellular carcinoma are chronic liver disease, cirrhosis and obesity; the main risk factors are viral hepatitis and excessive alcohol intake worldwide [1]. Chronic viral hepatitis infections, Hepatitis B and C, were indicated as the main causes of hepatic carcinogenicity and cirrhosis [1 - 4]. Because of this, the surface antigen of Hepatitis B (HBsAg) is the main marker of

---
* **Corresponding author Çağrı ÖNER:** Maltepe University, Medical Faculty, Department of Medical Biology and Genetics, İstanbul, Turkey; E-mail: cagri.oner@maltepe.edu.tr

Shazia Anjum (Ed.)

hepatic diseases and HCC. However, HBsAg is useful to determine the HCC, and it is not the only marker to detect HCC. Hepatitis B core antibody (anti-HBc) is another marker to detect HCC earlier.

Furthermore, sometimes HBsAg might be negative while anti-HBc is positive in HCC patients. HBV vaccination is important for reducing the risk of HCC [5]. The impact of hepatitis C on HCC development is observed in patients with cirrhosis and advanced fibrosis [6]. Infection with hepatitis B and C also increases the risk of HCC. Alcohol consumption is the other risk factor for HCC. As known previously, excessive alcohol consumption is the main reason for cirrhosis. Furthermore, HCC development occurs approximately in 40-50% of cirrhosis patients. So alcohol consumption can be the main risk factor for HCC [7, 8].

Hepatocellular carcinogenesis also appears without excessive alcohol consumption; it may arise in obesity, non-alcoholic fatty liver (NAFLD) and diabetes patients. The risk factors of these diseases are the risk factors of hepatocellular carcinogenesis directly. Glucose mechanism failure leads to the observation of diabetes in patients. These deficiencies in diabetic patients result in the pathologies/diseases of the liver, including cirrhosis, fatty liver, chronic hepatitis, and liver failure. Detecting HCC in diabetes patients is 3-4 times higher than in healthy individuals [9, 10]. Anti-inflammatory, proliferative signaling pathways and the related growth hormones cause hepatocellular carcinogenesis. The major genetic markers of diabetes are insulin-like growth hormone, insulin receptor substrate 1, α-fetoprotein (AFP) and des-γ-carboxyl prothrombin (DCP). The other factor which affects HCC occurrence is obesity. As is well known, hepatobiliary disorders, including NAFLD, steatosis, and cirrhosis, are brought on by obesity and can cause people to develop HCC [11].

There are toxins or compounds which lead to observing HCC. The most known compound is aflatoxin. This toxin is related and found in grains, corn, peanuts and soybeans. The carcinogenic effect of aflatoxin is observed in moisture and warm conditions. The amount of aflatoxin intake determines the risk of being hepatocellular carcinoma [1]. Furthermore, alcohol consumption and smoking are the major risk factors for HCC.

In the liver and related organs, there are some essential mechanisms for the survival of individuals. In this chapter, we focus on the carcinogenesis of hepatocellular carcinoma and the effect of natural compounds on hepatocellular carcinoma.

NATURAL COMPOUNDS AND THEIR USAGE IN HEPATOCELLULAR CARCINOMA

Coumarin and Coumarin Derivatives

Coumarins were originally isolated in the 18th century from tonka beans (*Dipteryx odorata Willd.*, Fabaceae), and used for various purposes [12, 13]. Coumarin is a natural compound of many plants and essential oils, including tonka beans, sweet clover, woodruff, oil of cassia, and lavender. Furthermore, its name derives from the *Coumarouna odorata* plant [14]. Coumarin is an odorless complex conjugated to sugars and acids, but is released by the action of acids, enzymes, or ultraviolet (UV) radiation [14]. Coumarin compounds have been used to treat various diseases as antispasmodics, especially in cancer, bums, brucellosis and rheumatic disease [14].

The molecular weight of Coumarin is approximately 146.15, and it is colorless with a characteristic odor. Its melting point is between 68-70°C, and its boiling point is 303°C. In chloroform, coumarin can have a UV absorption maximum of 272 nm. Moreover, it can be easily solved in ethanol, chloroform, distilled water and oils [14].

Coumarin is a member of the benzopyrone family, and can be classified into 4 subgroups: simple coumarins, furanocoumarins, pyranocoumarins and pyrone-substituted coumarins [13, 15, 16]. The hydroxylated, alkoxylated, and alkylated derivatives of coumarins include molecules like 7-hydroxycoumarin and 6,7-dihydroxycoumarin, which are simple coumarins. The difference between Furanocoumarins and Pyranocoumarins is the number of furan rings attached to the coumarin nucleus. Pyranocoumarins are analogous to furanocoumarins. 4-hydroxycoumarin, synthetic coumarin derivatives warfarin and benzopyrones are examples of coumarins substituting in the pyrone ring [13, 16].

Coumarin Metabolism in Cells

Initially, coumarin is metabolized in the cytochrome p450 system in cells. In this system, hydroxylation has occurred. The important and well-known coumarin hydroxylations are 7th and 3rd positions. If the hydroxylation is at the 7th position, it is called 7-hydroxycoumarin. If it is at the 3rd position, it is called 3-hydroxycoumarin. 3-hydroxxycoumarin is metabolized non-enzymatically. 0-hydroxyphenyllactic acid (OHPLA), 0-hydroxyphenylacetic acid (OHPAA) and glucuronide conjugate occurred as a result [14]. The activity of 7-hydroxycoumarin is greater in humans than in rodent microsomes. However, 3-hydroxycoumarin activity is observed highly in rodents [14].

Liposomes are also used for the encapsulation of coumarin. The slow release and slow metabolism of coumarin are the objectives of liposome encapsulation. 7-hydroxycoumarin is rapidly converted by conjugation to glucuronide in the gut and other tissues. All 7-hydroxycoumarin in plasma is absorbed from the gut and distributed to both organs with high blood flow and the extracellular matrix and intracellular structures of other tissues. 7-hydroxycoumarin is discarded by active renal tubular secretion, and this pathway is responsible for 90% of the initial coumarin in urine [14].

General Functions of Coumarins and Coumarin Derivatives

Coumarins are very useful in industry, especially in perfume, tobacco, paint and rubber industries. While 6-methylcoumarin is utilized as a flavor enhancer, 3,4-dihydroxycoumarin is specifically used in the perfume industry. 7-Hydroxycoumarin and its derivatives are important coumarins that are used as sun screens, fluorescent brighteners and florigenic enzyme substrates. 7-Amino-4-methylcoumarin and 4-methylumbelliferon are used as laser dyes. Two important coumarin derivatives are especially used in medicine. The first one is 4-Hydroxycoumarin. This coumarin derivative is a vitamin K antagonist and precursor of dicoumarol and warfarin. The second important coumarin derivative is amino methyl coumarin acetic acid (AMCA) which is used for labeling antibodies and lectins for staining [14].

Various natural and synthesized coumarin derivatives exhibit anti-tumor, inhibitory, anti-inflammatory, and antioxidant properties both *in vitro* and *in vivo*, according to studies on coumarins and their derivatives [12, 17]. Coumarin indicated cytotoxic effects against Human epithelial type 2 (Hep2) cells in a dose-dependent manner and also has characteristics of apoptosis as microvilli injury, extreme cytoplasmic vacuolization and nuclear fragmentation [18]. Since coumarin derivatives can inhibit growth in human cancer cell lines such as A549 (lung), ACHN (renal), H727 (lung), HL-60 (leukemia) and MCF-7 (breast) [19], they can have both cytostatic and cytotoxic properties [20, 21]. According to some clinical trials, the activity of coumarin derivatives was demonstrated as anti-proliferative activity in prostate cancer [22], malignant melanoma [23] and renal cell carcinoma [21, 24].

A high dose of 7-hydroxyl-4-methylcoumarin, which could be found in many Chinese herbs, inhibits the proliferation of the SMMC-7721 hepatocellular carcinoma cells. On the other hand, low concentrations of 7-hydroxyl-4-methylcoumarin trigger cell differentiation [25, 26]. Shen X. *et al.* produced a new coumarin derivative that is targeted against Microtubule Affinity-Regulating

Kinase 4 (MARK 4) which makes hepatocellular carcinoma cells more sensitive to an anticancer drug, Paclitaxel [27].

Fraxetin, esculetin, and daphnetin are some of the coumarin derivatives with inhibitory activity against cyclooxygenase and lipoxygenase [12, 28]. Glycycoumarin (GCM) is a representative coumarin derivative that includes a Chinese medical herbal, licorice, for HCC treatment [29, 30]. GCM has anti-viral [31] and anti-inflammatory effects [30, 32]. Licorice is known to have multiple biological functions, including anti-inflammatory, antivirus, anti-cancer, anti-spasmodic and hepatoprotective natural products [33]. Glycycoumarin contains licorice with favorable pharmacologic derivate *in vivo* [34]. In a study, GCM directly inactivated oncogenic kinase T-LAK cell-originated protein kinase and helped the activation of p53. As a result of this, inactivation by GCM cells was arrested during the cell cycle, and activation of cell death mechanisms *in vitro* and tumor reduction *in vivo* was observed [34].

Isofraxidin is another coumarin derivative with anti-stress, anti-fatigue, anti-gastric ulcer, and anti-depressive and anti-inflammatory effects [35]. Genistein is a natural component of coumarin and is thought to as a chemopreventive agent against especially hormonally regulated breast and prostate cancers [36]. Osthole is another type of coumarin. It is isolated from *Cnidium monnieri,* and it is reported that osthole might reduce the epithelial-mesenchymal transition (EMT) and induce apoptosis *via* inhibiting the cell cycle in various cancers [37 - 39].

Coumarin derivatives are composed of the main coumarin chain and some extra chemical structures such as monastrol, pyrazoline *etc.* In a study, coumarine derivative, which is formed with monastrol, caused to stimulate caspase 3 activation and inhibited cell growth in MCF-7 and MDA-MB-231 breast cancer cells [40]. A pyrazoline ring containing coumarin showed an anti-cancer and protective effect against HePG2 hepatocellular carcinoma cells [41]. Furthermore, in MHCC97 and HepG2 human hepatocellular carcinoma (HCC) cells, hydroxypyridinone-coumarin (HPC) is a useful coumarin derivative to decrease proliferation as a result of autophagy induction [42].

Genetic Markers of Coumarin and Coumarin Derivatives Treatment in HCC

Several metastatic genetic markers were determined after isofraxidin treatment to HuH-7 and HepG2 human hepatoma cell lines [35]. Matrix metalloproteinases (MMPs) are the major enzyme where an epithelial-mesenchymal transition occurs. MMP-7 was inhibited in hepatoma cells by isofraxidin treatment, and this inhibition occurred *via* the Extracellular Signal-Regulated Kinase 1/2 (ERK1/2) pathway. İsofraxidin inhibits ERK1/2 phosphorylation, and this causes degradation of activator protein-1 (AP-1) DNA binding activity, nuclear factor-kappa B (NF-k B) and inhibitory kappa B (Ik B), respectively [43].

Osthole is the most studied coumarin derivative in various cancer cases. It has many functions as EMT regulation, apoptotic process, and cell survival mechanisms like proliferation, growth and viability. Lın *et al.* determined that osthole triggers DNA damage, regulates adhesion *via* MMP-2 and MMP-9 expressions and effects cell division by downregulating cyclin B and cdc2 in hepatocellular carcinoma cells [44]. Another study aimed to determine the impact of both osthole and cisplatin treatment on CD133+ hepatocellular carcinoma cells and determined that osthole reduced AKT and Bad phosphorylation to decrease the amount of cytochrome C in CD133+ hepatocellular carcinoma cells. As a result of this reduction, cisplatin-induced mitochondrial apoptosis was developed, and osthole and cisplatin combinations provide to observe CD133+ on these hepatocellular carcinoma cells *via* the PTEN/AKT cascade [37]. In another study about the osthole effect, anti-proliferative and apoptotic impacts were determined on hepatocellular carcinoma cells. Furthermore, there wasn't any toxicity determined during osthole treatment by observing the expressions of Nf-kB and apoptotic genetic markers both *in vivo* and *in vitro* [45].

In a study for understanding the relationship between coumarin and the NF-kB pathway in HCC, a coumarin derivative, 7-Carbethoxyamino-2-oxo-2H-chomen-4-yl-methylpyrrolidine-1 carbodithioate (CPP), was synthesized. NF-kB is an important marker to understand the impacts of treated compounds on cells. NF-kB is a transcription factor and regulates the transcription of the genes involved in inflammation mechanisms [43]. In this study, cytotoxicity induction, suppression of DNA binding ability of NF-kB, cell migration and invasion induction were determined in HCC [12]. Furthermore, gene expression of NF-kB targeted genes, such as cyclin D1 and c-myc (proliferation), Bcl-2 (apoptosis), survivin (cell survival) and MMP-12 (metastasis), were inhibited after CPP treatment on HCC cells [12].

Glycycoumarin (GCM) treatment causes a significant reduction in hepatotoxicity. This cytotoxicity reduction mechanism depends on the relationship between Nrf2 (nuclear factor erythroid 2- related factor 2) and p38. *via* this pathway, GCM-related autophagy induction was observed on HCC cells *in vitro*. Furthermore, high expression of p62 causes Nrf2 upregulation in HCC [30].

Esculetin is another coumarin derivative, which has anticancer activity in various cancers such as human colon, breast, leukemia and cervical cancer by inhibiting proliferation through the Ras/ERK1/2 pathway [46 - 48]. Wang *et al.* indicated that esculetin increased Bax/Bcl-2 ratio, activated the caspase-dependent apoptotic pathway and induced the mitochondrial-mediated apoptosis pathway in HCC [46].

Pyranocoumarin decursin is another kind of coumarin, which is isolated from the roots of *Angelica gigas*. In both colon and bladder cancer cells, it inhibited the proliferation *via* Bax and Bcl-2 expressions in the apoptotic pathway [49].

Hydroxypyridinone-coumarin (HPC) is a coumarin derivative with antioxidant and protective properties [50]. Cui X. and Qin X. indicated that HPC treatment causes to increase Atg-5, beclin-1, Atg-3 and LC3B-II expressions related to autophagy in MHCC97 and HepG2 cells [42].

Curcumin and Curcumin Derivatives

Curcumin[(1E,6E)-1,7-bis(4-hydroxy-3-methoxyphenyl) hepta-1,6-diene- 3,5 - dione] is an natural compound which is extracted from *Curcuma longa* [51, 52]. Researches indicate that Curcumin has various negative impacts on proliferation, inflammation, angiogenesis and oxidation mechanisms [52 - 56]. Curcumin affects both genetic and epigenetic parameters of cells, especially investigated in cancer cells [57]. Curcumin is one of the most widely discovered pharmacological compounds in nanomedicine [58 - 60]. However, curcumin indicates pleiotropic activities of therapeutic concern, and its efficacy is limited due to its poor solubility in water, low stability under physiological conditions, and rapid metabolism [58].

In a study about tumor growth of xenograft nude mouse lung cancer model, curcumin was able to inhibit JAK2 activity and reduce tumor formations *via* JAK/STAT signaling cascade [61]. Furthermore, curcumin treatment effectively aborted Fas/FasL-mediated apoptosis and hypoxia-hypercapnia brain damage - induced brain edema [62]. According to the efficiency of curcumin derivatives, it was determined that nano-curcumin made out of pure curcumin with greater bioavailability; in the abolition of Treg cell growth induced by tumor shed TGF-β [63]. DNA methylation is the main therapeutic target in pancreatic cancer. The activity of novel curcumin analogues EF31 and UBS109 significantly inhibits the proliferation and cytosine methylation mechanisms of pancreatic cancer cells *via* targeting HSP-90 and NF-κB, leading to the downregulation of DNA methyltransferase-1 [64]. Another curcumin derivative, curcumin I (diferuloylmethane), protects neurons against oxidative damage by attenuation of phosphorylated p38 expression, caspase-3-activation, and toxic quinoprotein formation [65]. Furthermore, the neuroprotective effects of curcumin against oxygen-glucose deprivation/reoxygenation are mediated by peroxisome proliferator-activated receptor-γ (PPARγ) activation [66].

Tetrahydrocurcumin is a curcumin derivative, which is important in the gastrointestinal tract [67]. In a study, researchers wanted to compare the effects of tetrahydrocurcumin (THC) to curcumin on angiogenesis both *in vivo* and *in vitro*. They investigated that high doses of THC did not cause any cytotoxic effects, and both curcumin and THC share similar anti-angiogenic properties [68]. Due to the bioavailability of curcumin, curcumin glucuronide (CUR-G) and curcumin glucuronide/sulphate (CUR-G/S) were customized [69, 70]. CUR-G was observed as the major metabolite of CUR found in the plasma after oral administration in rats. In a comparison of the effects of CUR-G and curcumin in HepG2 hepatocellular carcinoma cells, it was found that CUR-G had less effects as the sight of the absorption rates [69]. EF24 [3,5-bis(2-flurobenzylidene) piperidin--one] is a synthetic curcumin derivative that supplies enhanced biological activity and bioavailability without increasing toxicity. EF24 activated the caspase-dependent apoptotic pathway and arrested the cell cycle and angiogenesis of liver cancer cells. As a result, EF24 showed anti-tumor activity on liver cancer cells [71]. A novel curcumin analog, CUR3d, reduced cellular proliferation *via* inhibition of the cell cycle (CDK2, CDK4, CDK5, CDK9, MDM2, MDM4 and TERT genes). Furthermore, CUR3d inhibited the epidermal and insulin-like growth receptors (EGFR, ERBB3, ERBB2, IGF1, IGF-1R, IGF2) expression in HepG2. Moreover, it attenuated the protein kinase-C family [72]. WZ35, a curcumin analog, promoted ROS-dependent JNK activation, thus WZ35 easily suppressed liver cancer cells' metastasis. Reversely, treatment of NAC and JNK inhibitor SP600125 and WZ35 synergistically could reduce MMP-2, MMP-9, and N-cadherin expressions and upregulated E-cadherin expression in liver cancer cells [73]. Another curcumin analog, EF25-(GSH)$_2$, activated the rate of apoptotic and non-apoptotic cell death mechanisms. Combined treatment with chloroquine, a late stage autophagy inhibitor, enhanced apoptosis and cytotoxicity [74]. Abdelmoaty *et al.* revealed that C0818, a novel curcumin derivative and targets Hsp90 protein, increased ROS-dependent cytotoxicity in hepatocellular carcinoma cells *in vitro* [75].

Curcumin has been proven to be effective in treating some cancers, particularly hepatocellular carcinoma cells. Since curcumin's bioavailability makes treatment challenging, some researchers have experimented with curcumin therapy with various combinations. Resveratrol and curcumin-treated Hepa1-6 hepatocellular carcinoma cells indicated that the synergistic effect of these two compounds caused an increase in intracellular reactive oxygen species (ROS) levels. This upregulation started the apoptosis mechanisms of cells [76]. In another study, metformin (a well-studied anti-diabetic drug) and curcumin combination was studied in HCC. Combined treatment of metformin and curcumin both upregulated the apoptotic mechanisms and suppressed metastasis and angiogenesis [77]. Piperine is an important plant alkaloid present in black pepper

(*Piper nigrum L.*) and long pepper (*Piper longum L.*). Furthermore, piperine can inhibit xenobiotic metabolizing enzymes and may exert an antioxidant effect by preventing free radical extinction and reducing glutathione consumption [78]. The synergistic effect of curcumin and piperine indicated that treatment downregulated the morphological, histopathological, biochemical, apoptotic and proliferative changes in the liver and serum DENA-induced HCC in rats [79]. *In vivo*, the combined treatment of curcumin with anti-Programmed cell Death-1 region decreased the HCC growth rate and rehabilitated the tumor microenvironment [80]. The synergistic effect of natural borneol and curcumin was observed, and natural borneol also triggers intracellular ROS overproduction and DNA damage with up-regulation of the expression level of phosphorylated ATM, BRCA1 and p53 in A375 human melanoma cells [81].

Genetic Markers of Curcumin and Curcumin Derivatives Treatment in HCC

UNC119 is a significant molecule that affects the cell cycle, growth, and proliferation. According to this acknowledgement, the relationship between curcumin and UNC119 was investigated. As a result of this study, curcumin downregulated UNC119 expression and also affected Wnt/β-catenin; TGF-β/epithelial-mesenchymal transition (EMT) molecules which are related to UNC119 [82]. Furthermore, CD147 (extracellular matrix metalloproteinase inducer; EMMPRIN) was suggested as the potential target of curcumin in hepatocellular carcinoma. Decreased levels of CD147 caused to increase in curcumin impact on hepatocellular carcinoma cells [83]. Xu *et al.* determined that curcumin cuts off the Wnt signaling by downregulating β-catenin, which suppresses the c-myc (transcription factor), vascular endothelial growth factor (VEGF) and cyclin D1 expressions (target genes of β-catenin) [84]. Epithelial-mesenchymal transition (EMT) is an important parameter for understanding cancer. To gain more insight into EMT, it is necessary to focus on hypoxia-inducible factor 1-alpha (HIF-1).In a recent study, HIF-1α was shown as a curcumin target in HepG2 hepatocellular carcinoma cells by inhibiting the expression of HIF-1α [85]. Turmeric curcumin inhibits Hepatitis C virus entry in primary human hepatocytes by affecting membrane fluency [86]. The reduced motility and decreased matrix metalloproteinase-9 expression were determined after SK-Hep-1, an invasive hepatocellular cancer cell line, was treated with curcumin [87]. The Wnt/β-catenin, VEGF, FGF, MAPK, and PI3K/AKT/mTOR cellular signaling pathways have an important role to understand the carcinogenesis mechanism of HCC [88]. Curcumin targets and inhibits the transcription factor nuclear factor (NF)-κB, MYC proto-oncogene (c-myc), apoptosis regulator (Bcl-2), nitric oxide synthase, cyclooxygenase-2, cyclin D1, matrix metalloproteinase-9 (MMP-9), tumor necrosis factor-α (TNF-α) and interleukins effectively in cancers [89, 90]. Furthermore, in various cancers, curcumin supplies antitumor effects *via* tumor growth factor-β, protein kinase B, and caspase-3 [88, 91, 92]. Moreover, curcumin also affects another apoptotic pathway which is called the extrinsic pathway. Curcumin treatment caused to increase Fas and FasL expression, and it continued with observing the high expression of caspase-3 and cleavage of PARP in Huh7 cells [93]. Curcumin may affect many cellular key features in cells. Mitochondrial molecules are also the targets of curcumin; as a result of this mechanism, endoplasmic reticulum stress and mitochondrial dysfunction occur in hepatocellular carcinoma cells [94]. Mitochondrial dysfunction indicates that curcumin might target the Ca pathway in cells. In a study, the Ca pathway was shown as a target of curcumin *via* endoplasmic reticulum stress and its hallmark GADD153 [95].

A study about HCC growth determined that curcumin targets Vascular Endothelial Growth Factor (VEGF) and PI3K/AKT signaling cascade both *in vitro* and *in vivo* [90]. Curcumin stimulates autophagy by activation of the Akt/ mTOR signaling cascade in cancer cells [96]. Furthermore, Shinojima *et al.* (2007) suggested that curcumin induces autophagy and inhibits the growth of malignant gliomas through the regulation of Akt and ERK signaling pathways [96]. In the DENA-induced HCC rat model study, a chemotherapeutic effect of curcumin was determined in terms of proliferation, angiogenesis and apoptosis [88]. In another study, the impact of curcumin was observed both *in vivo* and *in vitro*. The researchers indicated that curcumin treatment reduced alpha-fetoprotein (AFP) and serum aspartate aminotransferase (AST); induced serum albumin levels. Furthermore, not only reduced oxidative stress and apoptosis but also increased autophagy rate was determined as a result of curcumin treatment in the same research [97]. Induced pyroptosis and apoptosis rates were observed in the HePG2 hepatocellular carcinoma cell line as a result of curcumin treatment [98].

Curcumin has an impact on not only genetic features but also epigenetic markers. One of these epigenetic markers is non-coding RNAs. The well-known member of these non-coding RNAs is micro RNA (miRNA). miRNAs are 18-24 nucleotides in length and can inhibit mRNA transcription and translation in cells. Some researchers determined the possible relationship between miRNAs and curcumin in various cancers, especially hepatocellular carcinoma. Li *et al.* suggested that miR-21 inhibition affects the curcumin function positively. Inhibition of miR-21 caused to increase in curcumin activity, thus low proliferation rates and high apoptosis rates were observed *via* TGF-β1/Smad3 signaling cascade in hepatocellular carcinoma cells [99]. In another study, transfection of miR-200a and miR-200b caused to gain resistance to curcumin *via* Bcl-2, Bad and Bax genes in hepatocellular carcinoma cells [100]. Gender-determining region Y-related high-mobility group box 6 (SOX6) is the main target of miR-21-5p. Furthermore, a recent study indicates that the invasion, metastasis and proliferation of HCC cells might be regulated by curcumin *via* miR-21-5p and SOX6 [101].

Leaf *of Olea Europaea* and Its Extract

Olea europaea (OE), a small evergreen tree belonging to the Oleaceae family, is found predominantly in Mediterranean regions [102 - 104]. Different parts and products derived from this plant, such as fruits, alperujo, leaves, and oils, have been used as health enhancers since ancient times [105, 106]. After the advent of various positive properties of the Mediterranean diet, such as cardioprotective effects, a curiosity for OE and its byproducts has emerged [107].

The first studies on this subject were related to the fruit of the plant, the olive and the olive oil obtained from it. In later periods, the interest in research on affordable and easily available olive leaves increased due to the abundance of phenolic compounds.

Over the years, OE leaf extracts (OLE) have been used to enhance health and longevity. OE leaves have antioxidant, anti-hypertensive, anti-inflammatory, anti-microbial, anti-HIV, anti-atherosclerotic, anti-tumor, cardioprotective, and hypoglycemic properties [105, 108 - 117]. In addition, as a result of various studies conducted with different types of cancer, the anti-cancer and anti-proliferative properties of OLE were determined. Bouallagui *et al.* demonstrated the inhibition of Cyclin D and proliferation in luminal breast cancer cells (MCF-7 cells) by OLE [118]. It has been shown in various studies that OLE inhibited proliferation by inducing cell cycle arrest and apoptosis in human leukemic cell lines (HL-60, Jurkat cells and K562 cells) and melanoma B16 cell lines [117, 119 - 121]. OLE on the JIMT-1 breast cancer cell line led to a significant cell cycle arrest at the G1 phase by the inactivation of the MAPK-proliferation pathway at the extracellular signal-related kinase (ERK1/2) [122]. In a study investigating the effects of OLE on miRNAs in glioblastoma multiforme, it was determined that the use of OLE with temozolomide upregulates miR-181b, miR-153, miR-145, miR-137, and let-7d that are involved in cell cycle and apoptotic pathways [123].

Major Derivatives of Olea Europaea Leaf Extract and their Relationship with Various Types of Cancer

OLE has the highest level of bioactive compounds among the different structures/products of the plant (oleuropein ranges: 0.005 - 0.12% in olive oil, 1 - 14% in OLE, 0.87% in alperujo) [105, 106, 124]. Although the number of phytochemicals' in olive leaf extract may vary depending on various factors such as leaf harvesting season, climatic conditions, field stress and tree subspecies, it basically contains five groups of phenolic compounds as oleuropeosides/secoroids glycoside (oleuropein and verbascoside), flavones (luteolin-7-glucoside, apigenin-7-glucoside, diosmetin-7- glucoside, luteolin, and diosmetin), flavanols (rutin, quarcetin), flavan-3-ols (catechin) and simple phenols (tyrosol, hydroxytyrosol, vanillin, vanillic acid, gallic acid, *p*-hydroxybenzoic acid, *p*-coumaric acid, ferulic acid and caffeic acid) [103, 105, 125 - 129]. The anticancer effectiveness of OLE is thought to be the consequence of complex interactions among the biologically active components of the extract, cancer cells and conventional therapy [130]. In this section, oleuropein, hydroxytyrosol and luteolin OLE derivatives especially used in medicine, are emphasized.

Oleuropein, a phenolic secoroids glycoside with the chemical formula $C_{25}H_{32}O_{13}$, is one of the most active common compounds in OE leaves and fruit. It is also referred to as the coumarin-like components [109, 117, 124, 131, 132]. Oleuropein consists of hydroxytyrosol, elenolic acid and a glucose molecule with an oleosidic skeleton. Its molecular weight of it is approximately 540.5148 Da. Its melting point is 88°C [109, 133]. It has antioxidant [134], anti-inflammatory [135, 136], anti-viral [137], anti-bacterial [138, 139], anti-clastogenic [140] cardioprotective [141], hepatoprotective [142, 143], and antidiabetic effects [144 - 146]. Oleuropein is also defined as an anti-cancer, cytotoxic, anti-proliferative, apoptotic and anti-metastatic compound that prevents recurrent tumor growth and proliferation [144, 147, 148]. Oleuropein contributed to G2/M phase cell cycle arrest and cell death associated with JNK activation in a study on HeLa cells [132]. In studies conducted in MCF-7 and ER-negative breast cancer cells (SKBR3), it was determined that the use of oleuropein increased the expression levels of BAX and p53 and simultaneously suppressed Bcl2 [149, 150]. In another study conducted with A375 cells, it was determined that the use of 250 μM oleuropein decreased cell proliferation and inhibited the pAKT / mTOR pathway through the decrease in AKT/S6 phosphorylation [151]. Also as a result of an *in vivo* study in relation to skin damage caused by chronic ultraviolet B radiation, it was determined that administration of oleuropein at a dose of 25 mg/kg body weight to mice exposed to ultraviolet B radiation for 17 weeks significantly reduced tumor volumes [116].

Hydroxytyrosol (HT), 2-(3,4-dihydroxyphenyl)-ethanol, is a phenolic compound present in the leaf and fruit of OE. In addition, hydroxytyrosol is released by hydrolysis of secoroidss in OLE, such as oleuropein, in the stomach, absorbed by the small intestine by passive diffusion, and assembled in plasma, liver and urine depending on the quantity [152 - 154]. Molecular weight of hydroxytyrosol is 154.16 Da, and its melting point is around 55°C. It can be easily dissolved in water and polar organic solvents and easily oxidized in aqueous solutions [114, 153, 155, 156]. HT has antioxidant, antimicrobial, antiatherogenic, antithrombotic, anti-inflammatory, anti-HIV and anti-carcinogenic activity [153, 157 - 168].

In various studies, it has been reported that the use of HT at appropriate levels in normal and non-transformed cells *in vitro* inhibits excessive ROS production, reduces both cellular and DNA oxidative damage, and thus inhibits the formation and progression of tumorigenesis [154, 169, 170]. Also, several *in vivo* studies have reported that HT inhibits cancer development by activating the nuclear factor-E2-related factor-2/antioxidant responding element (Nrf2/ARE) pathway, resulting in increased transcription of both antioxidant enzymes and phase II detoxifying enzymes [171, 172]. Various *in vitro* studies with human promyelocytic leukemia HL60 and human colon carcinoma HT-29 cell lines have demonstrated that HT blocks the cell cycle through inhibition of CDK proteins and stimulation of CDK inhibitors, and triggers apoptosis by releasing cytochrome c, which activates the effector caspase-3 [160, 173 - 178]. In toxicology studies conducted on long-term and acute dose use, it was determined that the side effects of HT were not observed [179 - 181]. Concomitant usage of oleuropein and HT reduced inflammatory angiogenesis in cultured endothelial cells, through MMP-9 and COX-2 inhibition [182]. Some studies with oleuropein and HT demonstrated that 17 β-estradiol-mediated proliferation was reduced in MCF-7 breast cancer, and activation of GPER/GPR30 dependent pathways promoted apoptosis in ER-negative SKBR3 breast cancer cells [150, 183].

Luteolin (3',4',5,7-Tetrahydroxyflavone, $C_{15}H_{10}O_6$) is an important flavone found not only in OLE, but also in different fruits and vegetables such as celery, artichoke, green peppers, perilla leaves, chamomile, carrots, onion leaves, broccoli, and parsley [184 - 187]. Various studies have shown that luteolin has anti-inflammatory, anti-microbial, cardioprotective, anti-diabetic, anti-hypertension and antioxidant properties [188 - 191]. It has been demonstrated that luteolin is effective in cancer treatment due to its ability to modulate immune system-related transcription factors (NF-B, AP-1, and STAT3/IRF-1… *etc.*), which have physiological roles such as cell growth, differentiation, proliferation, and survival [186, 188]. In addition, oxidative stress also plays an important role in the pathophysiology of different types of cancer [192, 193]. In a study by Song *et al.* with the gastric cancer cell line, it was determined that the use of luteolin decreased the expression of Mcl-1, Survivin and Bcl-xl target genes of STAT3 and triggered apoptosis as a result of inhibiting signal transducer and activator of transcription 3 (STAT3) activation by promoting the interaction of STAT3 with SHP-1. In addition, they confirmed that luteolin inhibits tumor growth in their study with an *in vivo* gastric cancer cell xenograft mouse model [194]. In a study with the BGC-823 cell line, it was determined that luteolin caused the activation of caspases and increased cytochrome c level in the cytoplasm, decreased Bcl-2 level, ERK1/2 phosphorylation, p-PI3K, p-AKT and p-mTOR expression levels. The study demonstrated that luteolin triggers intrinsic apoptosis by causing a dual inhibition of MAPK and PI3K signaling pathways [195]. In the study with human myeloid leukemia cells, it was determined that luteolin inhibited proliferation and promoted apoptosis [196]. In addition, inhibition of cell invasion and anti-proliferative effects of luteolin have been determined by various studies [197, 198]. As a result of studies investigating the effects of luteolin treatment on Hs-746 T gastric cancer cells and HUVECs, it was determined that VEGF secretion decreased due to suppression of Notch1 expression and cell migration, proliferation and vasculogenic mimicry tubes were inhibited [199, 200]. Many kinds of tumors overexpress nuclear factor erythroid 2-related factor 2 (Nrf2), which promotes tumor development and imparts resistance to anticancer treatment. As a result of an *in vitro* study, luteolin has been identified as a potent inhibitor of Nrf2 [201].

OLE and OLE Derivatives in HCC

Both cell culture and animal experiments have been conducted to investigate the effects of OLE and its components in HCC. OLE had a strong anti-carcinogenic effect against the HepG2 cancer cell line according to a study that investigated the anticancer effect of olive leaf methanolic extract on breast, colon, hepatocellular, and cervical carcinoma cells and compared the results to the standard drug vinblastine [202]. In research employing H4IIE rat hepatoma cells and healthy liver clone-9 cells to investigate the apoptotic, genotoxic, cytotoxic, and oxidative effects of OLE, it was determined that OLE selectively promoted cytotoxicity in rat hepatoma cell lines and it did not cause cytotoxicity in healthy cells. This selectivity appears to be due to cancer cells' heightened ability to create reactive oxygen species (ROS). Furthermore, the findings suggest that OLEs can exacerbate apoptotic damage while also having anti-proliferative and pro-apoptotic actions on H4IIE cells [203].

In various studies with HepG2 cells, it was determined that the use of oleuropein inhibits cell proliferation and induces apoptosis in HCC [204, 205]. In a study by Yan *et al.*, it was determined that the use of oleuropein induced intrinsic apoptosis by increasing the expression of the BAX gene while decreasing the Bcl-2 gene expression [204]. The use of oleuropein in HepG2 cells was found to significantly suppress the PI3K/AKT signal cascade which is associated with proliferation, cell survival, invasion, and migration and plays a critical role in HCC pathogenesis by inhibiting AKT phosphorylation [204, 206, 207]. In another study, it was demonstrated that oleuropein activated Ca^{2+}-associated mitochondrial apoptosis by increasing cytosolic cytochrome c and cleaved caspase-9/caspase-3 levels and induced cell cycle arrest in HepG2 cells [208]. In a study targeting the pro-NGF/NGF signaling pathway in HepG2 cells, high doses of oleuropein decreased MMP-7 gene expression and NGF level while increasing proNGF level and caspase3 gene expression. In this study, the use of cisplatin and oleuropein together was evaluated, and it was determined that oleuropein has the ability to increase the antitumor activity of cisplatin, and this combination can improve the side effect of cisplatin by reducing the required dose in the treatment [205].

Yamada *et al.* indicated that the significantly and dose-dependently suppressed TGF-α-induced HCC cell migration by oleuropein and 3-hydroxytyrosol (3-HT) formed from the hydrolysis of the secoiridoid oleuropein [209].

HT inhibited cell proliferation through inhibition of fatty acid synthase activity in human HepG2 and Hep3B cell lines. In addition, antioxidant pathways in cells were stimulated by HT, preventing oxidative stress, and cellular IL-6 levels were decreased [210]. The administration of 1 and 5 μM HT in HepG2 cells inhibited the uncontrolled growth of cells by blocking invasion and triggering the apoptotic death pathway [211]. In an orthotopic model of human HCC *in vivo*, it has been shown that hydroxytyrosol (HT) induced G2/M cell cycle arrest and suppressed the activation of AKT and nuclear factor-kappa B (NF-κB) pathways that result in inhibition of proliferation and increased apoptosis in human HCC cells [212].

An *in vitro* study showed that luteolin induced apoptosis in human hepatoma HepG2 cells by activating JNK and p38 kinase, and Bax/Bak translocation of mitochondria [213]. In a study in which the effects of luteolin on human hepatoma cells were investigated both *in vitro* (HepG2, HLF, and HAK-1B cell lines) and *in vivo* (xenografted tumor model by HAK-1B hepatoma cells in nude mice), luteolin caused a decrease in Ser727 phosphorylation of STAT3 through inactivation of CDK5 and thus increased functional Fas/CD95 expression with caspase 8 activation. In addition, luteolin caused a decrease in the Tyr705 phosphorylation of STAT3, which caused a decrease in target gene products such as cyclin D1, survivin, Bcl-xl, and vascular endothelial growth factor. As a result of these studies, it has been stated that luteolin may lead to inhibit the pathways mediated by STAT3, such as survival, angiogenesis and cell cycle progression and proliferation, which are the basic features of cancer cells, and increase the susceptibility to apoptosis through the upregulation of Fas/CD95 [214]. It was shown that luteolin may suppress the development of liver cancer cells in a dose- and time-dependent way in research using various luteolin concentrations using liver cancer cell lines (SMMC-7721, BEL-7402) and normal liver cell lines (HL-7702). Luteolin induced apoptosis by decreasing the mitochondrial membrane potential of liver cancer cells as a result of increased Bax/Bcl-2 ratio and activating the caspase-3 cascade. Luteolin also arrested liver cancer cells cycle at the G1/S phase. The study also demonstrated that normal liver cells HL-7702 were not affected by luteolin treatment [215]. Luteolin arrested the cell cycle in the G1 phase and triggered apoptosis in HCC cells *via* TGF-β1, p53 and Fas/Fas-ligand signaling pathways [216]. In the drug combination study conducted in relation to luteolin, it was shown that luteolin can synergize the antitumor effects of 5-fluorouracil in HepG2 and Bel7402 cell lines, and this is more effective than the use of drugs alone. The combined use of both drugs inhibited cell growth *via* apoptosis. In addition, as a result of this combined drug administration, Bax/Bcl-2 ratios and p53 expressions were significantly increased and PARP cleavage was enhanced [217]. Luteolin enhanced the expression of ICAM-1, which has a tumor suppressor role by restricting cell proliferation and promoting differentiation, in a research examining the impact of luteolin on the expression of ICAM-1, LFA-3, and PCNA genes in the H22 hepatoma cell line. It reduced the expression of LFA-3 which plays a role as an oncogene in the formation and progression of liver cancer, and PCNA which is closely related to tumor angiogenesis, proliferation, invasion and metastasis [218]. In a xenograft model, luteolin induced cell death and tumor shrinkage in HepG2 cells. It also reduced NF-κB DNA-binding activity and promoted the release of reactive oxygen species (ROS), which mediate AMPK-NF-κB signaling [219]. In hepatocellular carcinoma (HCC), Wei-Jiunn *et al.* determined that luteolin inhibited both MAPK/ERKs and PI3K-Akt pathways by blocking the phosphorylation of c-Met, ERK, and Akt, and as a result, HGF-induced HepG2 cell invasion is aborted [198]. Various pathogenic alterations, including changes in antioxidant and liver marker enzyme levels, are detected in the DN-induced liver carcinogenesis process. In the DN-induced liver carcinogenesis model developed in BALB/c mice, luteolin restored these alterations. Luteolin also reduced the levels of α-fetoprotein and interferon-γ, both of which were elevated during carcinogenesis, while increased the increasing the decreased level of interleukin 2 [220].

Leaf of *Cynara Scolymus* (globe artichoke) and Its Extract

50- 150 cm tall perennial herbaceous plant *Cynara scolymus L.* (CS), known as globe artichoke, is a pharmacologically significant therapeutic plant of the Asteraceae family that is widely grown in Mediterranean regions [221, 222]. Ancient Egyptians, Greeks, and Romans used the CS as food and medicinal [223]. Although many sections of the CS (head, reservoir, inner parts, exterior parts, leaves, and stem) are utilized as herbal medicine, CS leaves and extracts (CSE) derived from leaves are the most commonly used in studies.

CS leaves and CSE have been utilized as hepatoprotective, choleretics, anti-HIV, anti-oxidative, diuretic, antifungal, and antibacterial agents in herbal medicine [221, 224 - 228].

In vivo and *in vitro* studies investigated the effects of CS and CSE on various types of cancer, and the leaf extract showed various anticancer effects, such as inhibiting angiogenesis and proliferation at various stages of carcinogenesis [226,

229, 230]. The research of CSE with the human breast cancer cell line MDA-MB231, which is estrogen receptor-negative, revealed that the extract activated apoptosis *via* mitochondrial and death receptor activation, along with caspase-9 and caspase-8 activation. An increase in the Bax/Bcl-2 ratio and up-regulation of the cyclin-dependent kinase inhibitor p21WAF1 was also identified, both of which are important parts of the apoptosis pathway. The treatment with CSEs significantly reduced cell motility and invasion abilities. A considerable reduction in the proteolytic activity of metalloproteinase-2 (MMP-2) protein, which is involved in the degradation of extracellular matrix components, was also discovered in the same study [231]. Mileo *et al.* reported that modest dosages of CSE therapy reduced human breast cancer cell proliferation *via* a caspase-independent mechanism in a separate investigation. Furthermore, it was discovered in this study that CSE treatment increased galactosidase (SA-β-gal) levels in MDA-MB231 cells and triggered the up-regulation of tumor suppressor genes. Furthermore, the extract triggered epigenetic alterations in total proteins *via* modifying DNA hypomethylation and lysine acetylation levels. According to the findings of the study, CSE therapy reduces breast cancer cell development by inducing premature senescence *via* epigenetic and ROS-mediated pathways [232]. CSE treatment decreased cell growth and proliferation, altered cell survival of MPM cell lines by inducing apoptosis, and hindered migration and invasion of cell lines, according to research with the human MPM cell lines MSTO-211H, NCI-H28, and MPP89. CSE treatment decreased cell growth and proliferation, altered cell survival of MPM cell lines by inducing apoptosis, and hindered migration and invasion of cell lines, according to research with the human MPM cell lines MSTO-211H, NCI-H28, and MPP89. The effects of CSE on tumorigenesis in mice were investigated *in vivo*, and it was revealed that xenographed tumors (MSTO-211H) produced from animals given the extract had considerably decreased Ki67 expression [233]. The effects of CSE on tumorigenesis in mice were investigated *in vivo*, and it was revealed that xenographed tumors (MSTO-211H) produced from animals given the extract had considerably decreased Ki67 expression [233]. In a study conducted with two different human colon cancer cell lines, HT-29 and RKO cell lines, in which the effect of CSEs on cell growth was examined, it was observed that artichoke leaf extracts can affect HT-29 and RKO colon cancer cells by inducing DNA fragmentation and activating the mitochondrial-dependent pathway of apoptosis, increasing the cells in the sub- G1 phase, and resulting in disruption of the cell cycle [234]. In the presence of CSE, pro-apoptotic (BAX) gene expression and a cell cycle inhibitor (p21$^{CIP/WAF1}$) gene expression were elevated in DLD1 colorectal cancer cells, whereas anti-apoptotic BCL-2 gene expression was suppressed. DLD1 cells died *via* apoptosis, according to DNA fragmentation data [235].

Major Derivatives of Cynara Scolymus Extract and their Relationship with Various types of Cancer

Cynara scolymus extract (CSE) contains phenolic acid derivatives [mono- and di-caffeoylquinic acid compounds: quinic acid and chlorogenoquinone, chlorogenic acid, neochlorogenic acids, gallic acid and 1,3-dicaffeoylquinic acid (cynarin)], flavonoids (luteolin, luteolin-7-O-glycoside, luteolin-7-O-rutinoside, apigenin), sesquiterpene glycosides (cynarascoloside A/B and cynarascoloside C), sesquiterpene lactones (cynaropicrin, grossheimin), triterpene saponins (cynarasaponin E, J, C, A/H and F/I), amino and fatty acids (hydroxyoctade-catrienoic acid, dihydroxy-octadecatrienoic acid, hydroxy-oxo-octadecatrienoic acid and tyrosyl-l-leucin, dihydroxy benzoic acid), inulin, vitamin C, vitamin K and some minerals such as calcium, iron, and zinc [223, 236 - 238].

Luteolin-7-O-glucoside (luteoloside; cynaroside, $C_{21}H_{20}O_{11}$) is a flavonoid that has anti-inflammatory, antioxidative and antibacterial and anticancer properties [239, 240]. In human oral cancer cells, the luteolin-7-O-glucoside suppresses cell migration and invasion through modulating MMP-2 production and the extracellular signal-regulated kinase pathway [241]. It is reported that luteoloside could inhibit the proliferation of colon cancer cells [240]. As a result of a study related to human chronic myeloid leukemia, it was stated that the inhibitory effect of luteoloside on K562 cell proliferation was associated with G2/M phase arrest and induction of apoptosis [242]. The luteoloside-induced apoptosis in Hela cells is mediated by both intrinsic and extrinsic mechanisms, and the effects of luteoloside may be regulated by mitogen-activated protein kinases and mTOR signaling pathways *via* p53, according to a study on cervical cancer [243].

Apigenin (4', 5, 7,-trihydroxyflavone, with molecular formula $C_{15}H_{10}O_5$) is an important flavonoid found in *Cynara scolymus*, *Olea europaea*, *Hypericum perforatum*, parsley, celery, and chamomile [244, 245]. Apigenin has antioxidant, anti-hyperglycemic, anti-inflammatory, antimutagenic, antiviral, and anti-apoptotic properties [246 - 249]. Apigenin promotes apoptosis in cancer cells *via* altering the expression of Bcl-2, Bax, STAT-3, and Akt proteins, according to various studies [250, 251]. Apigenin has also been reported to induce inhibition of metastasis and angiogenesis by interacting with signaling molecules in the ERK, JNK, and p38-activated protein kinase (MAPK) pathway [252]. Apigenin has been proposed as a chemotherapeutic agent because of its low intrinsic toxicity and impressive effects on normal and malignant cells, according to research comparing it to different flavonoids [253]. Furthermore, apigenin has been shown to reduce chemoresistance and radioresistance, as well as sensitize cancer cells to these treatments [254].

CSE and CSE Derivatives in HCC

The diethyl nitrosamine (DEN)-induced hepatocellular carcinoma study in Sprague–Dawley rats showed that application of 1 g of CSE had an ameliorating effect on DEN-induced changes of biochemical parameters, such as antioxidant enzymes, antioxidant enzymes, angiogenic growth factors, liver function enzymes and other substances produced by the liver [255]. In addition, treatment of HepG2 cells with CSE for 24 hours reduced cell viability in a dose-dependent manner and triggered apoptosis in HepG2 cells *via* annexin and caspase-3 activation [226]. In a study investigating the effects of silver nanoparticles synthesized using CSE on various cancer cells lines [colon carcinoma cells (HCT-116), hepatocellular carcinoma cells (HePG-2), breast carcinoma cells (MCF-7), and human cervical cancer cell (HeLa)], it was reported that Ag-CSE-NPs, which have the ability to enter cancer cells and penetrate to their small size without affecting healthy cells, show the highest inhibition in HepG2 cell line [256].

In a study, the effects of luteoloside against human hepatoma cells both *in vitro* (Hep3B, SNU-449, Huh-7, SMMC-7721, MHCC-LM3 and MHCC97-H) and *in vivo* (xenograft mice model with SMMC-7721 cells) have been investigated. Luteoloside was determined to significantly inhibit the proliferation, migration and invasive capacity of HCC cells *in vitro* and *in vivo*. In addition, the inhibitory effect of luteoloside on metastasis was observed *in vivo* in the male BALB/c-nu/nu mouse lung metastasis model. Decreased ROS levels caused by luteoloside resulted in decreased proteolytic cleavage of caspase-1 and inhibition of IL-1β, and decreased inflammatory expression of NLRP3. As a result of the study, it was stated that luteoloside showed its inhibitory effect on proliferation, invasion and metastasis of HCC cells through inhibition of NLRP3 inflammation [257]. The anti-proliferative effect of luteoloside on HepG2 cells was connected with G2/M phase cell cycle arrest by JNK activation, according to a study on luteoloside anti-proliferation on tumor cells and the biological mechanism of luteoloside cytotoxicity in HepG2 cells [258].

A study with HepG2, SMMC-7721, and Huh-7 cell lines determined that apigenin can induce G1 arrest in HepG2 in a dose-dependent manner [259]. In the HCC model induced by administration of 2-acetylaminofluorene (2-AAF) for 14 days following a single dose of diethyl nitrosamine (DEN), apigenin only reduced the mitochondrial membrane potential (MMP), reactive oxygen species (ROS) level, mitochondrial swelling, and cytochrome c excretion in cancerous hepatocytes. and increased caspase-3 activation [260]. In a study in which the human hepatoma cell lines Huh7 and Hep3B were examined *in vitro,* and the effects on the tumorigenicity of Huh7 cells were evaluated *in vivo*, it was determined that apigenin inhibited Huh7 cell proliferation, cell cycle, colony formation and cell invasion. In addition, apigenin reduced tumor growth, promoted tumor cell necrosis, decreased Ki67 expression, and increased Bax and Bcl-2 expression in xenograft tumors of Huh7 cells. As a result of the bioinformatic analysis of the miRNA transcriptome, it was determined that up-regulated miRNAs were associated with the hepatocellular carcinoma pathway, and down-regulated miRNAs were associated with the basic regulatory pathways defined as proteoglycans in the cancer pathway [261]. As a result of *in vitro* (SMMC-7721 and HepG2 cells) and *in vivo* (Xenograft mouse model with HepG2 cells) studies, apigenin administration inhibited tumor growth *in vitro* and *in vivo* through downregulation of H19 and reduced β-catenin expression, leading to inactivation of Wnt/β-catenin signaling [262].

CONCLUSION

Natural products or components are important substances for their therapeutic or protective properties. By the results of these studies in which natural products or components are used for treating various cancer, modern-day drugs have been discovered. Not only therapeutic but also the protective properties of these substances may help reduce the incidence of various cancer. The explained natural substances in this chapter are novel natural products, and are still being investigated and studied to understand the exact properties of hepatocellular cancer. With the developed studies, both genetic, biochemical and physiological effects of these components are investigated, and their effects on metabolism and cellular mechanisms, such as inflammation, apoptosis and vitality, are examined. Although cancer has become a common disease today, it is a disease known to increase survival with its early diagnosis. In particular, lifestyle and genetic background can prevent the emergence of this disease or reduce its effect. For this reason, the effects of these natural components should not be ignored in increasing the survival of individuals and ensuring the natural protection of their health.

CONSENT FOR PUBLICATION

Not applicable.

CONFLICT OF INTEREST

The author declares no conflict of interest, financial or otherwise.

ACKNOWLEDGEMENTS

Declared none.

REFERENCES

[1]   Balogh, J.; Victor, D., III; Asham, E.H.; Burroughs, S.G.; Boktour, M.; Saharia, A.; Li, X.; Ghobrial, M.; Monsour, H., Jr Hepatocellular carcinoma: A review. *J. Hepatocell. Carcinoma,* **2016,** *3,* 41-53.
       [http://dx.doi.org/10.2147/JHC.S61146] [PMID: 27785449]

[2]   Crissien, A.M.; Frenette, C. Current management of hepatocellular carcinoma. *Gastroenterol. Hepatol. (N. Y.),* **2014,** *10*(3), 153-161.
       [PMID: 24829542]

[3]   (IARC) IAfRoC. Monographs on the evaluation of carcinogenic risks to humans. *Hepatitis Viruses,* **1994,** *59,* 182-221.

[4]   Chen, G.; Lin, W.; Shen, F.; Iloeje, U.H.; London, W.T.; Evans, A.A. Past HBV viral load as predictor of mortality and morbidity from HCC and chronic liver disease in a prospective study. *Am. J. Gastroenterol,* **2006,** *101*(8), 1797-1803.
       [http://dx.doi.org/10.1111/j.1572-0241.2006.00647.x] [PMID: 16817842]

[5]   Hosaka, T.; Suzuki, F.; Kobayashi, M.; Seko, Y.; Kawamura, Y.; Sezaki, H.; Akuta, N.; Suzuki, Y.; Saitoh, S.; Arase, Y.; Ikeda, K.; Kobayashi, M.; Kumada, H. Long-term entecavir treatment reduces hepatocellular carcinoma incidence in patients with hepatitis B virus infection. *Hepatology,* **2013,** *58*(1), 98-107.
       [http://dx.doi.org/10.1002/hep.26180] [PMID: 23213040]

[6]   Lok, A.S.; Seeff, L.B.; Morgan, T.R.; di Bisceglie, A.M.; Sterling, R.K.; Curto, T.M.; Everson, G.T.; Lindsay, K.L.; Lee, W.M.; Bonkovsky, H.L.; Dienstag, J.L.; Ghany, M.G.; Morishima, C.; Goodman, Z.D. Incidence of hepatocellular carcinoma and associated risk factors in hepatitis C-related advanced liver disease. *Gastroenterology,* **2009,** *136*(1), 138-148.
       [http://dx.doi.org/10.1053/j.gastro.2008.09.014] [PMID: 18848939]

[7]   Hassan, M.M.; Hwang, L.Y.; Hatten, C.J.; Swaim, M.; Li, D.; Abbruzzese, J.L.; Beasley, P.; Patt, Y.Z. Risk factors for hepatocellular carcinoma: Synergism of alcohol with viral hepatitis and diabetes mellitus. *Hepatology,* **2002,** *36*(5), 1206-1213.
       [http://dx.doi.org/10.1053/jhep.2002.36780] [PMID: 12395331]

[8]   Turati, F.; Galeone, C.; Rota, M.; Pelucchi, C.; Negri, E.; Bagnardi, V.; Corrao, G.; Boffetta, P.; La Vecchia, C. Alcohol and liver cancer: A systematic review and meta-analysis of prospective studies. *Ann. Oncol,* **2014,** *25*(8), 1526-1535.
       [http://dx.doi.org/10.1093/annonc/mdu020] [PMID: 24631946]

[9]   Wong, R.J.; Cheung, R.; Ahmed, A. Nonalcoholic steatohepatitis is the most rapidly growing indication for liver transplantation in patients with hepatocellular carcinoma in the U.S. *Hepatology,* **2014,** *59*(6), 2188-2195.
       [http://dx.doi.org/10.1002/hep.26986] [PMID: 24375711]

[10]   Wang, C.; Wang, X.; Gong, G.; Ben, Q.; Qiu, W.; Chen, Y.; Li, G.; Wang, L. Increased risk of hepatocellular carcinoma in patients with diabetes mellitus: A systematic review and meta-analysis of cohort studies. *Int. J. Cancer,* **2012,** *130*(7), 1639-1648.
       [http://dx.doi.org/10.1002/ijc.26165] [PMID: 21544812]

[11]   Reddy, J.K.; Sambasiva Rao, M. Lipid metabolism and liver inflammation. II. Fatty liver disease and fatty acid oxidation. *Am. J. Physiol. Gastrointest. Liver Physiol,* **2006,** *290*(5), G852-G858.
       [http://dx.doi.org/10.1152/ajpgi.00521.2005] [PMID: 16603729]

[12]   Neelgundmath, M.; Dinesh, K.R.; Mohan, C.D.; Li, F.; Dai, X.; Siveen, K.S.; Paricharak, S.; Mason, D.J.; Fuchs, J.E.; Sethi, G.; Bender, A.; Rangappa, K.S.; Kotresh, O.; Basappa, Novel synthetic coumarins that targets NF-κB in Hepatocellular carcinoma. *Bioorg. Med. Chem. Lett,* **2015,** *25*(4), 893-897.
       [http://dx.doi.org/10.1016/j.bmcl.2014.12.065] [PMID: 25592709]

[13]   Lacy, A.; O'Kennedy, R. Studies on coumarins and coumarin-related compounds to determine their therapeutic role in the treatment of cancer. *Curr. Pharm. Des,* **2004,** *10*(30), 3797-3811.

[http://dx.doi.org/10.2174/1381612043382693] [PMID: 15579072]

[14]   Egan, D.; O'kennedy, R.; Moran, E.; Cox, D.; Prosser, E.; Thornes, R.D. The pharmacology, metabolism, analysis, and applications of coumarin and coumarin-related compounds. *Drug Metab. Rev,* **1990**, *22*(5), 503-529.
       [http://dx.doi.org/10.3109/03602539008991449] [PMID: 2078993]

[15]   Ojala, T., Ed. *Biological Screening of Plant Coumarins*; , **2001**.

[16]   G, K.; R, O.K. Coumarins: Biology, applications and mode of action. In: *The Chemistry and Occurrence of Coumarins*; R, O.K.; RD, T., Eds.; John Wiley & Sons: Chichester, **1997**; pp. 23-66.

[17]   Kontogiorgis, C.; Hadjipavlou-Litina, D. Biological evaluation of several coumarin derivatives designed as possible anti-inflammatory/antioxidant agents. *J. Enzyme Inhib. Med. Chem,* **2003**, *18*(1), 63-69.
       [http://dx.doi.org/10.1080/1475636031000069291] [PMID: 12751823]

[18]   Mirunalini, S.; Deepalakshmi, K.; Manimozhi, J. Antiproliferative effect of coumarin by modulating oxidant/antioxidant status and inducing apoptosis in Hep2 cells. *Biomed. Aging Pathol,* **2014**, *4*(2), 131-135.
       [http://dx.doi.org/10.1016/j.biomag.2014.01.006]

[19]   Marshall, M.E.; Kervin, K.; Benefield, C.; Umerani, A.; Albainy-Jenei, S.; Zhao, Q.; Khazaeli, M.B. Growth-inhibitory effects of coumarin (1,2-benzopyrone) and 7-hydroxycoumarin on human malignant cell lines *in vitro. J. Cancer Res. Clin. Oncol,* **1994**, *120*(S1) Suppl., S3-S10.
       [http://dx.doi.org/10.1007/BF01377114] [PMID: 7510710]

[20]   Benci, K.; Mandić, L.; Suhina, T.; Sedić, M.; Klobučar, M.; Kraljević Pavelić, S.; Pavelić, K.; Wittine, K.; Mintas, M. Novel coumarin derivatives containing 1,2,4-triazole, 4,5-dicyanoimidazole and purine moieties: synthesis and evaluation of their cytostatic activity. *Molecules,* **2012**, *17*(9), 11010-11025.
       [http://dx.doi.org/10.3390/molecules170911010] [PMID: 22971585]

[21]   Salem, M.; Marzouk, M.; El-Kazak, A. Synthesis and characterization of some new coumarins with *in vitro* antitumor and antioxidant activity and high protective effects against DNA damage. *Molecules,* **2016**, *21*(2), 249.
       [http://dx.doi.org/10.3390/molecules21020249] [PMID: 26907244]

[22]   Mohler, J.L.; Gomella, L.G.; Crawford, E.D.; Glode, L.M.; Zippe, C.D.; Fair, W.R.; Marshall, M.E. Phase II evaluation of coumarin (1,2-benzopyrone) in metastatic prostatic carcinoma. *Prostate,* **1992**, *20*(2), 123-131.
       [http://dx.doi.org/10.1002/pros.2990200208] [PMID: 1549551]

[23]   Thornes, R.D.; Daly, L.; Lynch, G.; Breslin, B.; Browne, H.; Browne, H.Y.; Corrigan, T.; Daly, P.; Edwards, G.; Gaffney, E.; Henley, J.; Healy, T.; Keane, F.; Lennon, F.; McMurray, N.; O'Loughlin, S.; Shine, M.; Tanner, A. Treatment with coumarin to prevent or delay recurrence of malignant melanoma. *J. Cancer Res. Clin. Oncol,* **1994**, *120*(S1) Suppl., S32-S34.
       [http://dx.doi.org/10.1007/BF01377122] [PMID: 8132701]

[24]   Marshall, M.E.; Butler, K.; Fried, A. Phase I evaluation of coumarin (1,2-benzopyrone) and cimetidine in patients with advanced malignancies. *Mol. Biother,* **1991**, *3*(3), 170-178.
       [PMID: 1768368]

[25]   Wu, X.Z.; Xie, G.R. Induced differentiation of hepatocellular carcinoma by natural products. *Afr. J. Tradit. Complement. Altern. Med,* **2008**, *5*(4), 325-331.
       [PMID: 20161953]

[26]   Pan, J.; Zhang, Q.; Zhao, C.; Zheng, R. Redifferentiation of human hepatoma cells induced by synthesized coumarin. *Cell Biol. Int,* **2004**, *28*(5), 329-333.
       [http://dx.doi.org/10.1016/j.cellbi.2004.02.002] [PMID: 15193276]

[27]   Shen, X.; Liu, X.; Wan, S.; Fan, X.; He, H.; Wei, R.; Pu, W.; Peng, Y.; Wang, C. Discovery of Coumarin as Microtubule Affinity-Regulating Kinase 4 Inhibitor That Sensitize Hepatocellular

Carcinoma to Paclitaxel. *Front Chem,* **2019**, *7*, 366.
[http://dx.doi.org/10.3389/fchem.2019.00366] [PMID: 31179271]

[28] Fylaktakidou, K.; Hadjipavlou-Litina, D.; Litinas, K.; Nicolaides, D. Natural and synthetic coumarin derivatives with anti-inflammatory/ antioxidant activities. *Curr. Pharm. Des,* **2004**, *10*(30), 3813-3833.
[http://dx.doi.org/10.2174/1381612043382710] [PMID: 15579073]

[29] Qiao, X.; Liu, C.F.; Ji, S.; Lin, X.H.; Guo, D.A.; Ye, M. Simultaneous determination of five minor coumarins and flavonoids in Glycyrrhiza uralensis by solid-phase extraction and high-performance liquid chromatography/electrospray ionization tandem mass spectrometry. *Planta Med,* **2014**, *80*(02/03), 237-242.
[http://dx.doi.org/10.1055/s-0033-1360272] [PMID: 24496986]

[30] Song, X.; Yin, S.; Huo, Y.; Liang, M.; Fan, L.; Ye, M.; Hu, H. Glycycoumarin ameliorates alcohol-induced hepatotoxicity *via* activation of Nrf2 and autophagy. *Free Radic. Biol. Med,* **2015**, *89*, 135-146.
[http://dx.doi.org/10.1016/j.freeradbiomed.2015.07.006] [PMID: 26169726]

[31] Adianti, M.; Aoki, C.; Komoto, M.; Deng, L.; Shoji, I.; Wahyuni, T.S. M.I.; Soetjipto, Fuchino, H.; Kawahara, N.; Hotta, H. Anti-hepatitis C virus compounds obtained from *Glycyrrhiza uralensis* and other *Glycyrrhiza* species. *Microbiol. Immunol,* **2014**, *58*(3), 180-187.
[http://dx.doi.org/10.1111/1348-0421.12127] [PMID: 24397541]

[32] Fu, Y.; Chen, J.; Li, Y.J.; Zheng, Y.F.; Li, P. Antioxidant and anti-inflammatory activities of six flavonoids separated from licorice. *Food Chem,* **2013**, *141*(2), 1063-1071.
[http://dx.doi.org/10.1016/j.foodchem.2013.03.089] [PMID: 23790887]

[33] Wang, Z.Y.; Nixon, D.W. Licorice and Cancer. *Nutr. Cancer,* **2001**, *39*(1), 1-11.
[http://dx.doi.org/10.1207/S15327914nc391_1] [PMID: 11588889]

[34] Song, X.; Yin, S.; Zhang, E.; Fan, L.; Ye, M.; Zhang, Y.; Hu, H. Glycycoumarin exerts anti-liver cancer activity by directly targeting T-LAK cell-originated protein kinase. *Oncotarget,* **2016**, *7*(40), 65732-65743.
[http://dx.doi.org/10.18632/oncotarget.11610] [PMID: 27582549]

[35] Yamazaki, T.; Tokiwa, T. Isofraxidin, a coumarin component from Acanthopanax senticosus, inhibits matrix metalloproteinase-7 expression and cell invasion of human hepatoma cells. *Biol. Pharm. Bull,* **2010**, *33*(10), 1716-1722.
[http://dx.doi.org/10.1248/bpb.33.1716] [PMID: 20930381]

[36] Constantinou, A.I.; Kamath, N.; Murley, J.S. Genistein inactivates bcl-2, delays the G2/M phase of the cell cycle, and induces apoptosis of human breast adenocarcinoma MCF-7 cells. *Eur. J. Cancer,* **1998**, *34*(12), 1927-1934.
[http://dx.doi.org/10.1016/S0959-8049(98)00198-1] [PMID: 10023317]

[37] Ye, J.; Sun, D.; Yu, Y.; Yu, J. Osthole resensitizes CD133[+] hepatocellular carcinoma cells to cisplatin treatment *via* PTEN/AKT pathway. *Aging (Albany NY),* **2020**, *12*(14), 14406-14417.
[http://dx.doi.org/10.18632/aging.103484] [PMID: 32673286]

[38] Wang, L.; Peng, Y.; Shi, K.; Wang, H.; Lu, J.; Li, Y.; Ma, C. Osthole inhibits proliferation of human breast cancer cells by inducing cell cycle arrest and apoptosis. *J. Biomed. Res,* **2015**, *29*(2), 132-138.
[PMID: 25859268]

[39] Wen, Y.C.; Lee, W.J.; Tan, P.; Yang, S.F.; Hsiao, M.; Lee, L.M.; Chien, M.H. By inhibiting snail signaling and miR-23a-3p, osthole suppresses the EMT-mediated metastatic ability in prostate cancer. *Oncotarget,* **2015**, *6*(25), 21120-21136.
[http://dx.doi.org/10.18632/oncotarget.4229] [PMID: 26110567]

[40] Sashidhara, K.V.; Avula, S.R.; Sharma, K.; Palnati, G.R.; Bathula, S.R. Discovery of coumarin–monastrol hybrid as potential antibreast tumor-specific agent. *Eur. J. Med. Chem,* **2013**, *60*, 120-127.

[http://dx.doi.org/10.1016/j.ejmech.2012.11.044] [PMID: 23287057]

[41]   Amin, K.M.; Abou-Seri, S.M.; Awadallah, F.M.; Eissa, A.A.M.; Hassan, G.S.; Abdulla, M.M. Synthesis and anticancer activity of some 8-substituted-7-methoxy-2H-chromen-2-one derivatives toward hepatocellular carcinoma HepG2 cells. *Eur. J. Med. Chem,* **2015**, *90*, 221-231. [http://dx.doi.org/10.1016/j.ejmech.2014.11.027] [PMID: 25461322]

[42]   Cui, X.; Qin, X. Hydroxypyridinone-Coumarin Inhibits the Proliferation of MHCC97 and HepG2 Human Hepatocellular Carcinoma Cells and Down-Regulates the Phosphoinositide-3 Kinase Pathway. *Med. Sci. Monit,* **2020**, *26*, e920785. [http://dx.doi.org/10.12659/MSM.920785] [PMID: 32218414]

[43]   Vallabhapurapu, S.; Karin, M. Regulation and function of NF-kappaB transcription factors in the immune system. *Annu. Rev. Immunol,* **2009**, *27*(1), 693-733. [http://dx.doi.org/10.1146/annurev.immunol.021908.132641] [PMID: 19302050]

[44]   Lin, Z.K.; Liu, J.; Jiang, G.Q.; Tan, G.; Gong, P.; Luo, H.F.; Li, H.M.; Du, J.; Ning, Z.; Xin, Y.; Wang, Z.Y. Osthole inhibits the tumorigenesis of hepatocellular carcinoma cells. *Oncol. Rep,* **2017**, *37*(3), 1611-1618. [http://dx.doi.org/10.3892/or.2017.5403] [PMID: 28184928]

[45]   Zhang, L.; Jiang, G.; Yao, F.; He, Y.; Liang, G.; Zhang, Y.; Hu, B.; Wu, Y.; Li, Y.; Liu, H. Growth inhibition and apoptosis induced by osthole, a natural coumarin, in hepatocellular carcinoma. *PLoS One,* **2012**, *7*(5), e37865. [http://dx.doi.org/10.1371/journal.pone.0037865] [PMID: 22662241]

[46]   Wang, J.; Lu, M.L.; Dai, H.L.; Zhang, S.P.; Wang, H.X.; Wei, N. Esculetin, a coumarin derivative, exerts *in vitro* and *in vivo* antiproliferative activity against hepatocellular carcinoma by initiating a mitochondrial-dependent apoptosis pathway. *Braz. J. Med. Biol. Res,* **2015**, *48*(3), 245-253. [http://dx.doi.org/10.1590/1414-431x20144074] [PMID: 25517918]

[47]   Duan, J; Shi, J; Ma, X; Xuan, Y; Li, P; Wang, H Esculetin inhibits proliferation, migration, and invasion of clear cell renal cell carcinoma cells. *Biomedicine & Pharmacotherapy,* **2020**, *125*, 110031. [http://dx.doi.org/10.1016/j.biopha.2020.110031]

[48]   Park, S.S.; Park, S.K.; Lim, J.H.; Choi, Y.H.; Kim, W.J.; Moon, S.K. Esculetin inhibits cell proliferation through the Ras/ERK1/2 pathway in human colon cancer cells. *Oncol. Rep,* **2011**, *25*(1), 223-230. [PMID: 21109980]

[49]   Kim, W.J.; Lee, S.J.; Choi, Y.D.; Moon, S.K. Decursin inhibits growth of human bladder and colon cancer cells *via* apoptosis, G1-phase cell cycle arrest and extracellular signal-regulated kinase activation. *Int. J. Mol. Med,* **2010**, *25*(4), 635-641. [PMID: 20198313]

[50]   Bistrović, A.; Krstulović, L.; Harej, A.; Grbčić, P.; Sedić, M.; Koštrun, S.; Pavelić, S.K.; Bajić, M.; Raić-Malić, S. Design, synthesis and biological evaluation of novel benzimidazole amidines as potent multi-target inhibitors for the treatment of non-small cell lung cancer. *Eur. J. Med. Chem,* **2018**, *143*, 1616-1634. [http://dx.doi.org/10.1016/j.ejmech.2017.10.061] [PMID: 29133046]

[51]   Zhang, J.Y.; Lin, M.T.; Zhou, M.J.; Yi, T.; Tang, Y.N.; Tang, S.L.; Yang, Z.J.; Zhao, Z.Z.; Chen, H.B. Combinational treatment of curcumin and quercetin against gastric cancer MGC-803 cells *in vitro*. *Molecules,* **2015**, *20*(6), 11524-11534. [http://dx.doi.org/10.3390/molecules200611524] [PMID: 26111180]

[52]   Wang, H.; Zhang, K.; Liu, J.; Yang, J.; Tian, Y.; Yang, C.; Li, Y.; Shao, M.; Su, W.; Song, N. Curcumin regulates cancer progression: focus on ncrnas and molecular signaling pathways. *Front. Oncol,* **2021**, *11*, 660712. [http://dx.doi.org/10.3389/fonc.2021.660712] [PMID: 33912467]

[53]   Chen, L.; Zhan, C.Z.; Wang, T.; You, H.; Yao, R. Curcumin inhibits the proliferation, migration,

invasion, and apoptosis of diffuse large b-cell lymphoma cell line by regulating MiR-21/VHL axis. *Yonsei Med. J, 2020, 61*(1), 20-29.
[http://dx.doi.org/10.3349/ymj.2020.61.1.20] [PMID: 31887796]

[54]   Siriviriyakul, P.; Chingchit, T.; Klaikeaw, N.; Chayanupatkul, M.; Werawatganon, D. Effects of curcumin on oxidative stress, inflammation and apoptosis in L-arginine induced acute pancreatitis in mice. *Heliyon, 2019, 5*(8), e02222.
[http://dx.doi.org/10.1016/j.heliyon.2019.e02222] [PMID: 31485503]

[55]   Gaikwad, D; Shewale, R; Patil, V; Mali, D; Gaikwad, U; Jadhav, N. Enhancement in *in vitro* anti-angiogenesis activity and cytotoxicity in lung cancer cell by pectin-PVP based curcumin particulates. *Int. J. Biol. Macromol, 2017, 104,* 656-664.

[56]   Yang, L.; Zheng, Z.; Qian, C.; Wu, J.; Liu, Y.; Guo, S.; Li, G.; Liu, M.; Wang, X.; Kaplan, D.L. Curcumin-functionalized silk biomaterials for anti-aging utility. *J. Colloid Interface Sci, 2017, 496,* 66-77.
[http://dx.doi.org/10.1016/j.jcis.2017.01.115] [PMID: 28214625]

[57]   Liu, Y.; Sun, H.; Makabel, B.; Cui, Q.; Li, J.; Su, C.; Ashby, C.R., Jr; Chen, Z.; Zhang, J. The targeting of non-coding RNAs by curcumin: Facts and hopes for cancer therapy (Review). *Oncol. Rep, 2019, 42*(1), 20-34.
[http://dx.doi.org/10.3892/or.2019.7148] [PMID: 31059075]

[58]   Singh, S.P.; Sharma, M.; Gupta, P.K. Cytotoxicity of curcumin silica nanoparticle complexes conjugated with hyaluronic acid on colon cancer cells. *Int. J. Biol. Macromol, 2015, 74,* 162-170.
[http://dx.doi.org/10.1016/j.ijbiomac.2014.11.037] [PMID: 25511568]

[59]   Yallapu, M.M.; Jaggi, M.; Chauhan, S.C. Curcumin nanoformulations: A future nanomedicine for cancer. *Drug Discov. Today, 2012, 17*(1-2), 71-80.
[http://dx.doi.org/10.1016/j.drudis.2011.09.009] [PMID: 21959306]

[60]   Liu, J.; Chen, S.; Lv, L.; Song, L.; Guo, S.; Huang, S. Recent progress in studying curcumin and its nano-preparations for cancer therapy. *Curr. Pharm. Des, 2013, 19*(11), 1974-1993.
[PMID: 23116308]

[61]   Wu, L.; Guo, L.; Liang, Y.; Liu, X.; Jiang, L.; Wang, L. Curcumin suppresses stem-like traits of lung cancer cells *via* inhibiting the JAK2/STAT3 signaling pathway. *Oncol. Rep, 2015, 34*(6), 3311-3317.
[http://dx.doi.org/10.3892/or.2015.4279] [PMID: 26397387]

[62]   Yu, L.; Fan, Y.; Ye, G.; Li, J.; Feng, X.; Lin, K.; Dong, M.; Wang, Z. Curcumin inhibits apoptosis and brain edema induced by hypoxia-hypercapnia brain damage in rat models. *Am. J. Med. Sci, 2015, 349*(6), 521-525.
[http://dx.doi.org/10.1097/MAJ.0000000000000457] [PMID: 25867253]

[63]   Hossain, D.M.S.; Panda, A.K.; Chakrabarty, S.; Bhattacharjee, P.; Kajal, K.; Mohanty, S.; Sarkar, I.; Sarkar, D.K.; Kar, S.K.; Sa, G. MEK inhibition prevents tumour-shed transforming growth factor- β -induced T-regulatory cell augmentation in tumour milieu. *Immunology, 2015, 144*(4), 561-573.
[http://dx.doi.org/10.1111/imm.12397] [PMID: 25284464]

[64]   Nagaraju, G.P.; Zhu, S.; Wen, J.; Farris, A.B.; Adsay, V.N.; Diaz, R.; Snyder, J.P.; Mamoru, S.; El-Rayes, B.F. Novel synthetic curcumin analogues EF31 and UBS109 are potent DNA hypomethylating agents in pancreatic cancer. *Cancer Lett, 2013, 341*(2), 195-203.
[http://dx.doi.org/10.1016/j.canlet.2013.08.002] [PMID: 23933177]

[65]   Meesarapee, B.; Thampithak, A.; Jaisin, Y.; Sanvarinda, P.; Suksamrarn, A.; Tuchinda, P.; Morales, N.P.; Sanvarinda, Y. Curcumin I mediates neuroprotective effect through attenuation of quinoprotein formation, p-p38 MAPK expression, and caspase-3 activation in 6-hydroxydopamine treated SH-SY5Y cells. *Phytother. Res, 2014, 28*(4), 611-616.
[http://dx.doi.org/10.1002/ptr.5036] [PMID: 23857913]

[66]   Liu, Z.J.; Liu, H.Q.; Xiao, C.; Fan, H.Z.; Huang, Q.; Liu, Y.H.; Wang, Y. Curcumin protects neurons against oxygen-glucose deprivation/reoxygenation-induced injury through activation of peroxisome

proliferator-activated receptor-γ function. *J. Neurosci. Res,* **2014**, *92*(11), 1549-1559.
[http://dx.doi.org/10.1002/jnr.23438] [PMID: 24975470]

[67]   Sugiyama, Y.; Kawakishi, S.; Osawa, T. Involvement of the β-diketone moiety in the antioxidative Mechanism of Tetrahydrocurcumin. *Biochem. Pharmacol,* **1996**, *52*(4), 519-525.
[http://dx.doi.org/10.1016/0006-2952(96)00302-4] [PMID: 8759023]

[68]   Yoysungnoen, P.; Wirachwong, P.; Changtam, C.; Suksamrarn, A.; Patumraj, S. Anti-cancer and anti-angiogenic effects of curcumin and tetrahydrocurcumin on implanted hepatocellular carcinoma in nude mice. *World J. Gastroenterol,* **2008**, *14*(13), 2003-2009.
[http://dx.doi.org/10.3748/wjg.14.2003] [PMID: 18395899]

[69]   Shoji, M.; Nakagawa, K.; Watanabe, A.; Tsuduki, T.; Yamada, T.; Kuwahara, S.; Kimura, F.; Miyazawa, T. Comparison of the effects of curcumin and curcumin glucuronide in human hepatocellular carcinoma HepG2 cells. *Food Chem,* **2014**, *151*, 126-132.
[http://dx.doi.org/10.1016/j.foodchem.2013.11.021] [PMID: 24423511]

[70]   Asai, A.; Miyazawa, T. Occurrence of orally administered curcuminoid as glucuronide and glucuronide/sulfate conjugates in rat plasma. *Life Sci,* **2000**, *67*(23), 2785-2793.
[http://dx.doi.org/10.1016/S0024-3205(00)00868-7] [PMID: 11105995]

[71]   Liu, H.; Liang, Y.; Wang, L.; Tian, L.; Song, R.; Han, T.; Pan, S.; Liu, L. *In vivo* and *in vitro* suppression of hepatocellular carcinoma by EF24, a curcumin analog. *PLoS One,* **2012**, *7*(10), e48075.
[http://dx.doi.org/10.1371/journal.pone.0048075] [PMID: 23118928]

[72]   Bhullar, K.S.; Jha, A.; Rupasinghe, H.P.V. Novel carbocyclic curcumin analog CUR3d modulates genes involved in multiple apoptosis pathways in human hepatocellular carcinoma cells. *Chem. Biol. Interact,* **2015**, *242*, 107-122.
[http://dx.doi.org/10.1016/j.cbi.2015.09.020] [PMID: 26409325]

[73]   Wang, L.; Han, L.; Tao, Z.; Zhu, Z.; Han, L.; Yang, Z.; Wang, H.; Dai, D.; Wu, L.; Yuan, Z.; Chen, T. The curcumin derivative WZ35 activates ROS-dependent JNK to suppress hepatocellular carcinoma metastasis. *Food Funct,* **2018**, *9*(5), 2970-2978.
[http://dx.doi.org/10.1039/C8FO00314A] [PMID: 29766185]

[74]   Zhou, T.; Ye, L.; Bai, Y.; Sun, A.; Cox, B.; Liu, D.; Li, Y.; Liotta, D.; Snyder, J.P.; Fu, H.; Huang, B. Autophagy and apoptosis in hepatocellular carcinoma induced by EF25-(GSH)2: A novel curcumin analog. *PLoS One,* **2014**, *9*(9), e107876.
[http://dx.doi.org/10.1371/journal.pone.0107876] [PMID: 25268357]

[75]   Abdelmoaty, A.A.A.; Zhang, P.; Lin, W.; Fan, Y.; Ye, S.; Xu, J. C0818, a novel curcumin derivative, induces ROS-dependent cytotoxicity in human hepatocellular carcinoma cells *in vitro via* disruption of Hsp90 function. *Acta Pharmacol Sin,* **2022**, *43*(2), 446-456.
[http://dx.doi.org/10.1038/s41401-021-00642-3] [PMID: 33824458]

[76]   Du, Q.; Hu, B.; an, H.M.; Shen, K.P.; Xu, L.; Deng, S.; Wei, M.M. Synergistic anticancer effects of curcumin and resveratrol in Hepa1-6 hepatocellular carcinoma cells. *Oncol. Rep,* **2013**, *29*(5), 1851-1858.
[http://dx.doi.org/10.3892/or.2013.2310] [PMID: 23446753]

[77]   Zhang, H.H.; Zhang, Y.; Cheng, Y.N.; Gong, F.L.; Cao, Z.Q.; Yu, L.G.; Guo, X.L. Metformin incombination with curcumin inhibits the growth, metastasis, and angiogenesis of hepatocellular carcinoma *in vitro* and *in vivo*. *Mol. Carcinog,* **2018**, *57*(1), 44-56.
[http://dx.doi.org/10.1002/mc.22718] [PMID: 28833603]

[78]   Mittal, R.; Gupta, R.L. *In vitro* antioxidant activity of piperine. *Methods Find. Exp. Clin. Pharmacol,* **2000**, *22*(5), 271-274.
[http://dx.doi.org/10.1358/mf.2000.22.5.796644] [PMID: 11031726]

[79]   Patial, V.; S, M.; Sharma, S.; Pratap, K.; Singh, D.; Padwad, Y.S. Synergistic effect of curcumin and piperine in suppression of DENA-induced hepatocellular carcinoma in rats. *Environ. Toxicol. Pharmacol,* **2015**, *40*(2), 445-452.

[http://dx.doi.org/10.1016/j.etap.2015.07.012] [PMID: 26278679]

[80]   Guo, L.; Li, H.; Fan, T.; Ma, Y.; Wang, L. Synergistic efficacy of curcumin and anti-programmed cell death-1 in hepatocellular carcinoma. *Life Sci,* **2021,** *279,* 119359.
[http://dx.doi.org/10.1016/j.lfs.2021.119359] [PMID: 33753114]

[81]   Chen, J.; Li, L.; Su, J.; Li, B.; Chen, T.; Wong, Y.S. Synergistic apoptosis-inducing effects on A375 human melanoma cells of natural borneol and curcumin. *PLoS One,* **2014,** *9*(6), e101277.
[http://dx.doi.org/10.1371/journal.pone.0101277] [PMID: 24971451]

[82]   Zhao, Z; Malhotra, A; Seng, WY Curcumin modulates hepatocellular carcinoma by reducing UNC119 expression. **2019,** *38*(3), 195-203.
[http://dx.doi.org/10.1615/JEnvironPatholToxicolOncol.2019029549]

[83]   Jia, L.; Wang, H.; Qu, S.; Miao, X.; Zhang, J. CD147 regulates vascular endothelial growth factor-A expression, tumorigenicity, and chemosensitivity to curcumin in hepatocellular carcinoma. *IUBMB Life,* **2008,** *60*(1), 57-63.
[http://dx.doi.org/10.1002/iub.11] [PMID: 18379992]

[84]   Xu, M.X.; Zhao, L.; Deng, C.; Yang, L.; Wang, Y.; Guo, T.; Li, L.; Lin, J.; Zhang, L. Curcumin suppresses proliferation and induces apoptosis of human hepatocellular carcinoma cells *via* the wnt signaling pathway. *Int. J. Oncol,* **2013,** *43*(6), 1951-1959.
[http://dx.doi.org/10.3892/ijo.2013.2107] [PMID: 24064724]

[85]   Duan, W.; Chang, Y.; Li, R.; Xu, Q.; Lei, J.; Yin, C.; Li, T.; Wu, Y.; Ma, Q.; Li, X. Curcumin inhibits hypoxia inducible factor-1α-induced epithelial-mesenchymal transition in HepG2 hepatocellular carcinoma cells. *Mol. Med. Rep,* **2014,** *10*(5), 2505-2510.
[http://dx.doi.org/10.3892/mmr.2014.2551] [PMID: 25216080]

[86]   Anggakusuma, Colpitts, C.C.; Schang, L.M.; Rachmawati, H.; Frentzen, A.; Pfaender, S. Turmeric curcumin inhibits entry of all hepatitis C virus genotypes into human liver cells. *Gut,* **2014,** *63*(7), 1137-1149.
[http://dx.doi.org/10.1136/gutjnl-2012-304299]

[87]   Lin, L.I.; Ke, Y.F.; Ko, Y.C.; Lin, J.K. Curcumin inhibits SK-Hep-1 hepatocellular carcinoma cell invasion *in vitro* and suppresses matrix metalloproteinase-9 secretion. *Oncology,* **1998,** *55*(4), 349-353.
[http://dx.doi.org/10.1159/000011876] [PMID: 9663426]

[88]   Abouzied, M.M.M.; Eltahir, H.M.; Abdel Aziz, M.A.; Ahmed, N.S.; Abd El-Ghany, A.A.; Abd El-Aziz, E.A.; Abd El-Aziz, H.O. Curcumin ameliorate DENA-induced HCC *via* modulating TGF-β, AKT, and caspase-3 expression in experimental rat model. *Tumour Biol,* **2015,** *36*(3), 1763-1771.
[http://dx.doi.org/10.1007/s13277-014-2778-z] [PMID: 25519685]

[89]   Kumar, P.; Kadakol, A.; Shasthrula, P.; Mundhe, N.; Jamdade, V.; Barua, C.; Gaikwad, A. Curcumin as an adjuvant to breast cancer treatment. *Anticancer. Agents Med. Chem,* **2015,** *15*(5), 647-656.
[http://dx.doi.org/10.2174/1871520615666150101125918] [PMID: 25553436]

[90]   Pan, Z.; Zhuang, J.; Ji, C.; Cai, Z.; Liao, W.; Huang, Z. Curcumin inhibits hepatocellular carcinoma growth by targeting VEGF expression. *Oncol. Lett,* **2018,** *15*(4), 4821-4826.
[http://dx.doi.org/10.3892/ol.2018.7988] [PMID: 29552121]

[91]   Zhang, C.Y.; Zhang, L.; Yu, H.X.; Bao, J.D.; Lu, R.R. Curcumin inhibits the metastasis of K1 papillary thyroid cancer cells *via* modulating E-cadherin and matrix metalloproteinase-9 expression. *Biotechnol. Lett,* **2013,** *35*(7), 995-1000.
[http://dx.doi.org/10.1007/s10529-013-1173-y] [PMID: 23474829]

[92]   Chen, W.C.; Lai, Y.A.; Lin, Y.C.; Ma, J.W.; Huang, L.F.; Yang, N.S.; Ho, C.T.; Kuo, S.C.; Way, T.D. Curcumin suppresses doxorubicin-induced epithelial-mesenchymal transition *via* the inhibition of TGF-β and PI3K/AKT signaling pathways in triple-negative breast cancer cells. *J. Agric. Food Chem,* **2013,** *61*(48), 11817-11824.
[http://dx.doi.org/10.1021/jf404092f] [PMID: 24236784]

[93] Wang, W.Z.; Li, L.; Liu, M.Y.; Jin, X.B.; Mao, J.W.; Pu, Q.H.; Meng, M.J.; Chen, X.G.; Zhu, J.Y. Curcumin induces FasL-related apoptosis through p38 activation in human hepatocellular carcinoma Huh7 cells. *Life Sci,* **2013**, *92*(6-7), 352-358.
[http://dx.doi.org/10.1016/j.lfs.2013.01.013] [PMID: 23352975]

[94] Cheng, C-Y.; Lin, Y-H.; Su, C-C. Curcumin inhibits the proliferation of human hepatocellular carcinoma J5 cells by inducing endoplasmic reticulum stress and mitochondrial dysfunction. *Int. J. Mol. Med,* **2010**, *26*(5), 673-678.
[http://dx.doi.org/10.3892/ijmm_00000513] [PMID: 20878089]

[95] Wang, WH; Chiang, IT; Ding, K; Chung, JG; Lin, WJ; Lin, S.S. Curcumin-induced apoptosis in human hepatocellular carcinoma j5 cells: critical role of ca(+2)-dependent pathway. *Evid. Based. Complement. Alternat. Med.,* **2012**, *2012*, 512907.
[http://dx.doi.org/10.1155/2012/512907]

[96] Shinojima, N.; Yokoyama, T.; Kondo, Y.; Kondo, S. Roles of the Akt/mTOR/p70S6K and ERK1/2 signaling pathways in curcumin-induced autophagy. *Autophagy,* **2007**, *3*(6), 635-637.
[http://dx.doi.org/10.4161/auto.4916] [PMID: 17786026]

[97] Elmansi, A.M.; El-Karef, A.A.; El-Shishtawy, M.M.; Eissa, L.A. Hepatoprotective effect of curcumin on hepatocellular carcinoma through autophagic and apoptic pathways. *Ann. Hepatol,* **2017**, *16*(4), 607-618.
[http://dx.doi.org/10.5604/01.3001.0010.0307] [PMID: 28611265]

[98] Liang, W.F.; Gong, Y.X.; Li, H.F.; Sùn, F.L.; Li, W.L.; Chen, D.Q.; Xie, D.P.; Ren, C.X.; Guo, X.Y.; Wang, Z.Y.; Kwon, T.; Sun, H.N. Curcumin activates ROS signaling to promote pyroptosis in hepatocellular carcinoma HepG2 cells. *In Vivo,* **2021**, *35*(1), 249-257.
[http://dx.doi.org/10.21873/invivo.12253] [PMID: 33402471]

[99] Li, J.; Wei, H.; Liu, Y.; Li, Q.; Guo, H.; Guo, Y.; Chang, Z. Curcumin inhibits hepatocellular carcinoma *via* regulating miR-21/TIMP3 axis. *Evid. Based Complement. Alternat. Med,* **2020**, *2020*, 1-13.
[http://dx.doi.org/10.1155/2020/2892917] [PMID: 32724322]

[100] Liang, H.H.; Wei, P.L.; Hung, C.S.; Wu, C.T.; Wang, W.; Huang, M.T.; Chang, Y.J. MicroRNA-200a/b influenced the therapeutic effects of curcumin in hepatocellular carcinoma (HCC) cells. *Tumour Biol,* **2013**, *34*(5), 3209-3218.
[http://dx.doi.org/10.1007/s13277-013-0891-z] [PMID: 23760980]

[101] Zhou, C.; Hu, C.; Wang, B.; Fan, S.; Jin, W. Curcumin suppresses cell proliferation, migration, and invasion through modulating miR-21-5p/ *SOX6* axis in hepatocellular carcinoma. *Cancer Biother. Radiopharm,* **2020**, cbr.2020.3734.
[http://dx.doi.org/10.1089/cbr.2020.3734] [PMID: 32757994]

[102] Ryan, D.; Antolovich, M.; Prenzler, P.; Robards, K.; Lavee, S. Biotransformations of phenolic compounds in *Olea europaea* L. *Sci. Hortic. (Amsterdam),* **2002**, *92*(2), 147-176.
[http://dx.doi.org/10.1016/S0304-4238(01)00287-4]

[103] Ghanbari, R.; Anwar, F.; Alkharfy, K.M.; Gilani, A.H.; Saari, N. Valuable nutrients and functional bioactives in different parts of olive (*Olea europaea* L.)-a review. *Int. J. Mol. Sci,* **2012**, *13*(3), 3291-3340.
[http://dx.doi.org/10.3390/ijms13033291] [PMID: 22489153]

[104] Castejón, M.L.; Montoya, T.; Alarcón-de-la-Lastra, C.; Sánchez-Hidalgo, M. Potential protective role exerted by secoiridoids from *Olea europaea* L. in cancer, cardiovascular, neurodegenerative, aging-related, and immunoinflammatory diseases. *Antioxidants,* **2020**, *9*(2), 149.
[http://dx.doi.org/10.3390/antiox9020149] [PMID: 32050687]

[105] El, S.N.; Karakaya, S. Olive tree (*Olea europaea*) leaves: potential beneficial effects on human health. *Nutr. Rev,* **2009**, *67*(11), 632-638.
[http://dx.doi.org/10.1111/j.1753-4887.2009.00248.x] [PMID: 19906250]

[106] Japón-Luján, R.; Luque-Rodríguez, J.M.; Luque de Castro, M.D. Dynamic ultrasound-assisted extraction of oleuropein and related biophenols from olive leaves. *J. Chromatogr. A,* **2006**, *1108*(1), 76-82.
[http://dx.doi.org/10.1016/j.chroma.2005.12.106] [PMID: 16442552]

[107] Torić, J.; Marković, A.K.; Brala, C.J.; Barbarić, M. Anticancer effects of olive oil polyphenols and their combinations with anticancer drugs. *Acta Pharm,* **2019**, *69*(4), 461-482.
[http://dx.doi.org/10.2478/acph-2019-0052] [PMID: 31639094]

[108] Susalit, E.; Agus, N.; Effendi, I.; Tjandrawinata, R.R.; Nofiarny, D.; Perrinjaquet-Moccetti, T.; Verbruggen, M. Olive (*Olea europaea*) leaf extract effective in patients with stage-1 hypertension: Comparison with Captopril. *Phytomedicine,* **2011**, *18*(4), 251-258.
[http://dx.doi.org/10.1016/j.phymed.2010.08.016] [PMID: 21036583]

[109] Nediani, C.; Ruzzolini, J.; Romani, A.; Calorini, L. Oleuropein, a bioactive compound from *Olea europaea* L., as a potential preventive and therapeutic agent in non-communicable diseases. *Antioxidants,* **2019**, *8*(12), 578.
[http://dx.doi.org/10.3390/antiox8120578] [PMID: 31766676]

[110] Lockyer, S.; Rowland, I.; Spencer, J.P.E.; Yaqoob, P.; Stonehouse, W. Impact of phenolic-rich olive leaf extract on blood pressure, plasma lipids and inflammatory markers: A randomised controlled trial. *Eur. J. Nutr,* **2017**, *56*(4), 1421-1432.
[http://dx.doi.org/10.1007/s00394-016-1188-y] [PMID: 26951205]

[111] Eidi, A.; Eidi, M.; Darzi, R. Antidiabetic effect of *Olea europaea* L. in normal and diabetic rats. *Phytother. Res,* **2009**, *23*(3), 347-350.
[http://dx.doi.org/10.1002/ptr.2629] [PMID: 18844257]

[112] Gonzalez, M.; Zarzuelo, A.; Gamez, M.; Utrilla, M.; Jimenez, J.; Osuna, I. Hypoglycemic activity of olive leaf. *Planta Med,* **1992**, *58*(6), 513-515.
[http://dx.doi.org/10.1055/s-2006-961538] [PMID: 1484890]

[113] Markin, D.; Duek, L.; Berdicevsky, I. *In vitro* antimicrobial activity of olive leaves. Antimikrobielle Wirksamkeit von Olivenblattern *in vitro. Mycoses,* **2003**, *46*(3-4), 132-136.
[http://dx.doi.org/10.1046/j.1439-0507.2003.00859.x] [PMID: 12870202]

[114] Pereira, A.; Ferreira, I.; Marcelino, F.; Valentão, P.; Andrade, P.; Seabra, R.; Estevinho, L.; Bento, A.; Pereira, J. Phenolic compounds and antimicrobial activity of olive (*Olea europaea* L. Cv. Cobrançosa) leaves. *Molecules,* **2007**, *12*(5), 1153-1162.
[http://dx.doi.org/10.3390/12051153] [PMID: 17873849]

[115] Lee-Huang, S.; Zhang, L.; Lin Huang, P.; Chang, Y.T.; Huang, P.L. Anti-HIV activity of olive leaf extract (OLE) and modulation of host cell gene expression by HIV-1 infection and OLE treatment. *Biochem. Biophys. Res. Commun,* **2003**, *307*(4), 1029-1037.
[http://dx.doi.org/10.1016/S0006-291X(03)01292-0] [PMID: 12878215]

[116] Kimura, Y.; Sumiyoshi, M. Olive leaf extract and its main component oleuropein prevent chronic ultraviolet B radiation-induced skin damage and carcinogenesis in hairless mice. *J. Nutr,* **2009**, *139*(11), 2079-2086.
[http://dx.doi.org/10.3945/jn.109.104992] [PMID: 19776181]

[117] Anter, J.; Fernández-Bedmar, Z.; Villatoro-Pulido, M.; Demyda-Peyras, S.; Moreno-Millán, M.; Alonso-Moraga, Á.; Muñoz-Serrano, A.; Luque de Castro, M.D. A pilot study on the DNA-protective, cytotoxic, and apoptosis-inducing properties of olive-leaf extracts. *Mutat. Res. Genet. Toxicol. Environ. Mutagen,* **2011**, *723*(2), 165-170.
[http://dx.doi.org/10.1016/j.mrgentox.2011.05.005] [PMID: 21620995]

[118] Bouallagui, Z.; Han, J.; Isoda, H.; Sayadi, S. Hydroxytyrosol rich extract from olive leaves modulates cell cycle progression in MCF-7 human breast cancer cells. *Food Chem. Toxicol,* **2011**, *49*(1), 179-184.
[http://dx.doi.org/10.1016/j.fct.2010.10.014] [PMID: 20955751]

[119] Samet, I; Han, J; Jlaiel, L; Sayadi, S.; Isoda, H. Olive (*Olea europaea*) leaf extract induces apoptosis and monocyte/macrophage differentiation in human chronic myelogenous leukemia K562 cells: insight into the underlying mechanism. *Oxidative Medicine and Cellular Longevity,* **2014**, *2014*

[120] Fares, R.; Bazzi, S.; Baydoun, S.E.; Abdel-Massih, R.M. The antioxidant and anti-proliferative activity of the Lebanese *Olea europaea* extract. *Plant Foods Hum. Nutr,* **2011**, *66*(1), 58-63.
[http://dx.doi.org/10.1007/s11130-011-0213-9] [PMID: 21318304]

[121] Mijatovic, S.A.; Timotijevic, G.S.; Miljkovic, D.M.; Radovic, J.M.; Maksimovic-Ivanic, D.D.; Dekanski, D.P.; Stosic-Grujicic, S.D. Multiple antimelanoma potential of dry olive leaf extract. *Int. J. Cancer,* **2011**, *128*(8), 1955-1965.
[http://dx.doi.org/10.1002/ijc.25526] [PMID: 20568104]

[122] Barrajón-Catalán, E.; Taamalli, A.; Quirantes-Piné, R.; Roldan-Segura, C.; Arráez-Román, D.; Segura-Carretero, A.; Micol, V.; Zarrouk, M. Differential metabolomic analysis of the potential antiproliferative mechanism of olive leaf extract on the JIMT-1 breast cancer cell line. *J. Pharm. Biomed. Anal,* **2015**, *105*, 156-162.
[http://dx.doi.org/10.1016/j.jpba.2014.11.048] [PMID: 25560707]

[123] Tunca, B.; Tezcan, G.; Cecener, G.; Egeli, U.; Ak, S.; Malyer, H.; Tumen, G.; Bilir, A. *Olea europaea* leaf extract alters microRNA expression in human glioblastoma cells. *J. Cancer Res. Clin. Oncol,* **2012**, *138*(11), 1831-1844.
[http://dx.doi.org/10.1007/s00432-012-1261-8] [PMID: 22722712]

[124] Ahmad Farooqi, A.; Fayyaz, S.; Silva, A.; Sureda, A.; Nabavi, S.; Mocan, A.; Nabavi, S.; Bishayee, A. Oleuropein and cancer chemoprevention: the link is hot. *Molecules,* **2017**, *22*(5), 705.
[http://dx.doi.org/10.3390/molecules22050705] [PMID: 28468276]

[125] Goulas, V.; Exarchou, V.; Troganis, A.N.; Psomiadou, E.; Fotsis, T.; Briasoulis, E.; Gerothanassis, I.P. Phytochemicals in olive-leaf extracts and their antiproliferative activity against cancer and endothelial cells. *Mol. Nutr. Food Res,* **2009**, *53*(5), 600-608.
[http://dx.doi.org/10.1002/mnfr.200800204] [PMID: 19194970]

[126] Araújo, M.; Prada, J.; Mariz-Ponte, N.; Santos, C.; Pereira, J.A.; Pinto, D.C.G.A.; Silva, A.M.S.; Dias, M.C. Antioxidant Adjustments of Olive Trees (*Olea Europaea*) under Field Stress Conditions. *Plants,* **2021**, *10*(4), 684.
[http://dx.doi.org/10.3390/plants10040684] [PMID: 33916326]

[127] Laguerre, M.; López Giraldo, L.J.; Piombo, G.; Figueroa-Espinoza, M.C.; Pina, M.; Benaissa, M.; Combe, A.; Rossignol Castera, A.; Lecomte, J.; Villeneuve, P. Characterization of olive-leaf phenolics by ESI-MS and evaluation of their antioxidant capacities by the CAT assay. *J. Am. Oil Chem. Soc,* **2009**, *86*(12), 1215-1225.
[http://dx.doi.org/10.1007/s11746-009-1452-x]

[128] Sabry, O.M. Beneficial health effects of olive leaves extracts. *J. Nat. Sci.Res.,* **2014**, *4*(19), 1-9.

[129] Talhaoui, N.; Taamalli, A.; Gómez-Caravaca, A.M.; Fernández-Gutiérrez, A.; Segura-Carretero, A. Phenolic compounds in olive leaves: Analytical determination, biotic and abiotic influence, and health benefits. *Food Res. Int,* **2015**, *77*, 92-108.
[http://dx.doi.org/10.1016/j.foodres.2015.09.011]

[130] Espeso, J.; Isaza, A.; Lee, J.Y.; Sörensen, P.M.; Jurado, P.; Avena-Bustillos, R.J.; Olaizola, M.; Arboleya, J.C. Olive leaf waste management. *Front. Sustain. Food Syst,* **2021**, *5*, 660582.
[http://dx.doi.org/10.3389/fsufs.2021.660582]

[131] Hassen, I.; Casabianca, H.; Hosni, K. Biological activities of the natural antioxidant oleuropein: Exceeding the expectation – A mini-review. *J. Funct. Foods,* **2015**, *18*, 926-940.
[http://dx.doi.org/10.1016/j.jff.2014.09.001]

[132] Yao, J.; Wu, J.; Yang, X.; Yang, J.; Zhang, Y.; Du, L. Oleuropein induced apoptosis in HeLa cells *via* a mitochondrial apoptotic cascade associated with activation of the c-Jun NH2-terminal kinase. *J.*

Pharmacol. Sci, **2014**, *125*(3), 300-311.
[http://dx.doi.org/10.1254/jphs.14012FP] [PMID: 25048019]

[133]   Soler-Rivas, C.; Espín, J.C.; Wichers, H.J. Oleuropein and related compounds. *J. Sci. Food Agric,* **2000**, *80*(7), 1013-1023.
[http://dx.doi.org/10.1002/(SICI)1097-0010(20000515)80:7<1013::AID-JSFA571>3.0.CO;2-C]

[134]   Jemai, H.; El Feki, A.; Sayadi, S. Antidiabetic and antioxidant effects of hydroxytyrosol and oleuropein from olive leaves in alloxan-diabetic rats. *J. Agric. Food Chem,* **2009**, *57*(19), 8798-8804.
[http://dx.doi.org/10.1021/jf901280r] [PMID: 19725535]

[135]   Giamarellos-Bourboulis, E.J.; Geladopoulos, T.; Chrisofos, M.; Koutoukas, P.; Vassiliadis, J.; Alexandrou, I.; Tsaganos, T.; Sabracos, L.; Karagianni, V.; Pelekanou, E.; Tzepi, I.; Kranidioti, H.; Koussoulas, V.; Giamarellou, H. Oleuropein: A novel immunomodulator conferring prolonged survival in experimental sepsis by *Pseudomonas aeruginosa. Shock,* **2006**, *26*(4), 410-416.
[http://dx.doi.org/10.1097/01.shk.0000226342.70904.06] [PMID: 16980890]

[136]   Giner, E.; Recio, M.C.; Ríos, J.L.; Giner, R.M. Oleuropein protects against dextran sodium sulfate-induced chronic colitis in mice. *J. Nat. Prod,* **2013**, *76*(6), 1113-1120.
[http://dx.doi.org/10.1021/np400175b] [PMID: 23758110]

[137]   Lee-Huang, S.; Huang, P.L.; Zhang, D.; Lee, J.W.; Bao, J.; Sun, Y.; Chang, Y.T.; Zhang, J.; Huang, P.L. Discovery of small-molecule HIV-1 fusion and integrase inhibitors oleuropein and hydroxytyrosol: Part I. Integrase inhibition. *Biochem. Biophys. Res. Commun,* **2007**, *354*(4), 872-878.
[http://dx.doi.org/10.1016/j.bbrc.2007.01.071] [PMID: 17275783]

[138]   Tranter, H.S.; Tassou, S.C.; Nychas, G.J. The effect of the olive phenolic compound, oleuropein, on growth and enterotoxin B production by *Staphylococcus aureus. J. Appl. Bacteriol,* **1993**, *74*(3), 253-259.
[http://dx.doi.org/10.1111/j.1365-2672.1993.tb03023.x] [PMID: 8468258]

[139]   Tassou, C.C.; Nychas, G.J.; Board, R.G. Effect of phenolic compounds and oleuropein on the germination of *Bacillus cereus* T spores. *Biotechnol. Appl. Biochem,* **1991**, *13*(2), 231-237.
[PMID: 1904245]

[140]   Benavente-García, O.; Castillo, J.; Lorente, J.; Alcaraz, M. Radioprotective effects *in vivo* of phenolics extracted from *Olea europaea* L. leaves against X-ray-induced chromosomal damage: comparative study *versus* several flavonoids and sulfur-containing compounds. *J. Med. Food,* **2002**, *5*(3), 125-135.
[http://dx.doi.org/10.1089/10966200260398152] [PMID: 12495584]

[141]   Manna, C.; Migliardi, V.; Golino, P.; Scognamiglio, A.; Galletti, P.; Chiariello, M.; Zappia, V. Oleuropein prevents oxidative myocardial injury induced by ischemia and reperfusion. *J. Nutr. Biochem,* **2004**, *15*(8), 461-466.
[http://dx.doi.org/10.1016/j.jnutbio.2003.12.010] [PMID: 15302080]

[142]   Domitrović, R.; Jakovac, H.; Marchesi, V.V.; Šain, I.; Romić, Ž.; Rahelić, D. Preventive and therapeutic effects of oleuropein against carbon tetrachloride-induced liver damage in mice. *Pharmacol. Res,* **2012**, *65*(4), 451-464.
[http://dx.doi.org/10.1016/j.phrs.2011.12.005] [PMID: 22214867]

[143]   Kim, SW; Hur, W; Li, TZ; Lee, YK; Choi, JE; Hong, SW Oleuropein prevents the progression of steatohepatitis to hepatic fibrosis induced by a high-fat diet in mice. *Experimental & Molecular Medicine,* **2014**, *46*(4), e92.
[http://dx.doi.org/10.1038/emm.2014.10]

[144]   Messeha, S.S.; Zarmouh, N.O.; Asiri, A.; Soliman, K.F.A. Gene Expression Alterations Associated with Oleuropein-Induced Antiproliferative Effects and S-Phase Cell Cycle Arrest in Triple-Negative Breast Cancer Cells. *Nutrients,* **2020**, *12*(12), 3755.
[http://dx.doi.org/10.3390/nu12123755] [PMID: 33297339]

[145]   Murotomi, K.; Umeno, A.; Yasunaga, M.; Shichiri, M.; Ishida, N.; Koike, T.; Matsuo, T.; Abe, H.; Yoshida, Y.; Nakajima, Y. Oleuropein-rich diet attenuates hyperglycemia and impaired glucose

tolerance in type 2 diabetes model mouse. *J. Agric. Food Chem,* **2015**, *63*(30), 6715-6722.
[http://dx.doi.org/10.1021/acs.jafc.5b00556] [PMID: 26165358]

[146] Hadrich, F.; Garcia, M.; Maalej, A.; Moldes, M.; Isoda, H.; Feve, B.; Sayadi, S. Oleuropein activated AMPK and induced insulin sensitivity in C2C12 muscle cells. *Life Sci,* **2016**, *151*, 167-173.
[http://dx.doi.org/10.1016/j.lfs.2016.02.027] [PMID: 26872981]

[147] Barzegar, F.; Zaefizadeh, M.; Yari, R.; Salehzadeh, A. Synthesis of nano-paramagnetic oleuropein to induce KRAS over-expression: A new mechanism to inhibit AGS cancer cells. *Medicina (Kaunas),* **2019**, *55*(7), 388.
[http://dx.doi.org/10.3390/medicina55070388] [PMID: 31330954]

[148] Bulotta, S.; Oliverio, M.; Russo, D.; Procopio, A. Biological Activity of Oleuropein and its Derivatives. In: *Natural Products: Phytochemistry, Botany and Metabolism of Alkaloids, Phenolics and Terpenes*; Ramawat, K.G.; Mérillon, J-M., Eds.; Springer Berlin Heidelberg: Berlin, Heidelberg, **2013**; pp. 3605-3638.
[http://dx.doi.org/10.1007/978-3-642-22144-6_156]

[149] Hassan, Z.K.; Elamin, M.H.; Omer, S.A.; Daghestani, M.H.; Al-Olayan, E.S.; Elobeid, M.A.; Virk, P. Oleuropein induces apoptosis *via* the p53 pathway in breast cancer cells. *Asian Pac. J. Cancer Prev,* **2013**, *14*(11), 6739-6742.
[http://dx.doi.org/10.7314/APJCP.2013.14.11.6739] [PMID: 24377598]

[150] Chimento, A.; Casaburi, I.; Rosano, C.; Avena, P.; De Luca, A.; Campana, C.; Martire, E.; Santolla, M.F.; Maggiolini, M.; Pezzi, V.; Sirianni, R. Oleuropein and hydroxytyrosol activate GPER/ GPR30-dependent pathways leading to apoptosis of ER-negative SKBR3 breast cancer cells. *Mol. Nutr. Food Res,* **2014**, *58*(3), 478-489.
[http://dx.doi.org/10.1002/mnfr.201300323] [PMID: 24019118]

[151] Ruzzolini, J.; Peppicelli, S.; Andreucci, E.; Bianchini, F.; Scardigli, A.; Romani, A.; la Marca, G.; Nediani, C.; Calorini, L. Oleuropein, the main polyphenol of *Olea europaea* leaf extract, has an anti-cancer effect on human BRAF melanoma cells and potentiates the cytotoxicity of current chemotherapies. *Nutrients,* **2018**, *10*(12), 1950.
[http://dx.doi.org/10.3390/nu10121950] [PMID: 30544808]

[152] Rodríguez-Morató, J.; Boronat, A.; Kotronoulas, A.; Pujadas, M.; Pastor, A.; Olesti, E.; Pérez-Mañá, C.; Khymenets, O.; Fitó, M.; Farré, M.; de la Torre, R. Metabolic disposition and biological significance of simple phenols of dietary origin: hydroxytyrosol and tyrosol. *Drug Metab. Rev,* **2016**, *48*(2), 218-236.
[http://dx.doi.org/10.1080/03602532.2016.1179754] [PMID: 27186796]

[153] Vilaplana-Pérez, C.; Auñón, D.; García-Flores, L.A.; Gil-Izquierdo, A. Hydroxytyrosol and potential uses in cardiovascular diseases, cancer, and AIDS. *Front. Nutr,* **2014**, *1*, 18.
[http://dx.doi.org/10.3389/fnut.2014.00018] [PMID: 25988120]

[154] Bernini, R.; Merendino, N.; Romani, A.; Velotti, F. Naturally occurring hydroxytyrosol: synthesis and anticancer potential. *Curr. Med. Chem,* **2013**, *20*(5), 655-670.
[http://dx.doi.org/10.2174/092986713804999367] [PMID: 23244583]

[155] Benavente-García, O.; Castillo, J.; Lorente, J.; Ortuño, A.; Del Rio, J.A. Antioxidant activity of phenolics extracted from *Olea europaea* L. leaves. *Food Chem,* **2000**, *68*(4), 457-462.
[http://dx.doi.org/10.1016/S0308-8146(99)00221-6]

[156] Somova, L.I.; Shode, F.O.; Ramnanan, P.; Nadar, A. Antihypertensive, antiatherosclerotic and antioxidant activity of triterpenoids isolated from *Olea europaea*, subspecies africana leaves. *J. Ethnopharmacol,* **2003**, *84*(2-3), 299-305.
[http://dx.doi.org/10.1016/S0378-8741(02)00332-X] [PMID: 12648829]

[157] Gómez-Acebo, E.; Pertejo, J.A.; Calles, D.A. Topical use of hydroxytyrosol and derivatives for the prevention of HIV infection. Google Patents, 2012.

[158] Granados-Principal, S.; Quiles, J.L.; Ramirez-Tortosa, C.; Camacho-Corencia, P.; Sanchez-Rovira, P.;

Vera-Ramirez, L.; Ramirez-Tortosa, M.C. Hydroxytyrosol inhibits growth and cell proliferation and promotes high expression of sfrp4 in rat mammary tumours. *Mol. Nutr. Food Res,* **2011**, *55*(S1) Suppl. 1, S117-S126.
[http://dx.doi.org/10.1002/mnfr.201000220] [PMID: 21120994]

[159]   Granados-Principal, S.; Quiles, J.L.; Ramirez-Tortosa, C.L.; Sanchez-Rovira, P.; Ramirez-Tortosa, M.C. Hydroxytyrosol: from laboratory investigations to future clinical trials. *Nutr. Rev,* **2010**, *68*(4), 191-206.
[http://dx.doi.org/10.1111/j.1753-4887.2010.00278.x] [PMID: 20416016]

[160]   Ragione, F.D.; Cucciolla, V.; Borriello, A.; Pietra, V.D.; Pontoni, G.; Racioppi, L.; Manna, C.; Galletti, P.; Zappia, V. Hydroxytyrosol, a natural molecule occurring in olive oil, induces cytochrome c-dependent apoptosis. *Biochem. Biophys. Res. Commun,* **2000**, *278*(3), 733-739.
[http://dx.doi.org/10.1006/bbrc.2000.3875] [PMID: 11095977]

[161]   Zrelli, H.; Matsuoka, M.; Kitazaki, S.; Zarrouk, M.; Miyazaki, H. Hydroxytyrosol reduces intracellular reactive oxygen species levels in vascular endothelial cells by upregulating catalase expression through the AMPK–FOXO3a pathway. *Eur. J. Pharmacol,* **2011**, *660*(2-3), 275-282.
[http://dx.doi.org/10.1016/j.ejphar.2011.03.045] [PMID: 21497591]

[162]   Richard, N.; Arnold, S.; Hoeller, U.; Kilpert, C.; Wertz, K.; Schwager, J. Hydroxytyrosol is the major anti-inflammatory compound in aqueous olive extracts and impairs cytokine and chemokine production in macrophages. *Planta Med,* **2011**, *77*(17), 1890-1897.
[http://dx.doi.org/10.1055/s-0031-1280022] [PMID: 21830187]

[163]   Killeen, M.J.; Linder, M.; Pontoniere, P.; Crea, R. NF-κβ signaling and chronic inflammatory diseases: exploring the potential of natural products to drive new therapeutic opportunities. *Drug Discov. Today,* **2014**, *19*(4), 373-378.
[http://dx.doi.org/10.1016/j.drudis.2013.11.002] [PMID: 24246683]

[164]   Dell'Agli, M.; Maschi, O.; Galli, G.V.; Fagnani, R.; Dal Cero, E.; Caruso, D.; Bosisio, E. Inhibition of platelet aggregation by olive oil phenols *via* cAMP-phosphodiesterase. *Br. J. Nutr,* **2008**, *99*(5), 945-951.
[http://dx.doi.org/10.1017/S0007114507837470] [PMID: 17927845]

[165]   Petroni, A.; Blasevich, M.; Salami, M.; Papini, N.; Montedoro, G.F.; Galli, C. Inhibition of platelet aggregation and eicosanoid production by phenolic components of olive oil. *Thromb. Res,* **1995**, *78*(2), 151-160.
[http://dx.doi.org/10.1016/0049-3848(95)00043-7] [PMID: 7482432]

[166]   Léger, C.L.; Carbonneau, M.A.; Michel, F.; Mas, E.; Monnier, L.; Cristol, J.P.; Descomps, B. A thromboxane effect of a hydroxytyrosol-rich olive oil wastewater extract in patients with uncomplicated type I diabetes. *Eur. J. Clin. Nutr,* **2005**, *59*(5), 727-730.
[http://dx.doi.org/10.1038/sj.ejcn.1602133] [PMID: 15798774]

[167]   Visioli, F.; Caruso, D.; Grande, S.; Bosisio, R.; Villa, M.; Galli, G.; Sirtori, C.; Galli, C. Virgin Olive Oil Study (VOLOS): vasoprotective potential of extra virgin olive oil in mildly dyslipidemic patients. *Eur. J. Nutr,* **2005**, *44*(2), 121-127.
[http://dx.doi.org/10.1007/s00394-004-0504-0] [PMID: 15309433]

[168]   Goya, L.; Mateos, R.; Bravo, L. Effect of the olive oil phenol hydroxytyrosol on human hepatoma HepG2 cells. *Eur. J. Nutr,* **2007**, *46*(2), 70-78.
[http://dx.doi.org/10.1007/s00394-006-0633-8] [PMID: 17200875]

[169]   Fabiani, R.; Rosignoli, P.; De Bartolomeo, A.; Fuccelli, R.; Servili, M.; Montedoro, G.F.; Morozzi, G. Oxidative DNA damage is prevented by extracts of olive oil, hydroxytyrosol, and other olive phenolic compounds in human blood mononuclear cells and HL60 cells. *J. Nutr,* **2008**, *138*(8), 1411-1416.
[http://dx.doi.org/10.1093/jn/138.8.1411] [PMID: 18641183]

[170]   Guo, W.; An, Y.; Jiang, L.; Geng, C.; Zhong, L. The protective effects of hydroxytyrosol against UVB-induced DNA damage in HaCaT cells. *Phytother. Res,* **2010**, *24*(3), 352-359.

[http://dx.doi.org/10.1002/ptr.2943] [PMID: 19610043]

[171] Zhu, L.; Liu, Z.; Feng, Z.; Hao, J.; Shen, W.; Li, X.; Sun, L.; Sharman, E.; Wang, Y.; Wertz, K.; Weber, P.; Shi, X.; Liu, J. Hydroxytyrosol protects against oxidative damage by simultaneous activation of mitochondrial biogenesis and phase II detoxifying enzyme systems in retinal pigment epithelial cells. *J. Nutr. Biochem,* **2010,** *21*(11), 1089-1098.
[http://dx.doi.org/10.1016/j.jnutbio.2009.09.006] [PMID: 20149621]

[172] Zou, X.; Feng, Z.; Li, Y.; Wang, Y.; Wertz, K.; Weber, P.; Fu, Y.; Liu, J. Stimulation of GSH synthesis to prevent oxidative stress-induced apoptosis by hydroxytyrosol in human retinal pigment epithelial cells: Activation of Nrf2 and JNK-p62/SQSTM1 pathways. *J. Nutr. Biochem,* **2012,** *23*(8), 994-1006.
[http://dx.doi.org/10.1016/j.jnutbio.2011.05.006] [PMID: 21937211]

[173] Della Ragione, F.; Cucciolla, V.; Borriello, A.; Della Pietra, V.; Manna, C.; Galletti, P.; Zappia, V. Pyrrolidine dithiocarbamate induces apoptosis by a cytochrome c-dependent mechanism. *Biochem. Biophys. Res. Commun,* **2000,** *268*(3), 942-946.
[http://dx.doi.org/10.1006/bbrc.2000.2161] [PMID: 10679310]

[174] Della Ragione, F.; Cucciolla, V.; Criniti, V.; Indaco, S.; Borriello, A.; Zappia, V. Antioxidants induce different phenotypes by a distinct modulation of signal transduction. *FEBS Lett,* **2002,** *532*(3), 289-294.
[http://dx.doi.org/10.1016/S0014-5793(02)03683-9] [PMID: 12482581]

[175] Fabiani, R.; De Bartolomeo, A.; Rosignoli, P.; Servili, M.; Montedoro, G.F.; Morozzi, G. Cancer chemoprevention by hydroxytyrosol isolated from virgin olive oil through G1 cell cycle arrest and apoptosis. *Eur. J. Cancer Prev,* **2002,** *11*(4), 351-358.
[http://dx.doi.org/10.1097/00008469-200208000-00006] [PMID: 12195161]

[176] Fabiani, R.; De Bartolomeo, A.; Rosignoli, P.; Servili, M.; Selvaggini, R.; Montedoro, G.F.; Di Saverio, C.; Morozzi, G. Virgin olive oil phenols inhibit proliferation of human promyelocytic leukemia cells (HL60) by inducing apoptosis and differentiation. *J. Nutr,* **2006,** *136*(3), 614-619.
[http://dx.doi.org/10.1093/jn/136.3.614] [PMID: 16484533]

[177] Fabiani, R.; Rosignoli, P.; De Bartolomeo, A.; Fuccelli, R.; Morozzi, G. Inhibition of cell cycle progression by hydroxytyrosol is associated with upregulation of cyclin-dependent protein kinase inhibitors p21(WAF1/Cip1) and p27(Kip1) and with induction of differentiation in HL60 cells. *J. Nutr,* **2008,** *138*(1), 42-48.
[http://dx.doi.org/10.1093/jn/138.1.42] [PMID: 18156402]

[178] Guichard, C.; Pedruzzi, E.; Fay, M.; Marie, J-C.; Braut-Boucher, F.; Daniel, F.; Grodet, A.; Gougerot-Pocidalo, M.A.; Chastre, E.; Kotelevets, L.; Lizard, G.; Vandewalle, A.; Driss, F.; Ogier-Denis, E. Dihydroxyphenylethanol induces apoptosis by activating serine/threonine protein phosphatase PP2A and promotes the endoplasmic reticulum stress response in human colon carcinoma cells. *Carcinogenesis,* **2006,** *27*(9), 1812-1827.
[http://dx.doi.org/10.1093/carcin/bgl009] [PMID: 16524888]

[179] D'Angelo, S.; Manna, C.; Migliardi, V.; Mazzoni, O.; Morrica, P.; Capasso, G.; Pontoni, G.; Galletti, P.; Zappia, V. Pharmacokinetics and metabolism of hydroxytyrosol, a natural antioxidant from olive oil. *Drug Metab. Dispos,* **2001,** *29*(11), 1492-1498.
[PMID: 11602527]

[180] Christian, M.S.; Sharper, V.A.; Hoberman, A.M.; Seng, J.E.; Fu, L.; Covell, D.; Diener, R.M.; Bitler, C.M.; Crea, R. The toxicity profile of hydrolyzed aqueous olive pulp extract. *Drug Chem. Toxicol,* **2004,** *27*(4), 309-330.
[http://dx.doi.org/10.1081/DCT-200039714] [PMID: 15573469]

[181] Auñon-Calles, D.; Canut, L.; Visioli, F. Toxicological evaluation of pure hydroxytyrosol. *Food Chem. Toxicol,* **2013,** *55,* 498-504.
[http://dx.doi.org/10.1016/j.fct.2013.01.030] [PMID: 23380205]

[182] Scoditti, E.; Calabriso, N.; Massaro, M.; Pellegrino, M.; Storelli, C.; Martines, G.; De Caterina, R.; Carluccio, M.A. Mediterranean diet polyphenols reduce inflammatory angiogenesis through MMP-9 and COX-2 inhibition in human vascular endothelial cells: A potentially protective mechanism in atherosclerotic vascular disease and cancer. *Arch. Biochem. Biophys,* **2012**, *527*(2), 81-89.
[http://dx.doi.org/10.1016/j.abb.2012.05.003] [PMID: 22595400]

[183] Sirianni, R.; Chimento, A.; De Luca, A.; Casaburi, I.; Rizza, P.; Onofrio, A.; Iacopetta, D.; Puoci, F.; Andò, S.; Maggiolini, M.; Pezzi, V. Oleuropein and hydroxytyrosol inhibit MCF-7 breast cancer cell proliferation interfering with ERK1/2 activation. *Mol. Nutr. Food Res,* **2010**, *54*(6), 833-840.
[http://dx.doi.org/10.1002/mnfr.200900111] [PMID: 20013881]

[184] Chen, Z.; Kong, S.; Song, F.; Li, L.; Jiang, H. Pharmacokinetic study of luteolin, apigenin, chrysoeriol and diosmetin after oral administration of Flos Chrysanthemi extract in rats. *Fitoterapia,* **2012**, *83*(8), 1616-1622.
[http://dx.doi.org/10.1016/j.fitote.2012.09.011] [PMID: 22999990]

[185] Lim, S.H.; Jung, S.K.; Byun, S.; Lee, E.J.; Hwang, J.A.; Seo, S.G.; Kim, Y.A.; Yu, J.G.; Lee, K.W.; Lee, H.J. Luteolin suppresses UVB-induced photoageing by targeting JNK1 and p90 ^{RSK2}. *J. Cell. Mol. Med,* **2013**, *17*(5), 672-680.
[http://dx.doi.org/10.1111/jcmm.12050] [PMID: 23551430]

[186] Imran, M.; Rauf, A.; Abu-Izneid, T.; Nadeem, M.; Shariati, M.A.; Khan, I.A.; Imran, A.; Orhan, I.E.; Rizwan, M.; Atif, M.; Gondal, T.A.; Mubarak, M.S. Luteolin, a flavonoid, as an anticancer agent: A review. *Biomed. Pharmacother,* **2019**, *112*, 108612.
[http://dx.doi.org/10.1016/j.biopha.2019.108612] [PMID: 30798142]

[187] Miean, K.H.; Mohamed, S. Flavonoid (myricetin, quercetin, kaempferol, luteolin, and apigenin) content of edible tropical plants. *J. Agric. Food Chem,* **2001**, *49*(6), 3106-3112.
[http://dx.doi.org/10.1021/jf000892m] [PMID: 11410016]

[188] Aziz, N.; Kim, M.Y.; Cho, J.Y. Anti-inflammatory effects of luteolin: A review of *in vitro, in vivo*, and *in silico* studies. *J. Ethnopharmacol,* **2018**, *225*, 342-358.
[http://dx.doi.org/10.1016/j.jep.2018.05.019] [PMID: 29801717]

[189] Seelinger, G.; Merfort, I.; Schempp, C. Anti-oxidant, anti-inflammatory and anti-allergic activities of luteolin. *Planta Med,* **2008**, *74*(14), 1667-1677.
[http://dx.doi.org/10.1055/s-0028-1088314] [PMID: 18937165]

[190] Wall, C; Lim, R; Poljak, M; Lappas, M. Dietary flavonoids as therapeutics for preterm birth: luteolin and kaempferol suppress inflammation in human gestational tissues *in vitro*. *Oxid. Med. Cell. Longev,* **2013**, *2013*.
[http://dx.doi.org/10.1155/2013/485201]

[191] Zang, Y.; Igarashi, K.; Li, Y. Anti-diabetic effects of luteolin and luteolin-7- *O* -glucoside on KK- *A y* mice. *Biosci. Biotechnol. Biochem,* **2016**, *80*(8), 1580-1586.
[http://dx.doi.org/10.1080/09168451.2015.1116928] [PMID: 27170065]

[192] Balamurugan, K.; Karthikeyan, J. Evaluation of the antioxidant and anti-inflammatory nature of luteolin in experimentally induced hepatocellular carcinoma. *Biomedicine & Preventive Nutrition,* **2012**, *2*(2), 86-90.
[http://dx.doi.org/10.1016/j.bionut.2012.01.002]

[193] Jelic, M.; Mandic, A.; Maricic, S.; Srdjenovic, B. Oxidative stress and its role in cancer. *J. Cancer Res. Ther,* **2021**, *17*(1), 22-28.
[http://dx.doi.org/10.4103/jcrt.JCRT_862_16] [PMID: 33723127]

[194] Song, S.; Su, Z; Xu, H; Niu, M; Chen, X; Min, H Luteolin selectively kills STAT3 highly activated gastric cancer cells through enhancing the binding of STAT3 to SHP-1. *Cell Death & Disease,* **2017**, *8*(2), e2612.

[195] Lu, X.; Li, Y.; Li, X.; Aisa, H.A. Luteolin induces apoptosis *in vitro* through suppressing the MAPK

and PI3K signaling pathways in gastric cancer. *Oncol. Lett,* **2017,** *14*(2), 1993-2000.
[http://dx.doi.org/10.3892/ol.2017.6380] [PMID: 28789432]

[196] Ko, W.G.; Kang, T.H.; Lee, S.J.; Kim, Y.C.; Lee, B.H. Effects of luteolin on the inhibition of proliferation and induction of apoptosis in human myeloid leukaemia cells. *Phytother. Res,* **2002,** *16*(3), 295-298.
[http://dx.doi.org/10.1002/ptr.871] [PMID: 12164283]

[197] Lee, L-T.; Huang, Y-T.; Hwang, J-J.; Lee, P.P.; Ke, F-C.; Nair, M.P.; Kanadaswam, C.; Lee, M.T. Blockade of the epidermal growth factor receptor tyrosine kinase activity by quercetin and luteolin leads to growth inhibition and apoptosis of pancreatic tumor cells. *Anticancer Res,* **2002,** *22*(3), 1615-1627.
[PMID: 12168845]

[198] Lee, W.J.; Wu, L.F.; Chen, W.K.; Wang, C.J.; Tseng, T.H. Inhibitory effect of luteolin on hepatocyte growth factor/scatter factor-induced HepG2 cell invasion involving both MAPK/ERKs and PI3K–Akt pathways. *Chem. Biol. Interact,* **2006,** *160*(2), 123-133.
[http://dx.doi.org/10.1016/j.cbi.2006.01.002] [PMID: 16458870]

[199] Zang, M.; Hu, L.; Zhang, B.; Zhu, Z.; Li, J.; Zhu, Z.; Yan, M.; Liu, B. Luteolin suppresses angiogenesis and vasculogenic mimicry formation through inhibiting Notch1-VEGF signaling in gastric cancer. *Biochem. Biophys. Res. Commun,* **2017,** *490*(3), 913-919.
[http://dx.doi.org/10.1016/j.bbrc.2017.06.140] [PMID: 28655612]

[200] Zang, M.; Hu, L.; Fan, Z.; Wang, H.; Zhu, Z.; Cao, S.; Wu, X.; Li, J.; Su, L.; Li, C.; Zhu, Z.; Yan, M.; Liu, B. Luteolin suppresses gastric cancer progression by reversing epithelial-mesenchymal transition *via* suppression of the Notch signaling pathway. *J. Transl. Med,* **2017,** *15*(1), 52.
[http://dx.doi.org/10.1186/s12967-017-1151-6] [PMID: 28241766]

[201] Tang, X.; Wang, H.; Fan, L.; Wu, X.; Xin, A.; Ren, H.; Wang, X.J. Luteolin inhibits Nrf2 leading to negative regulation of the Nrf2/ARE pathway and sensitization of human lung carcinoma A549 cells to therapeutic drugs. *Free Radic. Biol. Med,* **2011,** *50*(11), 1599-1609.
[http://dx.doi.org/10.1016/j.freeradbiomed.2011.03.008] [PMID: 21402146]

[202] Nashwa, M.F.; Abdel-Aziz, M. Efficiency of olive (*Olea europaea* L.) leaf extract as antioxidant and anticancer agents. *J Agroaliment Processes Technol,* **2014,** *20*(1), 46-53.

[203] Bektay, M.Y.; Güler, E.M.; Gökçe, M.; Kiziltaş, M.V. Investigation of the Genotoxic, Cytotoxic, Apoptotic, and Oxidant Effects of Olive Leaf Extracts on Liver Cancer Cell Lines. *Turkish J. Phramaceutic Sci.,* **2021,** *18*(6), 781-789.
[http://dx.doi.org/10.4274/tjps.galenos.2021.03271] [PMID: 34979739]

[204] Yan, C.M.; Chai, E.Q.; Cai, H.Y.; Miao, G.Y.; Ma, W. Oleuropein induces apoptosis *via* activation of caspases and suppression of phosphatidylinositol 3-kinase/protein kinase B pathway in HepG2 human hepatoma cell line. *Mol. Med. Rep,* **2015,** *11*(6), 4617-4624.
[http://dx.doi.org/10.3892/mmr.2015.3266] [PMID: 25634350]

[205] Sherif, I.O.; Al-Gayyar, M.M.H. Oleuropein potentiates anti-tumor activity of cisplatin against HepG2 through affecting proNGF/NGF balance. *Life Sci,* **2018,** *198,* 87-93.
[http://dx.doi.org/10.1016/j.lfs.2018.02.027] [PMID: 29476769]

[206] Dimri, M.; Satyanarayana, A. Molecular Signaling Pathways and Therapeutic Targets in Hepatocellular Carcinoma. *Cancers (Basel),* **2020,** *12*(2), 491.
[http://dx.doi.org/10.3390/cancers12020491] [PMID: 32093152]

[207] Whittaker, S.; Marais, R.; Zhu, A.X. The role of signaling pathways in the development and treatment of hepatocellular carcinoma. *Oncogene,* **2010,** *29*(36), 4989-5005.
[http://dx.doi.org/10.1038/onc.2010.236] [PMID: 20639898]

[208] Cheng, J.S.; Chou, C.T.; Liu, Y.Y.; Sun, W.C.; Shieh, P.; Kuo, D.H.; Kuo, C.C.; Jan, C.R.; Liang, W.Z. The effect of oleuropein from olive leaf (*Olea europaea*) extract on Ca^{2+} homeostasis, cytotoxicity, cell cycle distribution and ROS signaling in HepG2 human hepatoma cells. *Food Chem.*

Toxicol, **2016**, *91*, 151-166.
[http://dx.doi.org/10.1016/j.fct.2016.03.015] [PMID: 27016494]

[209] Yamada, N.; Matsushima-Nishiwaki, R.; Masue, A.; Taguchi, K.; Kozawa, O. Olive oil polyphenols suppress the TGF-α-induced migration of hepatocellular carcinoma cells. *Biomed. Rep,* **2019**, *1*(1), 1-5.
[http://dx.doi.org/10.3892/br.2019.1215] [PMID: 31258902]

[210] Tutino, V.; Caruso, M.G.; Messa, C.; Perri, E.; Notarnicola, M. Antiproliferative, antioxidant and anti-inflammatory effects of hydroxytyrosol on human hepatoma HepG2 and Hep3B cell lines. *Anticancer Res,* **2012**, *32*(12), 5371-5377.
[PMID: 23225439]

[211] Giordano, E.; Davalos, A.; Nicod, N.; Visioli, F. Hydroxytyrosol attenuates tunicamycin-induced endoplasmic reticulum stress in human hepatocarcinoma cells. *Mol. Nutr. Food Res,* **2014**, *58*(5), 954-962.
[http://dx.doi.org/10.1002/mnfr.201300465] [PMID: 24347345]

[212] Zhao, B.; Ma, Y.; Xu, Z.; Wang, J.; Wang, F.; Wang, D.; Pan, S.; Wu, Y.; Pan, H.; Xu, D.; Liu, L.; Jiang, H. Hydroxytyrosol, a natural molecule from olive oil, suppresses the growth of human hepatocellular carcinoma cells *via* inactivating AKT and nuclear factor-kappa B pathways. *Cancer Lett,* **2014**, *347*(1), 79-87.
[http://dx.doi.org/10.1016/j.canlet.2014.01.028] [PMID: 24486741]

[213] Lee, H.J.; Wang, C.J.; Kuo, H.C.; Chou, F.P.; Jean, L.F.; Tseng, T.H. Induction apoptosis of luteolin in human hepatoma HepG2 cells involving mitochondria translocation of Bax/Bak and activation of JNK. *Toxicol. Appl. Pharmacol,* **2005**, *203*(2), 124-131.
[http://dx.doi.org/10.1016/j.taap.2004.08.004] [PMID: 15710173]

[214] Selvendiran, K.; Koga, H.; Ueno, T.; Yoshida, T.; Maeyama, M.; Torimura, T.; Yano, H.; Kojiro, M.; Sata, M. Luteolin promotes degradation in signal transducer and activator of transcription 3 in human hepatoma cells: An implication for the antitumor potential of flavonoids. *Cancer Res,* **2006**, *66*(9), 4826-4834.
[http://dx.doi.org/10.1158/0008-5472.CAN-05-4062] [PMID: 16651438]

[215] Ding, S.; Hu, A.; Hu, Y.; Ma, J.; Weng, P.; Dai, J. Anti-hepatoma cells function of luteolin through inducing apoptosis and cell cycle arrest. *Tumour Biol,* **2014**, *35*(4), 3053-3060.
[http://dx.doi.org/10.1007/s13277-013-1396-5] [PMID: 24287949]

[216] Yee, S.B.; Choi, H.J.; Chung, S.W.; Park, D.H.; Sung, B.; Chung, H.Y.; Kim, N.D. Growth inhibition of luteolin on HepG2 cells is induced *via* p53 and Fas/Fas-ligand besides the TGF-β pathway. *Int. J. Oncol,* **2015**, *47*(2), 747-754.
[http://dx.doi.org/10.3892/ijo.2015.3053] [PMID: 26096942]

[217] Xu, H.; Yang, T.; Liu, X.; Tian, Y.; Chen, X.; Yuan, R.; Su, S.; Lin, X.; Du, G. Luteolin synergizes the antitumor effects of 5-fluorouracil against human hepatocellular carcinoma cells through apoptosis induction and metabolism. *Life Sci,* **2016**, *144*, 138-147.
[http://dx.doi.org/10.1016/j.lfs.2015.12.002] [PMID: 26656468]

[218] Niu, J.X.; Guo, H.P.; Gan, H.M.; Bao, L.D.; Ren, J.J. Effect of luteolin on gene expression in mouse H22 hepatoma cells. *Genet. Mol. Res,* **2015**, *14*(4), 14448-14456.
[http://dx.doi.org/10.4238/2015.November.18.7] [PMID: 26600503]

[219] Hwang, J-T.; Park, O.J.; Lee, Y.K.; Sung, M.J.; Hur, H.J.; Kim, M.S.; Ha, J.H.; Kwon, D.Y. Anti-tumor effect of luteolin is accompanied by AMP-activated protein kinase and nuclear factor-κB modulation in HepG2 hepatocarcinoma cells. *Int. J. Mol. Med,* **2011**, *28*(1), 25-31.
[http://dx.doi.org/10.3892/ijmm.2011.667] [PMID: 21468539]

[220] Zhang, Q.; Yang, J.; Wang, J. Modulatory effect of luteolin on redox homeostasis and inflammatory cytokines in a mouse model of liver cancer. *Oncol. Lett,* **2016**, *12*(6), 4767-4772.
[http://dx.doi.org/10.3892/ol.2016.5291] [PMID: 28101223]

[221] Lattanzio, V.; Kroon, P.A.; Linsalata, V.; Cardinali, A. Globe artichoke: A functional food and source of nutraceutical ingredients. *J. Funct. Foods,* **2009**, *1*(2), 131-144.
[http://dx.doi.org/10.1016/j.jff.2009.01.002]

[222] Mehmetçik, G.; Özdemirler, G.; Koçak-Toker, N.; Çevikbaş, U.; Uysal, M. Effect of pretreatment with artichoke extract on carbon tetrachloride-induced liver injury and oxidative stress. *Exp. Toxicol. Pathol,* **2008**, *60*(6), 475-480.
[http://dx.doi.org/10.1016/j.etp.2008.04.014] [PMID: 18583118]

[223] Negro, D.; Montesano, V.; Grieco, S.; Crupi, P.; Sarli, G.; De Lisi, A.; Sonnante, G. Polyphenol compounds in artichoke plant tissues and varieties. *J. Food Sci,* **2012**, *77*(2), C244-C252.
[http://dx.doi.org/10.1111/j.1750-3841.2011.02531.x] [PMID: 22251096]

[224] Gebhardt, R. Anticholestatic activity of flavonoids from artichoke (*Cynara scolymus L.*) and of their metabolites. *Med. Sci. Monit,* **2001**, *7* Suppl. 1, 316-320.
[PMID: 12211745]

[225] Speroni, E.; Cervellati, R.; Govoni, P.; Guizzardi, S.; Renzulli, C.; Guerra, M.C. Efficacy of different *Cynara scolymus* preparations on liver complaints. *J. Ethnopharmacol,* **2003**, *86*(2-3), 203-211.
[http://dx.doi.org/10.1016/S0378-8741(03)00076-X] [PMID: 12738088]

[226] Miccadei, S.; Venere, D.D.; Cardinali, A.; Romano, F.; Durazzo, A.; Foddai, M.S.; Fraioli, R.; Mobarhan, S.; Maiani, G. Antioxidative and apoptotic properties of polyphenolic extracts from edible part of artichoke (*Cynara scolymus L.*) on cultured rat hepatocytes and on human hepatoma cells. *Nutr. Cancer,* **2008**, *60*(2), 276-283.
[http://dx.doi.org/10.1080/01635580801891583] [PMID: 18444161]

[227] Robinson, W.E., Jr; Reinecke, M.G.; Abdel-Malek, S.; Jia, Q.; Chow, S.A. Inhibitors of HIV-1 replication that inhibit HIV integrase. *Proc. Natl. Acad. Sci. USA,* **1996**, *93*(13), 6326-6331.
[http://dx.doi.org/10.1073/pnas.93.13.6326] [PMID: 8692814]

[228] Rondanelli, M.; Monteferrario, F.; Perna, S.; Faliva, M.A.; Opizzi, A. Health-promoting properties of artichoke in preventing cardiovascular disease by its lipidic and glycemic-reducing action. *Monaldi Arch. Chest Dis,* **2013**, *80*(1), 17-26.
[http://dx.doi.org/10.4081/monaldi.2013.87] [PMID: 23923586]

[229] Mileo, AM; Miccadei, S. Polyphenols as modulator of oxidative stress in cancer disease: new therapeutic strategies. *Oxid. Med. Cell. Longev,* **2016**, *2016*, 6475624.
[http://dx.doi.org/10.1155/2016/6475624]

[230] Sokkar, H.H.; Abo Dena, A.S.; Mahana, N.A.; Badr, A. Artichoke extracts in cancer therapy: do the extraction conditions affect the anticancer activity? *Future J.Pharmaceutic. Sci.,* **2020**, *6*(1), 78.
[http://dx.doi.org/10.1186/s43094-020-00088-0]

[231] Mileo, A.M.; Di Venere, D.; Linsalata, V.; Fraioli, R.; Miccadei, S. Artichoke polyphenols induce apoptosis and decrease the invasive potential of the human breast cancer cell line MDA-MB231. *J. Cell. Physiol,* **2012**, *227*(9), 3301-3309.
[http://dx.doi.org/10.1002/jcp.24029] [PMID: 22170094]

[232] Mileo, AM; Di Venere, D; Abbruzzese, C; Miccadei, S. Long term exposure to polyphenols of artichoke (*Cynara scolymus* L.) exerts induction of senescence driven growth arrest in the MDA-MB231 human breast cancer cell line. *Oxid. Med. Cell. Longev,* **2015**, *2015*, 363827.
[http://dx.doi.org/10.1155/2015/363827]

[233] Pulito, C.; Mori, F.; Sacconi, A.; Casadei, L.; Ferraiuolo, M.; Valerio, M.C.; Santoro, R.; Goeman, F.; Maidecchi, A.; Mattoli, L.; Manetti, C.; Di Agostino, S.; Muti, P.; Blandino, G.; Strano, S. *Cynara scolymus* affects malignant pleural mesothelioma by promoting apoptosis and restraining invasion. *Oncotarget,* **2015**, *6*(20), 18134-18150.
[http://dx.doi.org/10.18632/oncotarget.4017] [PMID: 26136339]

[234] Villarini, M.; Acito, M.; di Vito, R.; Vannini, S.; Dominici, L.; Fatigoni, C.; Pagiotti, R.; Moretti, M.

Pro-Apoptotic Activity of Artichoke Leaf Extracts in Human HT-29 and RKO Colon Cancer Cells. *Int. J. Environ. Res. Public Health,* **2021**, *18*(8), 4166.
[http://dx.doi.org/10.3390/ijerph18084166] [PMID: 33920761]

[235] Simsek, E.N.; Uysal, T. *In vitro* investigation of cytotoxic and apoptotic effects of *Cynara L.* species in colorectal cancer cells. *Asian Pac. J. Cancer Prev,* **2013**, *14*(11), 6791-6795.
[http://dx.doi.org/10.7314/APJCP.2013.14.11.6791] [PMID: 24377607]

[236] Sümer, E.; Senturk, G.E.; Demirel, Ö.U.; Yesilada, E. Comparative biochemical and histopathological evaluations proved that receptacle is the most effective part of *Cynara scolymus* against liver and kidney damages. *J. Ethnopharmacol,* **2020**, *249*, 112458.
[http://dx.doi.org/10.1016/j.jep.2019.112458] [PMID: 31809787]

[237] El Sayed, A.M.; Hussein, R.; Motaal, A.A.; Fouad, M.A.; Aziz, M.A.; El-Sayed, A. Artichoke edible parts are hepatoprotective as commercial leaf preparation. *Rev. Bras. Farmacogn,* **2018**, *28*(2), 165-178.
[http://dx.doi.org/10.1016/j.bjp.2018.01.002]

[238] Elmosallamy, A.; Abdel-Hamid, N.; Srour, L.; Hussein, S.A.A. Identification of polyphenolic compounds and hepatoprotective activity of artichoke (*Cynara scolymus L.*) edible part extracts in rats. *Egypt. J. Chem,* **2020**, *63*(6), 2273-2285.

[239] Seelinger, G.; Merfort, I.; Wölfle, U.; Schempp, C. Anti-carcinogenic effects of the flavonoid luteolin. *Molecules,* **2008**, *13*(10), 2628-2651.
[http://dx.doi.org/10.3390/molecules13102628] [PMID: 18946424]

[240] Baskar, A.A.; Ignacimuthu, S.; Michael, G.P.; Al Numair, K.S. Cancer chemopreventive potential of luteolin-7-O-glucoside isolated from *Ophiorrhiza mungos* Linn. *Nutr. Cancer,* **2011**, *63*(1), 130-138.
[http://dx.doi.org/10.1080/01635581.2010.516869] [PMID: 21161823]

[241] Velmurugan, B.K.; Lin, J.T.; Mahalakshmi, B.; Chuang, Y.C.; Lin, C.C.; Lo, Y.S.; Hsieh, M.J.; Chen, M.K. Luteolin-7-O-Glucoside Inhibits Oral Cancer Cell Migration and Invasion by Regulating Matrix Metalloproteinase-2 Expression and Extracellular Signal-Regulated Kinase Pathway. *Biomolecules,* **2020**, *10*(4), 502.
[http://dx.doi.org/10.3390/biom10040502] [PMID: 32224968]

[242] Shao, J.L.; Liang, H.R.; Dai, J.X. Luteoloside inhibits proliferation of human chronic myeloid leukemia K562 cells by inducing G2/M phase cell cycle arrest and apoptosis. *Trop. J. Pharm. Res,* **2016**, *15*(1), 39-45.
[http://dx.doi.org/10.4314/tjpr.v15i1.6]

[243] Shao, J.; Wang, C.; Li, L.; Liang, H.; Dai, J.; Ling, X.; Tang, H. Luteoloside Inhibits Proliferation and Promotes Intrinsic and Extrinsic Pathway-Mediated Apoptosis Involving MAPK and mTOR Signaling Pathways in Human Cervical Cancer Cells. *Int. J. Mol. Sci,* **2018**, *19*(6), 1664.
[http://dx.doi.org/10.3390/ijms19061664] [PMID: 29874795]

[244] Salehi, B.; Venditti, A.; Sharifi-Rad, M.; Kręgiel, D.; Sharifi-Rad, J.; Durazzo, A.; Lucarini, M.; Santini, A.; Souto, E.; Novellino, E.; Antolak, H.; Azzini, E.; Setzer, W.; Martins, N. The therapeutic potential of apigenin. *Int. J. Mol. Sci,* **2019**, *20*(6), 1305.
[http://dx.doi.org/10.3390/ijms20061305] [PMID: 30875872]

[245] Shukla, S.; Gupta, S. Apigenin: A promising molecule for cancer prevention. *Pharm. Res,* **2010**, *27*(6), 962-978.
[http://dx.doi.org/10.1007/s11095-010-0089-7] [PMID: 20306120]

[246] Yang, C.S.; Landau, J.M.; Huang, M.T.; Newmark, H.L. Inhibition of carcinogenesis by dietary polyphenolic compounds. *Annu. Rev. Nutr,* **2001**, *21*(1), 381-406.
[http://dx.doi.org/10.1146/annurev.nutr.21.1.381] [PMID: 11375442]

[247] Fidelis, Q.C.; Faraone, I.; Russo, D.; Aragão Catunda-Jr, F.E.; Vignola, L.; de Carvalho, M.G.; de Tommasi, N.; Milella, L. Chemical and Biological insights of *Ouratea hexasperma* (A. St.-Hil.) Baill.: A source of bioactive compounds with multifunctional properties. *Nat. Prod. Res,* **2019**, *33*(10), 1500-

1503.
[http://dx.doi.org/10.1080/14786419.2017.1419227] [PMID: 29338358]

[248] Villa-Rodriguez, J.A.; Kerimi, A.; Abranko, L.; Tumova, S.; Ford, L.; Blackburn, R.S.; Rayner, C.; Williamson, G. Acute metabolic actions of the major polyphenols in chamomile: An *in vitro* mechanistic study on their potential to attenuate postprandial hyperglycaemia. *Sci. Rep*, **2018**, *8*(1), 5471.
[http://dx.doi.org/10.1038/s41598-018-23736-1] [PMID: 29615674]

[249] Lim, R.; Barker, G.; Wall, C.A.; Lappas, M. Dietary phytophenols curcumin, naringenin and apigenin reduce infection-induced inflammatory and contractile pathways in human placenta, foetal membranes and myometrium. *Mol. Hum. Reprod,* **2013**, *19*(7), 451-462.
[http://dx.doi.org/10.1093/molehr/gat015] [PMID: 23475986]

[250] Seo, H.S.; Choi, H.S.; Kim, S.R.; Choi, Y.K.; Woo, S.M.; Shin, I.; Woo, J.K.; Park, S.Y.; Shin, Y.C.; Ko, S.K. Apigenin induces apoptosis *via* extrinsic pathway, inducing p53 and inhibiting STAT3 and NFκB signaling in HER2-overexpressing breast cancer cells. *Mol. Cell. Biochem,* **2012**, *366*(1-2), 319-334.
[http://dx.doi.org/10.1007/s11010-012-1310-2] [PMID: 22527937]

[251] Karmakar, S.; Davis, K.A.; Choudhury, S.R.; Deeconda, A.; Banik, N.L.; Ray, S.K. Bcl-2 inhibitor and apigenin worked synergistically in human malignant neuroblastoma cell lines and increased apoptosis with activation of extrinsic and intrinsic pathways. *Biochem. Biophys. Res. Commun,* **2009**, *388*(4), 705-710.
[http://dx.doi.org/10.1016/j.bbrc.2009.08.071] [PMID: 19695221]

[252] Peng, Q.; Deng, Z.; Pan, H.; Gu, L.; Liu, O.; Tang, Z. Mitogen-activated protein kinase signaling pathway in oral cancer. *Oncol. Lett,* **2018**, *15*(2), 1379-1388.
[http://dx.doi.org/10.3892/ol.2017.7491] [PMID: 29434828]

[253] Madunić, J.; Madunić, I.V.; Gajski, G.; Popić, J.; Garaj-Vrhovac, V. Apigenin: A dietary flavonoid with diverse anticancer properties. *Cancer Lett,* **2018**, *413*, 11-22.
[http://dx.doi.org/10.1016/j.canlet.2017.10.041] [PMID: 29097249]

[254] Ahmed, S.A.; Parama, D.; Daimari, E.; Girisa, S.; Banik, K.; Harsha, C.; Dutta, U.; Kunnumakkara, A.B. Rationalizing the therapeutic potential of apigenin against cancer. *Life Sci,* **2021**, *267*, 118814.
[http://dx.doi.org/10.1016/j.lfs.2020.118814] [PMID: 33333052]

[255] Metwally, N.S.; Kholeif, T.E.; Ghanem, K.Z.; Farrag, A.R.; Ammar, N.M.; Abdel-Hamid, A.H. The protective effects of fish oil and artichoke on hepatocellular carcinoma in rats. *Eur. Rev. Med. Pharmacol. Sci,* **2011**, *15*(12), 1429-1444.
[PMID: 22288304]

[256] Al-Radadi, N.S. Artichoke (*Cynara scolymus L.*,) mediated rapid analysis of silver nanoparticles and their utilisation on the cancer cell treatments. *J. Comput. Theor. Nanosci,* **2018**, *15*(6), 1818-1829.
[http://dx.doi.org/10.1166/jctn.2018.7317]

[257] Fan, S.; Wang, Y.; Lu, J.; Zheng, Y.; Wu, D.; Li, M.; Hu, B.; Zhang, Z.; Cheng, W.; Shan, Q. Luteoloside suppresses proliferation and metastasis of hepatocellular carcinoma cells by inhibition of NLRP3 inflammasome. *PLoS One,* **2014**, *9*(2), e89961.
[http://dx.doi.org/10.1371/journal.pone.0089961] [PMID: 24587153]

[258] Hwang, Y.J.; Lee, E.J.; Kim, H.R.; Hwang, K.A. Molecular mechanisms of luteolin-7-O-glucos-de-induced growth inhibition on human liver cancer cells: G2/M cell cycle arrest and caspase-independent apoptotic signaling pathways. *BMB Rep,* **2013**, *46*(12), 611-616.
[http://dx.doi.org/10.5483/BMBRep.2013.46.12.133] [PMID: 24257119]

[259] Li, Y.; Cheng, X.; Chen, C.; Huijuan, W.; Zhao, H.; Liu, W.; Xiang, Z.; Wang, Q. Apigenin, a flavonoid constituent derived from P. villosa, inhibits hepatocellular carcinoma cell growth by CyclinD1/CDK4 regulation *via* p38 MAPK-p21 signaling. *Pathol. Res. Pract,* **2020**, *216*(1), 152701.
[http://dx.doi.org/10.1016/j.prp.2019.152701] [PMID: 31780054]

[260] Seydi, E, R; Rasekh, H; Salimi, A; Mohsenifar, Z; Pourahmad, J Selective toxicity of apigenin on cancerous hepatocytes by directly targeting their mitochondria. *Anti-Cancer Agents in Medicinal Chemistry,* **2016**, *16*(12), 1576-1586.
[http://dx.doi.org/10.2174/1871520616666160425110839]

[261] Wang, S.M.; Yang, P.W.; Feng, X.J.; Zhu, Y.W.; Qiu, F.J.; Hu, X.D.; Zhang, S.H. Apigenin inhibits the growth of hepatocellular carcinoma cells by affecting the expression of microRNA transcriptome. *Front. Oncol,* **2021**, *11*, 657665.
[http://dx.doi.org/10.3389/fonc.2021.657665] [PMID: 33959508]

[262] Pan, F.; Zheng, Y.B.; Shi, C.J.; Zhang, F.; Zhang, J.; Fu, W. H19-Wnt/β-catenin regulatory axis mediates the suppressive effects of apigenin on tumor growth in hepatocellular carcinoma. *Eur. J. Pharmacol,* **2021**, *893*, 173810.
[http://dx.doi.org/10.1016/j.ejphar.2020.173810] [PMID: 33345859]

CHAPTER 3

Herbal Drug Substitution (*Abhava-Pratinidhi Dravya*): A Key to Stopping Economic Adulteration of Botanical Ingredients

Arun Shivakumar[1], Atul Namdeorao Jadhav[1,*], Ashok Basti Krishnaiah[2] and **Rangesh Paramesh[3]**

[1] *Himalaya Global Research Center FZ LLC, Dubai Science Park, Al Barsha, Dubai, UAE*

[2] *Research and Development Center, Himalaya Wellness Company, Bengaluru, Karnataka, India*

[3] *Manal Family Office Holdings Ltd., Dubai International Financial Centre, Dubai, UAE*

Abstract: Dwindling of natural resources coupled with the rising demand for several botanical ingredients in the Indian subcontinent and global market has led to scarcity and extensive adulteration. This may result in altered safety and efficacy of several single and polyherbal Ayurvedic formulations. Foreseeing this, Ayurveda experts have decided to use alternate herbal ingredients with similar properties. Such ingredients are known as *Pratinidhi* (a substitute) and are used in medicinal preparations. Because of the unavailability of a particular herb or the availability of the herb at a prohibitive cost, the usage of substitutes is necessary. This concept of substitution of herbs in Ayurvedic medicines is quite an elaborate and popular practice. In commerce, there are some predominant herbs whose substitutes or adulterants are also being traded. These substitutes belong to the same or different genera or cultivar species and may or may not have similar phytochemical constituents. This also relates to the use mentioned in the authoritative texts of Ayurveda and their modern pharmacological responses and safety. Ayurvedic system of medicine has an in-depth biochemical classification of herbs, based on which substitutes can be deduced. In addition, ancient texts have mentioned alternate herbs for some key ingredients.

In the present article, we are discussing commercially significant herbs, *viz. Ativisha*, *Bala*, *Guduchi* and *Vidanga*. These herbs have diverse clinical usage in Ayurveda and are reported to have properties such as immunomodulatory, anti-pyretic, anti-oxidant and anthelmintic. Based on this concept, the development of standard protocols for highly traded botanical ingredients will help the healthcare industry to meet the quality standards for medicinal products. Using substitute herbs will majorly reduce the overexploitation of natural resources and help bring balance to the ecosystem.

[*] **Corresponding author Atul Namdeorao Jadhav:** Himalaya Global Research Center FZ-LLC, Dubai Science Park, Al Barsha, Dubai, UAE; T: +9714 277 6008, Fax: +9714 277 6009; E-mail: dr.atul@himalayawellness.com

Shazia Anjum (Ed.)

Keywords: Adulterant, *Ativisha*, *Bala*, Bioactive Constituent, Endangered Herbs, *Guduchi*, Herbal Trade, Herbal Medicine, IUCN, Pharmacology, Phytochemical Constitution, *Pratinidhi*, Substitute, *Vidanga*.

1. INTRODUCTION

The usage of herbal medicines for the management of the health and wellness of mankind is gaining interest globally. According to the latest WHO report, 80% of the world's population relies on herbal medicine, resulting in a new trend of integration of alternative and complementary medicine into mainstream healthcare systems gradually [1, 2]. National Health Interview Survey 2012 reveals that more than 56% of the US population suffers from chronic conditions, of which 22% of the population depends on herbal therapies [3]. Medicinal plants contain many phytoconstituents with potential therapeutic value, *viz.* flavonoids, polyphenols, saponins, glycosides, tannins, alkaloids and terpenoids [4]. They exhibit a unique mode of action with very few or no side effects, even after prolonged usage, unlike conventional medicine [5]. Herbal medicines are widely used for the treatment of chronic diseases and also for maintaining the health of the elderly, which is of utmost concern. A clinical study conducted in Turkey in both urban and rural populations with diabetes mellitus, hypertension and hyperlipidemia found that most of the patients believed herbal medicine to be effective (68.3% good effect, 11.1% minor effect) and had no adverse effects (85.7%) [6]. A survey conducted in Thailand for the treatment of arthritis, asthma, cancer, cardiac failure, stroke, coronary artery disease, cardiac arrhythmias, chronic obstructive pulmonary disease (COPD), diabetes mellitus and hypertension revealed that the herbs used for the treatment included herbs such as *Andrographis paniculata (Burm.f.)* Nees, *Curcuma longa* L., *Zingiber officinale* Roscoe, *Boesenbergia rotunda*, *Aloe vera* (L) Burm.f. and *Centella asiatica* (L.) Urb [7]. A comprehensive study involving 1601 participants, both from urban (47.5%) and rural areas (52.5%), was conducted in Vietnam to evaluate the use of herbal medicine in the treatment of chronic medical conditions. Stomach and intestinal diseases (39.6%); followed by gout and other musculoskeletal conditions such as chronic backache (23.8%) and arthritis (22.1%); hypertension (19.6%); cardiovascular disorders (9.6%); liver diseases (9.1%); migraine or frequent headaches (6.9%); diabetes mellitus (6.2%); dyslipidaemia (6.2%); kidney diseases (6.0%); asthma (4.0%), cancer (2.9%), thyroid diseases (2.5%); mental disorders (2.1%); COPD (0.9%); Parkinson's disease (0.7%); and epilepsy (0.3%), were treated with herbal medicines [8]. The global trend for research on herbal ingredients has been increasing exponentially over a decade, with India and China leading in publishing research articles, that is, around 800 to 1100 articles per year [9]. The International Union for Conservation of Nature (IUCN) Red List of Threatened Species is the world's most comprehensive source for information on the global extinction and risk status of plant and animal species. It is estimated that more than 115,291 plant species have not been evaluated by the IUCN Red List of Threatened Species™ [10]. Threat and extinction of these medicinal herbs force us to adopt the concept of drug substitution, *i.e.*, *Abhava-pratinidhi dravya*, which is well documented (in 15th- and 16th-century literature) and practiced in Ayurvedic medicine [11]. The principle of *Abhava-pratinidhi dravya* describes using potential alternative herbs in clinical practice by an Ayurvedic physician without compromising safety and efficacy.

2. ECONOMICS OF HERBAL TRADE & ADULTERATION PRACTICES

The herbal industry is estimated to be at about US100$ billion with a consistent annual growth rate of 15% [12]. Herbal trade includes essential oils, extracts, phytopharmaceuticals, gums, spices used in medicine and tannins for pharmaceutical use and cosmetics. The global export market of medicinal plants is contributed majorly by five countries: China (27.1%), Hong Kong (7.6%), USA (7%), India (6.5%) and Germany (6.1%) [13]. The US Food and Drug Administration regulates botanical ingredients and finished products under separate regulations under the Dietary Supplement Health and Education Act of 1994 (DSHEA). "Economically motivated adulteration" (EMA) is defined as the "fraudulent, intentional omission, substitution or addition of a substance in a product to increase the apparent value of the product or reduce the cost of its production, *i.e.*, for economic gain." The American Botanical Council is continually upgrading the American Botanical Council, the American Herbal Pharmacopoeia and the University of Mississippi's National Center for Natural Products Research Botanical Adulterants Programs, which emphasize both accidental and intentional adulteration of botanical ingredients. These programs are commended by Canada, which involve herbal experts from universities, industry and government bodies to establish quality control for possible adulterants and identify the availability of official or unofficial analytical methods to help detect these adulterants [14].

Adulteration of botanical ingredients may be accidental or intentional for financial gains. Species-level adulteration ranges from 21% (in the case of *Crocus sativus* L.) to 80% (in the case of *Berberis asiatica* Roxb. Ex DC.) [15]. The growing demand for supplements for weight management necessitates herbal supplement manufacturers to add non-plant-derived compounds into the products to compete in the market. A detailed study conducted in Iran on weight management products available in the market has shown that for weight loss, sibutramine, laxative medicines (phenolphthalein) and appetite suppressants (amfepramone) are used in herbal preparations. In the case of herbal medicines, usually, 2 to 3 tablets are prescribed per day. Consuming these synthetic compounds beyond their daily consumption limits may result in severe side effects and even cause sudden death, which is a serious concern for human health [16]. The limited availability of authentic plants imposes adulteration, which could be a substandard herb like *Hypericum patulum* Thumb, substituting *Hypericum perforatum* L [17]. The WHO member countries have proposed 11 challenges in establishing safe and efficacious herbal medicine. Of these 11, lack of research data, lack of financial research support, and lack of mechanisms to monitor the safety of traditional and complementary medicine are the top 3 concerns mentioned in the WHO global report on traditional and complementary medicine, 2019 [18]. These concerns, along with an increase in the adulteration of herbal medicines, urge the regulators to find ways to develop alternative medicines that can deliver the optimum efficacy and safety.

3. CONCEPT OF *ABHAVA-PRATINIDHI DRAVYAS*

The problem of non-availability or extinction of certain medicinal plants possibly existed in earlier times as well, even before the globalization of Ayurveda and the industrial mass production of herbal medicines. Similarly, in Ayurvedic medical practice, the substitution of raw materials is very common when any prescribed herb is not available for the preparation of medicinal products. Further, many times, substitutes are deliberately selected and rationally used to bring about the desired effect.

As per *Dravyaguna Vijnana* (the science of ingredients and their properties in Ayurveda), each herb is classified based on (a) *Rasa* (taste), (b) *Guna* (quality), (c) *Veerya* (efficacy), (d) *Vipaka* (post-digestive state), (e) *Prabhava* (specific efficacy) and (f) *Karma* (pharmacological activity). When the desired herb is unavailable, it is allowed to be substituted with an herb that has the same effect and properties, which is called as *Abhava-Pratinidhi Dravya*. The principles of *Abhava-Pratinidhi Dravya, i.e.*, suggestions on the use of substitutes, have been mentioned in authoritative Ayurvedic texts like *Charaka Samhitā* and *Astanga Hridaya* [19]. Further, in *Charaka Samhitā* [4th chapter of *Sūtra Sthāna*], it is mentioned that "a wise physician need not stick to the list of herbs mentioned in the books for treatment purposes; instead, he can opt for other herbs that have similar properties and activities", thus giving the liberty to select appropriate substitutes as a solution to address the unavailability of primary medicinal plants. Interestingly, this concept is accepted by Ayurvedic practitioners and put into practice for various reasons, including similarity, easy availability and cost-effectiveness.

Abhava-Pratinidhi Dravya has been discussed in detail in other Ayurvedic lexicons, such as *Bhavaprakasha, Yogaratnakara* and *Bhaishajya Ratnavali.* They have also listed more than 100 herbs with suitable alternatives, *e.g.*, *Alhagi camelorum* DC. [*Duralabha*] in place of *Fagonia cretica* L. [*Dhanvyasa*], *Saussurea lappa* [*Kushta*] in place of *Valeriana wallichii* [*Tagara*] and *Inula racemose* Hook.f. [*Pushkaramula*] in place of *Saussurea lappa* [*Kushtha*]. Fascinatingly, a herb can have more than one alternative, *e.g.*, *Plumbago zeylanica* L. [*Chitraka*] can be replaced with *Baliospermum montanum* (Willd.) Müll.Arg. [*Danti*] and/or alkali of *Achyranthes aspera* L. [*Apamarga kshara*]. This list of substitutes may differ from one lexicon to another, *e.g.*, for *Aconitum heterophyllum* Wall. Ex Royle [*Ativisha*], *Cyperus scariosus* R.Br. [*Nagarmotha*] is a substitute as per *Bhavaprakasha* & *Bhaishajya Ratnavali*, while *Terminalia chebula* Retz. [*Haritaki*] can be a substitute as per *Yogaratnakara* texts. Replacing actual herbs with substitutes is recommended in some authoritative texts and the Ayurvedic Formulary of India, wherein the official list of substitutes for *Ashtavarga dravyas* is mentioned.

Interestingly, the substitution of herbs has also been practiced in the Unani system of medicine, within its own principles. However, the major difference is that Ayurveda does not recommend substitution for main or principal ingredients, whereas in Unani, there is no such distinction. Strikingly, substitutes sometimes have greater outcomes than that primary herbs. For example, the rhizome of *Costus speciosus* (J. Koenig) Sm. recognized as *Kebuka* is also sometimes sold for use in the name *Langali* [*Gloriosa superba* L.], but its action on the uterus is more potent than that of *Langali* [20].

In the present chapter, we shall discuss some of the prominent herbs Table **1** used in commerce, their substitutes as suggested in Ayurveda and commercial substitutes/adulterants.

3.1. *Ativisha* [Himalayan Aconite or Atis]

3.1.1. Introduction

Ativisha is dried, tuberous roots of *Aconitum heterophyllum* Wall. ex Royle [Family: Ranunculaceae]. *Ativisha* is also known as *Shuklakanda* in Sanskrit as its roots are white. From ancient times, this plant has been used in many formulations in Ayurveda, and it is popularly known as *Shishubhaishajya* due to its extensive use in pediatric formulations, used both externally as well as internally to treat various ailments. It is highly preferred in the management of dysentery [*Amatisara*], fever and digestive disorders in children. The tubers of *A. heterophyllum* are bitter and help cool the body. *Charaka Samhitā* mentions the use of the tuberous roots in internal formulations in the treatment of fever, rheumatic conditions and loss of vitality. Further, it is reported to be useful in treating urinary tract infections, diarrhea and inflammation. It is also used as an expectorant and for hepatoprotective activity.

Table 1. Herbs of commercial importance and their substitute/adulterants.

Herb [Sanskrit Name]	Botanical Names of Plants Used for Medicine	Pharmacological Reported Activities	Botanical Names used as a Substitute	Commercial Adulterants/Substitutes
Ativisha	*Aconitum heterophyllum* Wall. ex Royle	Hepatoprotective, antidiarrheal, expectorant, diuretic, and carminative anti-flatulent [23]	*Cyperus rotundus* L.	*Cyperus scariosus* R.Br., *Cryptocoryne spiralis* (Retz.)Fisch. ex Wydler, *Cherophyllum villosm* Wall.
Bala	*Sida cordifolia* L.	Anti-inflammatory, anti-ulcerogenic, cardioprotective tonic, hepatoprotective, antidiabetic [68]	*Sida rhombifolia* L.	*Sida cordata* (Burm.f.) Borss.Waalk., *Sida acuta* Burm.f., *Sida urens* L., *Sida canariensis* Willd. and *Abutilon Indicum*(L.) Sweet
Guduchi	*Tinospora cordifolia* (Willd.) Miers	Immunomodulatory, anti-diabetic, hepatoprotective, anti-pyretic, anti-arthritic [50-52]	*Tinospora sinensis* (Lour.) Merr	*Tinospora crispa* (L.) Hook.f. & Thomson
Vidanga	*Embelia ribes* Burm.f.	Anthelmintic, anti-microbial, anti-fertility, anti-diabetic [88-94]	*Embelia tsjeriam-cottam* (Roem. & Schult.)	*Myrsine Africana* L. and *Maesa indica* (Roxb.) A. DC.

Some Ayurvedic texts mention 2 varieties of the root based on color, *viz. Ativisha* in white [*Shukla*] and *Prativisha* in black [*Shyamaa*]. However, in *Charaka Samhitā, Ativisha* and *Prativisha* are considered synonyms of the same herb. Further, in current practice, only the white variety is used [21]. The pure and genuine roots have short starchy fractures and are bitter, without producing any acidity and tingling sensation on the tongue. It is one of the main ingredients of Ayurvedic formulations like *Ativishadi Churna, Baala Chaturbhadrika Churna, Sudarshana Churna* and *Shiva Gulika* [22].

A. heterophyllum is one of the most widely used medicinal plants in many herbal preparations as per the Ayurvedic Formulary of India. It is widely used even in the Chinese and Bhutanese systems of medicine [23]. The herb belongs to the Ranunculaceae family [crowfoot-habitat in swamps of most species] and is distributed in the western Himalayas, Kashmir, Uttarakhand, Sikkim and Nepal, mainly in high altitudes between 2500 and 4000 m. This species is highly toxic, hence termed as the "Queen of all poisons" [24]. *A. heterophyllum* is a red-listed plant as per the IUCN, which has a critically endangered species status [25].

3.1.2. Chemistry and Pharmacology

Alkaloids are the major class of chemical constituents present in this herb, ranging from 0.20% to 2.49% (Aconites). Atisine alone contributes to 0.14% to 0.37% [26], and other alkaloids such as heterophyllinine-A, heterophyllinine-B, dihydroatisine, lycoctonine [27], 6-dehydroacetylsepaconitine and 13-hydroxylappaconitine [28] are also present. This species possesses hepatoprotective, antidiarrheal, expectorant, diuretic, anti-phlegmatic, anti-pyretic and analgesic, anti-oxidant, alexipharmic, anodyne, anti-atrabilious, anti-flatulent, anti-periodic and carminative properties [23].

3.1.3. Commercial Demand and Supply

The herb is estimated to have the consumption of about 127.65MT/Year by the Indian herbal industries, whereas the annual trade is about 100 to 200MT/Year at a value ranging between 3500 and 10,500 ₹/kg, which is considered to be one of the high commercially valued herbs [29]. The National Medicinal Plant Board (NMPB) has prioritized this herb and placed it under the subsidized plant category in India to promote its cultivation, and has provided a 75% subsidy for cultivators [30].

3.1.4. Potential Substitute, Chemistry And Pharmacology

The high trade value and limited availability of *A. heterophyllum* force the herbal industry to use possible substitutes. *Cyperus rotundus* L., *Cyperus scariosus* R.Br. and *Cryptocoryne spiralis* (Retz.) Fisch. ex Wydler are available substitutes described in Ayurvedic texts. In the 16th century, *A. heterophyllum* was not easily available, and hence it was replaced with *C. rotundus* in prescriptions as both herbs are used for alleviating cough and digestive disorders [31].

C. rotundus is a weed commonly found in rice fields and watercourses, and it belongs to the Cyperaceae family. It grows in Asian countries (*e.g.*, India, China, Bhutan and Pakistan) and tropical, subtropical and temperate regions globally

[32]. The chemical constituents present are cyperotundone, cyperol, α-cyperolone, β-cyperone, camphene, ρ-cymol, calcium, copaene, cyperene, cyperenone, rotundene, cyperolone, caryophyllene, *d*-copadiene, *d*-epoxyguaiene, isocyperol, selinatriene, isokobusone, patchoulenone, kobusone, limonene, linoleic-acid, linolenic-acid, mustakone, myristic acid, oleanolic acid, oleic acid, β-pinene, rotundenol, rotundone, α-rotunol, β-rotunol, β-selinene, sitosterol, stearic acid, sugeonol and sugetriol [33]. This herb possesses anti-inflammatory and anti-ulcer properties [34], and is indicated in the treatment of malaria, pyresis, diarrhea, diabetes, inflammation and stomach and bowel disorders [35]. The annual consumption is about 886.69MT/Year with a trade value of 25 to 30 ₹/kg [29].

C. scariosus (commonly known as *nagarmotha*) is a weed that belongs to the Cyperaceae family and is found in damp places in West Bengal, Uttar Pradesh and East and southern parts of India. It is also found in in Madagascar, Indo-Malaysia and Australia [32]. High-Performance Thin-Layer Chromatography (HPTLC) and Gas Chromatography-Mass Spectroscopy (GCMS) analyses of solvent extracts of *C. scariosus* showed that the majority of chemical compounds present are the same as that in *C. rotundus* [36], *viz.* cyperene, cyperenone, rotundene, longifolin, caryophylline oxide and longiverbenon [37]. Essential oils such as citral, α-pinene, β-pinene, D-limonene and germacrene D are also present. *C. scariosus* exhibits anti-microbial, anti-oxidant, anti-cancer [38], anti-hyper-glycemic, anti-depressant, anti-nociceptive, immunosuppressant and hepato-protective [39] activities. The estimated annual trade is about 200 to 500MT/Year, with a trade value of about 25 to 30 ₹/kg [29].

C. spiralis belongs to the Araceae family and is found in marshy areas with stagnant water. It is distributed in Karnataka, Tamil Nadu, Kerala, Maharashtra and a few parts of Bangladesh [40]. The GCMS analysis revealed the presence of neomenthol, *cis-α* santalol, santalol, α-santalol, bicyclo (2.2.1) heptane and 2-methyl-3-methylene-2-(4-methyl-3-pentenyl)-, (1*S*-exo) [41]. The rhizome of this plant is used as an antidiarrheal [42], and phytochemical and pharmacological activities of *C. spiralis* are about 84.6% similar to those present in *A. hetero-phylum*, hence it is widely used in Siddha medicine as "native Ativisha" [43].

The roots of *Cherophyllum villosm* Wall. [Apiaceae], sold in the market by the name *Mitha Patisa*, are sometimes mistakenly supplied in place of genuine material in Amritsar and other North Indian markets. The roots of *C. villosm* are long, cylindrical, gradually tapering and grayish white [44].

3.1.5. Recommendations

A. heterophyllum is one of the highly traded medicinal plants, and its limited availability has driven the need to search for its possible substitute. Many studies are conducted to evaluate the chemo-profiling and biological activities of possible substitutes.

It is pertinent to note that the *Rasapanchaka* (Ayurvedic principles of drug action)—*rasa* (taste), *guna* (properties), *veerya* (potency), *vipaka* (taste after digestion), *prabhava* (unique action) and *karma* (pharmacological action)—attributes of *Musta* are similar to that of *Ativisha*. Both have a bitter and pungent taste, are easily digestible, retain pungency after digestion and pacify *kapha* and *pitta* doshas. Further, they are prescribed to increase digestive fire and indicted fever and diarrhea; thus, this is a classic example to scientifically justify the concept of *Pratinidhi Dravya* to substitute any herb/ingredient in the preparation of medicine in case of non-availability with another similarly potent drug having similar *rasa, guna, veerya, vipaka* and *karma* as specified in Ayurveda. *C. rotundus* is considered a potentially favorable substitute.

3.2. Guduchi [Giloe]

3.2.1. Introduction

Tinospora cordifolia (Willd.) Miers is one of the highly traded herbs in the Indian system of medicine. The term "*Guduchi*" or "*Giloe*" means the one that protects the body. The origin of this herb is described in ancient classical texts as "*Amrita*", which means from the drops of divine nectar. The potent activity of this herb as an antimicrobial fascinates to term as "Herbal antibiotics" [45].

The aqueous extract of *T. cordifolia*, also called as Indian Quinine, is very efficacious in treating various types of fevers, and its therapeutic strength lies in its immunomodulatory and detoxifying properties. This plant possesses restorative and alterative properties, hence it is a significant rejuvenator (*Rasayana*) and is recommended in the treatment of certain diseases under the group as a preventive as well as a curative.

In the earlier Ayurvedic literature, only one variety of *Guduchi* is described. However, *Dhanvantari Nighantu* [one of the Ayurvedic lexicons] subsequently introduced two varieties of *Guduchi—Guduchi* and *Kandodbhava Guduchi*. This variety (*Kandodbhava Guduchi*) is identified as *Tinospora sinensis* (Lour.) Merr.

Further, one more renowned Ayurvedic physician Mr Gangadhara mentioned about *Padma Guduchi* in his commentary, which is nothing but *T. sinensis* (Lour.) Merr [46].

This plant is one of the parts of several important Ayurvedic formulations, including *Guduchyadi Churna, Guduchyadi Kvatha* and *Amrtarista* [21].

It is recommended that the stem of this plant should preferably be used when it is green and fresh. If storage is desired, the stems should be collected during the rainy season, dried in shade and then stored.

T. cordifolia belongs to the family Menispermaceae and is a climber, which is widely used in Ayurveda, Siddha, Unani, Folk, Homeopathy and Sowa Rigpa. The herb is found in India, Sri Lanka and Bangladesh, and it is found in tropical areas in India, ascending to an altitude of 300m [32].

3.2.2. Chemistry and Pharmacology

Phenolics, alkaloids and glycosides are the major class of chemical constituents present in *T. cordifolia*. The major terpenoids present in *T. cordifolia* are tinosporide, furanolactone diterpene, furanolactone clerodane diterpene, furanoid diterpene, tinosporaside, ecdysterone makisterone, phenylpropene disaccharides cordifolioside A, B and C, cordifoliside D and E, tinocordioside, cordioside and palmatosides C and F. Alkaloids such as tinosporine, magnoflorine, berberine, choline [47], syringin [48], cordifolioside A (0.1 to 0.7%w/w) [49] and syringin are responsible for the immunomodulatory, anti-cancer, anti-diabetic, anti-toxin (found to reverse the toxicity caused by aflatoxins), anti-oxidant, anti-HIV, anti-osteoporotic, cardioprotective, hepato-protective and antidiarrheal activities [50]. Treatment for SARS CoV-2 with *Guduchi* helped effectively manage abnormal fever episodes, recover renal damage and manage edema caused due to SARS CoV-2 [51]. It is a potential neuro-regenerative against glutamate-induced excitotoxicity [52].

3.2.3. Commercial Demand and Supply

The annual trade volume of *T. cordifolia* stem is 1000 to 1500MT/Year and traded at 35 to 40 ₹/kg. The estimated annual consumption is more than 3700MT by large- and small-scale industries, including ayurvedic practitioners [29].

3.2.4. Potential Substitute, Chemistry and Pharmacology

T. cordifolia is substituted with *T. sinensis* and *T. crispa* [53]. More than 20% of the *T. cordifolia* is adulterated with a closely related species, *T. sinensis* [54]. *T. sinensis* is a large woody climber that belongs to the Menispermaceae family and is found in South and Southeast Asia, mainly in India, China, Nepal, Sri Lanka, Bangladesh, Myanmar to Thailand, Vietnam and Cambodia. *T. sinensis* can be differentiated from the authentic species by its large tomentose leaves, uniseriate multicellular type of trichome present on young stems and on both surfaces of the leaves, watery latex, prominent scattered oval shape lenticels, the stomatal index and difference in the area of the stomatal aperture [55]. The major chemical constituents present are tinosporine A, tinodinorlignoside A, 1-acetyltinos-inenoside D, 1-acetyltinosinenoside E [56], tinosporide A, tinosporin B [57], tinosineside, tinocordifolioside, malabaroliode, tinosporaside, 1-deacetyltin-osporaside, 4-hydroxyl-heptadec-6-enoic acid, cordicoside, synergin, palmatine, diosgenin, daucasterol, columbin, β-sitosterol, hydroxyecdysone and berberine [55]. *T. sinensis* has anti-inflammatory, anthelmintic, anti-ulcer and immuno-modulatory [55] properties. It is used in the treatment of Alzheimer's disease. The commercial annual demand for *T. sinensis* is more than 100MT [58].

T. crispa belongs to the Menispermaceae family and is a large woody succulent climbing shrub found in India (Arunachal Pradesh, Assam and West Bengal), Cambodia, China, Indonesia, Malaysia, Philippines and Thailand [59]. The significant morphoanatomical difference is the secretory head, which is ellipsoid in *T. cordifolia* and ovoid-sub globose in *T. crispa* [60]. The major alkaloids present in *T. crispa* are *N*-formyl asimilobine 2-*O*-β-D-glucopyranoside, *N*-formylasimilobine 2-*O*-β-D-glucopyranosyl-(1→2)-β-D-glucopyranoside, tinos-corside A, *N*-formyldehydroanonaine, *N*-formylnornuciferine, *N*-demethyl-*N*-formyldehydronornuciferine, magnoflorine, paprazine, *N*-transferuloyltyramine and cytidine [61]. It is widely used in the treatment of diabetes mellitus [62], jaundice, rheumatic disorders and hypertension. It has anti-inflammatory, cardioprotective and immunomodulatory properties [63, 64].

3.2.5. Recommendations

According to Ayurveda, *T. sinensis* (Syn. *T. malabarica*) is a substitute for *Guduchi*. *T. sinensis* (Syn. *T. malabarica*) belongs to the same family and has similar Ayurvedic pharmacodynamics (*Rasapanchaka*) as that of *Guduchi*, in terms of *rasa* (*tikta, kashaya*), *guna* (*guru, snigdha*), *virya* (*usna*), *vipaka* (*madhura*) and *karma* (pacifies all the three *doshas*) attributes.

There are a few quality control tools that help differentiate the species. HPTLC is a simple, economical and widely accepted quality control tool for evaluating adulteration. Chemical fingerprinting helps distinguish between herbs based on the chemical compounds present in them [60]. Liquid Chromatography-Mass Spectrometry helps identify chemical compounds present in them, such as furanoditerpenes (*e.g.*, borapetosides B, C and F). Other HPLC methods help identify 20β-hydroxyecdysone, cordioside, tinospraside and columbin (a key marker), which aid in differentiating *T. crispa* from other species [65, 66]. During the COVID-19 pandemic, there was a sudden increase in the demand for *Guduchi*, which led to the use of all three species in commerce. A recent study reported the occurrence of liver damage due to the use of *Giloe* herb. However, based on the current understanding, it might be because of the consumption of *T. crispa* [67]. Quantifying both alkaloidal and non-alkaloidal constituents of the species can be a good quality control tool [48]. In normal circumstances, *T. cordifolia* is available in optimum amounts, and a substitute is required in exceptional situations like the COVID-19 pandemic.

3.3. Bala

3.3.1. Introduction

In Ayurvedic medicine, *Sida cordifolia* L. is popularly known as "*Bala*" and country mallow. It belongs to the Malvaceae family. *Bala* means "strength". It is a rejuvenating ingredient in *Vata* disorders (especially for nervous conditions). Its stem and roots are strong, which contributes to its strengthening property. Further, *Bala* is used as a primary ingredient in various massage oils for treating arthritis, nervous system disorders and stroke. It is the principal ingredient of Ayurvedic formulations like Balarishta, Balaadi Kvatha, Balaadya Ghrita and Chandana Balaa Lakshaditaila [46].

It is also used in the treatment of a wide range of illnesses in western countries like China and Brazil [68]. In Ayurvedic literature, it is indicated to be used as an astringent, aphrodisiac, emollient and tonic. It is also used in the treatment of respiratory system and urinary system-related disorders [69].

3.3.2. Chemistry and Pharmacology

Various phytochemical reports indicated the presence of alkaloids, flavonoids, ecdysteroids and fatty acids in *Sida cordifolia* L. The roots have been reported to contain alkaloids (*e.g.*, β-phenethylamines and tryptamines) and quinazoline alkaloids (*e.g.*, vacisine). However, the reports on the presence of ephedrine and cryptolepine are not consistent. *S. cordifolia* is reported to have anti-inflammatory, analgesic, anti-pyretic, anti-ulcerogenic, cardioprotective and hepatoprotective activities. In addition, the plant also has antidiabetic, anti-hypercholesterolemic, anti-oxidant, anti-proliferative and wound-healing properties [68].

3.3.3. Commercial Demand and Supply

In the herbal drug industry, this herb is commonly traded with the name "*Bala*", and all prominent species like *Sida acuta* Burm.f., *Sida cordifolia* L. and *Sida rhombifolia* L. are traded with the same name. Based on the occurrence of the plant in particular regions, along with corroboration of field operating principles by the traders and herbal industry, the quantity of each species is deciphered. Basis this, the annual demand for *S. cordifolia* is reported to be 2000MT. This herb is in demand, but has limited supplies of other related herbs in commerce like *S. rhombifolia* (up to 2000MT) and *S. acuta* (up to 200MT) [29]. The availability of all three species is not critical [58]. However, as many allied species of *S. cordifolia* are used as "*Bala*", there is a need to develop a resource base of these species that meet botanical identification and standardization protocol [29].

3.3.4. Potential Substitute, Chemistry and Pharmacology

In several Ayurvedic literatures, there are different opinions on the botanical identity of "*Bala*". One of the authentic books in Ayurveda—*Bhavaprakasha Nighantu*—mentions four varieties, and *Dhanavantari Nighantu* mentions five varieties [70].

A review of *Sida* species that are found in India, China, Africa, and American countries reported about 142 chemical constituents, including 23 alkaloids, 19 flavonoids, 16 ecdysteroids, 5 terpenoids, 4 tocopherols, 3 lignans, 4 coumarins and other compounds [71]. In 2015, Subramanya *et al* studied polyphenol contents and anti-oxidant activity of methanolic extracts of eight *Sida* species collected from the western ghats of India. The species that were studied were *S. acuta, S. cordata, S. cordifolia, S. indica, S. mysorensis, S. retusa, S. rhombifolia* and *S. spinosa*. Among these, *S. cordifolia* was found to have a higher anti-oxidant effect [70]. In 2008, a pharmacognostic and analytical study on ecdysteroids in various *Sida* species, *viz. S. rhombifolia, S. cordifolia, S. cordata, S. acuta, S. urens* and *S. canariensis,* showed the presence of certain ecdysteroids in varying concentrations, whereas *S. hermaphrodita* showed none [72].

The closely traded "*Bala*" variety is *S. rhombifolia*, which is referred to as

"*Mahabala*" in Ayurvedic text [70]. Our phytochemical studies in the past on the plant showed the presence of ecdysone and its derivatives [73]. The *n*-hexanes and ethyl acetate extracts of the herb showed significant anti-inflammatory and anti-cholinesterase activities from the hexane extract and anti-oxidant activity from the ethyl acetate extract [74]. The seed extract from one of the subspecies *S. retusa* is shown to have chemopreventive and hepatoprotective effects in rats, ratifying its traditional use [75].

Various *Sida* species are mostly named after their leaf shape. In this case, the leaves are acute shaped and hence the name *S. acuta*. The extracts of aerial parts of *S. acuta* have been shown to have antiplasmodial and antimalarial activities [76]. The acetone extract of the aerial part has analgesic effect and can reduce diabetes-related inflammation in mice. The leaf extract showed hypoglycemic and hypolipidemic effects on alloxan-induced diabetic rats [77].

Abutilon Indicum is also known as "*Atibala*" in Ayurveda and belongs to the Malvaceae family. Along with *S. cordifolia* ("*Bala*"), it is called "*Dwaya Bala*" (Twin Bala) [78]. Traditionally, it has been reported beneficial as an aphrodisiac, anti-diabetic, nervine tonic and diuretic. It is known to contain several phytochemicals, including carbohydrates, phytosterols, flavonoids and phenolics [79, 80]. It is shown to have some important pharmacological activities like hepatoprotective, wound-healing, immunomodulatory and hypoglycemic activities [79].

3.3.5. Recommendations

The plant *Bala* (*S. cordifolia*), the other three species discussed above, and another commonly substituted plant *A. indicum* have the same *Rasapanchaka* attributes—*madhura* (*i.e.*, sweet) in taste (*rasa*), *guru, snigdha, picchila* properties (*guna*), cold (*i.e.*, sheeta) in potency (*virya*), *madhura* in *vipaka* (taste after digestion)—and pacify *vata* and *pitta doshas*.

Currently, in commerce, *S. rhombifolia* and *S. acuta* are also used as "*Bala*" in addition to *S. cordifolia*. These species are sometimes used interchangeably. Also, among these other herbs from Malvaceae family, *A. indicum* is known to be used as a substitute. These herbs have been studied individually for their phytochemical constituents and pharmacological actions. Some of the actions of these herbs are similar; however, their phytochemical compositions reveal diverse chemistry. In one of the studies done by us, we found that there is diversity in ecdysone content in various *Sida* species and flavonoids [72, 73]. This concludes that the phytochemical composition and their pharmacological actions are not completely understood.

3.4. Vidanga

3.4.1. Introduction

Vidanga (Embelia ribes Burm. f.) is one of the ancient herbs popularly used not only in Ayurvedic medicine but also in the Unani and Siddha systems of medicine. It is an important Ayurvedic herb used for many years to treat multiple health conditions and is a renowned herb for treating digestive disorders, especially those characterized by abdominal bloating caused by helminths. In addition, it is prescribed for dyspepsia, colic pain, cough and asthma. It is also used as an emetic. It is a part of several important formulations like *Vidangadi Churna*, *Vidangarishta* and *Vidangadi Lauha*, which are very useful in the management of gastrointestinal disorders [21].

Vidanga is known as *Embelia ribes* Burm. f. and belongs to the Myrsinaceae family. It is also commonly known as false black pepper. *E. ribes* is a woody climber and an Indo-Malaysian species found in India, Sri Lanka, Singapore, Malaysia and South China. In India, it is found in the central Himalayas, Arunachal Pradesh, Assam, Maharashtra, Andhra Pradesh, Karnataka, Kerala and Tamil Nadu [32].

3.4.2. Chemistry and Pharmacology

E. ribes contains 56 compounds, including 16 phenolics, 16 flavonoids, 4 coumarins, 5 fatty acids and 15 other compounds [81, 82]. Embelin is one of the major phytoconstituents in *E. ribes*, ranging from 1.0 to 5.08%w/w [83, 84]. Other phytoconstituents present are vilagin [85], embelinol, embeliaribyl ester, embeliol [86], homoembelin and vidangin [87]. The fruits of *Vidanga* are used for its potent anthelmintic activity and are termed as *krimigna* in Ayurveda [88]. Embelin has shown antiviral activity against influenza virus A and B [89]. *E. ribes* helps in wound healing [90] and is used in treating inflammatory bowel disease [91]. It also exhibits antibacterial, anticancer, hepatitis C protease inhibition [92], antifertility [93], anti-diabetic [94] and inhibition of the SARS-CoV-2 Mpro protease activities [95].

3.4.3. Commercial Demand and Supply

The health benefits of *E. ribes* bring more revenue for farmers. The annual trade is estimated as 100 to 200MT and traded at 450 to 550 ₹/kg. Whereas the estimated consumption by large- and small-scale herbal industries is about 772.98MT annually, which leads to economic adulteration [29]. The natural cultivation of *E. ribes* to supply the demand is very challenging due to fragmented populations, which results in inbreeding, development of abortive embryos, and also slow germination of fertile seeds due to their smaller size. The other mode of artificial regeneration makes it even more challenging due to its poor rooting from stem cuttings and seed viability, and low rate of germination, so eventually leading to overexploitation [96]. The NMPB set up by the Government of India to promote the medicinal plants sector identified fruits of *E. ribes* on the "Priority Species List" for large-scale cultivation and also red-listed due to its overexploitation [97].

3.4.4. Potential Substitute, Chemistry and Pharmacology

Commercially available *Vidanga* is heavily adulterated with many similar-looking substances. The high demand and very limited availability of *E. ribes* compel us to search for substitutes without compromising the safety and efficacy of the drug. The search for possible substitutes based on literature leads to the use of *Embelia tsjeriam-cottam* (Roem. & Schult.), *Myrsine Africana* L. and *Maesa indica* (Roxb.) A. DC. as possible substitutes and adulterants for *E. ribes* [98].

One of the most predominant substitutes used for *E. ribes* is *E. tsjeriam-cottam*, which is a climber that belongs to the Myrsinaceae family and is commonly known as *Vidanga*. This climber is observed in India, Myanmar and Sri Lanka at an altitude of 1600m [32]. *E. tsejeriam-cottam* contains embelin as one of the major chemical constituents ranging from 1.09 to 5.21%w/w [99], phenol, *2,4-bis*(*1,1*-Dimethylethyl), neophytadiene, squalene, moretenol [100], christembin, resinoids, vilangin, gallic acid, vanillic acid and salicylic acid [101]. *E. tsejeriam-cottam* shows antimycotic, antibacterial, cytotoxic [102] and anthelmintic activities [97]. *E. tsejeriam-cottam* is the most traded for *E. ribes* due to the presence of embelin in higher quantities and the same biological activities. The trade value is estimated to be around 500 to 600 ₹/kg, and the annual trade is around 500–1000MT [29].

M. Africana is a shrub that belongs to the Myrsinaceae family and is known as the Cape Myrtle, African boxwood and Thakisa [103]. This shrub is widely used in Ayurveda, Unani and Chinese system of medicines. This species is globally distributed across Africa, Arabia, Afghanistan, Pakistan, India, Nepal and China. Within India, it is found in Jammu & Kashmir, Himachal Pradesh, Uttar Pradesh, Assam and Meghalaya at an altitude of 300–2700m [32]. Embelin is one of the major chemical constituents in *M. africana* and contributes around 2.1 to 4.4%w/w [104]. Quercitol [105], myrsinoside A, myrsinoside B [106], myrsine [107] are the other phytoconstituents present in it. The potential pharmacological activities of this herb are anthelmintic [108], anti-oxidant, anti-inflammatory, antiwrinkle [109] and antispasmodic [110]. The annual trade is estimated to be around <10MT and is traded in the name *chapra* [29, 111].

M. indica belongs to the Myrsinaceae family and is commonly known as wild berry [112]. This shrub is globally found across Indo-Malaysia and Pakistan. In India, it is reported in Karnataka, Kerala, Maharashtra and Tamil Nadu [113]. Very few literatures are available on the chemical constituents present in the seeds of *M. indica*; of them, kiritiquinone [114], quercetin and quercetin-3-rhamnoside [115] are a few. *M. indica* exhibits antibacterial, radical scavenging, anti-oxidant and anti-diabetic activities [112]. There is not much evidence about the trade of this species.

3.4.5. Recommendations

E. ribes and *E. tsjeriam-cottam* are known as *Vidanga* and *Vidanga bheda*, respectively, in Ayurveda and are valuable anthelmintics (*krmighna*). Further, *Rasapanchaka* is also the same in both as explained in Ayurveda texts, *i.e.*, *Katu* and *Kashaya* in taste; have *laghu, ruksha* and *tikshna* properties; hot in potency; and pacifies/mitigates *kapha* and *vata*.

Vidanga is widely known for its anthelmintic property and is termed as *Krimighna*. A study was conducted to evaluate anthelmintic properties with a potential substitute. All the *Vidanga* substitute species, such as *E. tsjeriam-cottam, M. africana* L and *M. indica*, were subjected to study using *Caenorhabditis elegans* as a model system. The seeds of these species were extracted in ethyl acetate along with embelin and kiritquinone (one of the active constituents in *E. ribes*). The activity of *E. tsjeriam-cottam* was comparable with *E. ribes,* whereas other species showed relatively less activity, *i.e.*, *M. africana* L. followed by *M. indica*. The crude extracts showed 2-3 times higher activity compared with pure active molecules. This demonstrates *E. tsjeriam-cottam* could be a potential substitute for *E. ribes* and also helps in the protection of the endangered species [97].

The bioactive metabolite profiling of *Vidanga* species was done using HPLC to identify their common metabolites. This has a major impact on selecting a suitable substitute for *E. ribes* [104]. Furthermore, further studies are required to establish concrete evidence for evaluating the possible substitute. Many studies have been done on the chemical profiling of these herbs, whereas molecular evaluation for correlating their genetic similarity will provide detailed evidence of the expression of secondary metabolites.

CONCLUSION

In Ayurveda, herbs have been classified based on scientific evidence. The principle of herb substitution is based on the quality, activity and clinical evidence that add credence to its favor of the scientific approach. However, for a modern researcher, these are jigsaw puzzles that are yet to be completely comprehended. In the present chapter, we have tried to understand the connectivity between *Abhavapratinidhi dravya* and the present-day commercial substitutes for some commercially important herbal ingredients.

In the case of *Ativisha,* the herbs used in commerce are not Ayurveda-mentioned substitutes but similar herbs. Interestingly, the authentic Ayurvedic substitute herb is *C. rotundus,* which belongs to Cyperaceae family as against *A. heterophyllum* of Ranunculaceae family. This indicates that Ayurvedic substitution goes beyond the routine pharmacognostic understanding of the herb or even the habit of the herb. *C. rotundus* is clinically used by Ayurvedic physicians due to its availability and ease of handling. This throws a big challenge for phytochemists and pharmacologists to understand the Ayurvedic approach.

The other popular herb we reviewed here is *Bala, S. cordifolia,* which has several species from *Sida* genus that are mostly differentiated by the leaf structure. As per Ayurvedic texts, four herbs are considered—*Balachatustaya-Bala: S. cordifolia*; *Mahabala: S. rhombifolia*; *Atibala: A. indicum*; and *Nagabala: S. veronicaefolia* (syn. *Sida cordata*). These herbs have different clinical usage, except *Bala* and *Mahabala* have similar usage. The word *Bala* means that which increases strength, and *Mahabala* is that which can increase strength to a further extent. From a phytochemical perspective, one can ponder if a higher concentration of ecdysone and derivatives in *S. rhombifolia* should have been named *Mahabala*? However, no substitute is mentioned for *Bala* in the available Ayurveda texts, but it allows the use of *Mahabala* in place of *Bala*. However, in commerce, all the *Sida* species seem to be used as *Bala*. *Atibala* (*A. indicum*) has also been found to be used in commerce as *Bala*. This indicates that the commercial use of these herbs is interchangeable and is not necessarily precise. This warrants a proper commercial identification tool and develops understanding in the user community.

In the case of *Guduchi*, Ayurveda recommends *T. sinensis* (*Syn. T. malabarica*) as a substitute, which belongs to the same family and has similar pharmacognostic features and chemical composition. It is the same in the case of *Vidanga*, where *E. ribes* is the authentic species, and Ayurveda recommends the use of *E. tsjeriam-cottam* as a substitute. Embelin, the principal component of *E. ribes*, is also the main constituent in *E. tsjeriam-cottam*. In both these traded species, a thorough, detailed phytopharmacological study should be undertaken to guide trade.

In summary, the herbs of commerce reviewed here indicate an incomplete understanding of the *rasa, guna, virya* and *vipaka* of the herbs vs. their phytochemical constitution. Substitution of herbs is the need of the hour, with many medicinal plants becoming endangered. The essential criteria for substitution are the pharmacological activity rather than morphology or phytoconstituents. It is pertinent to note that Ayurveda has warned that the substitution is permissible only for polyherbal/multi-component formulas and not permitted for single-drug preparation. Substitution of herbs has achieved many goals, though the basic idea was to provide an herb with a similar therapeutic effect as that of the authentic herb. This underlines that our understanding of how herbs act and how they should be identified from the ethnopharmacological perspective needs a lot of in-depth studies.

CONSENT FOR PUBLICATION

Not applicable.

CONFLICT OF INTEREST

The authors declare no conflict of interest, financial or otherwise.

ACKNOWLEDGEMENTS

Declared none.

REFERENCES

[1]   Agyei-Baffour, P.; Kudolo, A.; Quansah, D.Y.; Boateng, D. Integrating herbal medicine into mainstream healthcare in Ghana: clients' acceptability, perceptions and disclosure of use. *BMC Complement. Altern. Med.,* **2017**, *17*(1), 1-9.
[http://dx.doi.org/10.1186/s12906-017-2025-4] [PMID: 29191194]

[2]   Ahmad Khan, M.S.; Ahmad, I. Herbal Medicine: Current Trends and Future Prospects. *In New Look to Phytomedicine,* Mohd Sajjad Ahmad Khan, Iqbal Ahmad, D. C., Ed.; Academic press. **2019**, 3-13.

[3]   Falci, L.; Shi, Z.; Greenlee, H. Multiple Chronic Conditions and Use of Complementary and Alternative Medicine Among US Adults: Results From the 2012 National Health Interview Survey. *Prev. Chronic Dis.,* **2016**, *13*(5), 1-13.
[http://dx.doi.org/10.5888/pcd13.150501] [PMID: 27149072]

[4]   Nontokozo, Z. Msomi, M. B. C. S. Herbal Medicine. *Herbal Medicine.,* **2019**. 215-227.

[5]   Wegener, T. Patterns and Trends in the Use of Herbal Products, Herbal Medicine and Herbal Medicinal Products. *Int. J. Complement. Altern. Med.,* **2017**, *9*(6).
[http://dx.doi.org/10.15406/ijcam.2017.09.00317]

[6]   Tulunay, M.; Aypak, C.; Yikilkan, H.; Gorpelioglu, S. Herbal medicine use among Turkish patients with chronic diseases. *J. Intercult. Ethnopharmacol.,* **2015**, *4*(3), 217-220.
[http://dx.doi.org/10.5455/jice.20150623090040] [PMID: 26401410]

[7]   Peltzer, K.; Pengpid, S. The use of herbal medicines among chronic disease patients in Thailand: a cross-sectional survey. *J. Multidiscip. Healthc.,* **2019**, *12*, 573-582.
[http://dx.doi.org/10.2147/JMDH.S212953] [PMID: 31413584]

[8]   Peltzer, K.; Nguyen Huu, T.; Bach Ngoc, N.; Pengpid, S. The Use of Herbal Remedies and Supplementary Products among Chronic Disease Patients in Vietnam. *Stud. Ethno-Med.*, **2017**, *11*(2), 137-145.
        [http://dx.doi.org/10.1080/09735070.2017.1305230]

[9]   Salmerón-Manzano, E.; Garrido-Cardenas, J.A.; Manzano-Agugliaro, F. Worldwide Research Trends on Medicinal Plants. *Int. J. Environ. Res. Public Health,* **2020**, *17*(10), 3376.
        [http://dx.doi.org/10.3390/ijerph17103376] [PMID: 32408690]

[10]   Bachman, S.P.; Field, R.; Reader, T.; Raimondo, D.; Donaldson, J.; Schatz, G.E.; Lughadha, E.N. Progress, challenges and opportunities for Red Listing. *Biol. Conserv.*, **2019**, *234*(February), 45-55.
        [http://dx.doi.org/10.1016/j.biocon.2019.03.002]

[11]   Venkatasubramanian, P.; Nagarajan, M.; Kuruvilla, G.R.; Kumar, K.S. Abhava pratinidhi dravya: A comparative phytochemistry of Ativisha, Musta and related species. *J. Ayurveda Integr. Med.*, **2015**, *6*(1), 53-63.
        [http://dx.doi.org/10.4103/0975-9476.146550] [PMID: 25878466]

[12]   Gomes, A. Market Analysis 2020. *6th World Congress on Medicinal Plants and Marine Drugs.*, **2020**.

[13]   Tripathi, H. RAM, S.; Kumar, S.; Khan, F. International Trade in Medicinal and Aromatics Plants: A Case Study of Past 18 Years. *Curr. Res. Med. Aromat. Plants,* **2017**, *39*(1), 1-17.

[14]   Anonymous, https://www.herbalgram.org/

[15]   Srirama, R.; Santhosh Kumar, J.U.; Seethapathy, G.S.; Newmaster, S.G.; Ragupathy, S.; Ganeshaiah, K.N.; Uma Shaanker, R.; Ravikanth, G. Species Adulteration in the Herbal Trade: Causes, Consequences and Mitigation. *Drug Saf.,* **2017**, *40*(8), 651-661.
        [http://dx.doi.org/10.1007/s40264-017-0527-0] [PMID: 28389979]

[16]   Khazan, M.; Hedayati, M.; Kobarfard, F.; Askari, S.; Azizi, F. Identification and determination of synthetic pharmaceuticals as adulterants in eight common herbal weight loss supplements. *Iran. Red Crescent Med. J.,* **2014**, *16*(3), e15344.
        [http://dx.doi.org/10.5812/ircmj.15344] [PMID: 24829782]

[17]   Sagar, P.K. Adulteration and Ubstitution in Endangered, ASU Herbal Medicinal Plants of India, Their Legal Status, Scientific Screening of Active Phytochemical Constituents. *Int. J. Pharm. Sci. Res.,* **2014**, *5*(9), 4023-4039.

[18]   Anonymous, *WHO Global Report on Traditional and Complementary Medicine 2019,* **2019**.

[19]   Vaidyanath, R. Astanga Hrdaya of Vagbhata SUTRA-STHANA; Chauhhamba Subharati Prakashan: Delhi, **2013**.

[20]   Garg S. Introduction, Substitute and Adulterant Plants; Periodical Experts Book Agency: Delhi, **1992**.

[21]   Anonymous. The Ayurvedic Pharmacopoeia of India, Part 1.; Department of AYUSH, Government of India: New Delhi, **1999**, 99.

[22]   Gogte, V.M. Ayurvedic Pharmacology & Therapeutic Uses of Medicinal Plants (Dravyaguna Vignyan), 1st edition Bharatiya Vidya Bhavan: Mumbai **2000**.

[23]   Paramanick, D.; Panday, R.; Shukla, S.S.; Sharma, V. Primary Pharmacological and Other Important Findings on the Medicinal Plant "*Aconitum Heterophyllum*" (Aruna). *J. Pharmacopuncture,* **2017**, *20*(2), 89-92.
        [http://dx.doi.org/10.3831/KPI.2017.20.011] [PMID: 30087784]

[24]   Paramanick, D.; Sharma, N.; Parveen, N.; Patel, N.; Keshri, M. Keshri., M.; Panday, R.; Shukla, S. S.; Sharma, V. A Review Article on Ayurvedic/ Herbal Plant "ARUNA" (*Aconitum Heterophyllum*). *Int. J. Adv. Res. (Indore),* **2017**, *5*(2), 319-325.
        [http://dx.doi.org/10.21474/IJAR01/3150]

[25]   Jeelani, S.M.; Siddique, M.A.A.; Rani, S. Variations of Morphology, Ecology and Chromosomes of

Aconitum Heterophyllum Wall., an Endangered Alpine Medicinal Plant in Himalayas. *Firenze Univ. Press,* **2016**, *68*(4), 294-305.

[26]   Malhotra, N.; Kumar, V.; Sood, H.; Singh, T.R.; Chauhan, R.S. Multiple genes of mevalonate and non-mevalonate pathways contribute to high aconites content in an endangered medicinal herb, *Aconitum heterophyllum* Wall. *Phytochemistry,* **2014**, *108*, 26-34.
[http://dx.doi.org/10.1016/j.phytochem.2014.08.025] [PMID: 25239552]

[27]   Nisar, M.; Obaidullah, ; Ahmad, M.; Wadood, N.; Lodhi, M.A.; Shaheen, F.; Choudhary, M.I. New diterpenoid alkaloids from *Aconitum heterophyllum Wall* : Selective butyrylcholinestrase inhibitors. *J. Enzyme Inhib. Med. Chem.,* **2009**, *24*(1), 47-51.
[http://dx.doi.org/10.1080/14756360801906202] [PMID: 18615279]

[28]   Ahmad, M.; Ahmad, W.; Ahmad, M.; Zeeshan, M.; Obaidullah, ; Shaheen, F. Norditerpenoid alkaloids from the roots of *Aconitum heterophyllum* Wall with antibacterial activity. *J. Enzyme Inhib. Med. Chem.,* **2008**, *23*(6), 1018-1022.
[http://dx.doi.org/10.1080/14756360701810140] [PMID: 18608773]

[29]   Goraya GS, Ved DK. Medicinal Plants in India : An Assessment of their Demand and Supply. National Medicinal Plants Board, Ministry of AYUSH, Government of India, New Delhi and Indian Council of Forestry Research & Education, Dehradun. Naonal Medicinal Plants Board, Ministry of AYUSH; 2017.

[30]   https://nmpb.nic.in/content/prioritised-list-medicinal-plants-cultivation

[31]   Venkatasubramanian, P.; Kumar, K.S.; Nagarajan, M.; Kuruvilla, G.R. Pharmacology of Ativisha, Musta and their substitutes. *J. Ayurveda Integr. Med.,* **2015**, *6*(2), 121-133.
[http://dx.doi.org/10.4103/0975-9476.146551] [PMID: 26167002]

[32]   http://envis.frlht.org/tr_bot_search (accessed Apr 14, 2021).

[33]   Kamala, A.; Middha, S. K.; Karigar, C. S. Plants in Traditional Medicine with Special Reference to Cyperus Rotundus L.: A Review. 3 Biotech, 2018, 8 (7), 309.
[http://dx.doi.org/10.1007/s13205-018-1328-6]

[34]   Ahmad, M.; MahayRookh, ; Rehman, A.B.; Muhammad, N.; Amber, ; Younus, M.; Wazir, A. Assessment of anti-inflammatory, anti-ulcer and neuro-pharmacological activities of *Cyperus rotundus* Linn. *Pak. J. Pharm. Sci.,* **2014**, *27*(6 Spec No.), 2241-2246.
[PMID: 26045387]

[35]   Peerzada, A.M.; Ali, H.H.; Naeem, M.; Latif, M.; Bukhari, A.H.; Tanveer, A. Cyperus rotundus L.: Traditional uses, phytochemistry, and pharmacological activities. *J. Ethnopharmacol.,* **2015**, *174*, 540-560.
[http://dx.doi.org/10.1016/j.jep.2015.08.012] [PMID: 26297840]

[36]   Botlagunta, M.; Kakarla, L.; Katragadda, S.B. Morphological and chemoprofile (liquid chromatography-mass spectroscopy and gas chromatography-mass spectroscopy) comparisons of Cyperus scariosus R. Br and *Cyperus rotundus* L. *Pharmacogn. Mag.,* **2015**, *11*(44) Suppl. 3, 439.
[http://dx.doi.org/10.4103/0973-1296.168975] [PMID: 26929579]

[37]   Kumar, A.; Niranjan, A.; Lehri, A.; Srivastava, R.K.; Tewari, S.K. Effect of Geographical Climatic Conditions on Yield, Chemical Composition and Carbon Isotope Composition of Nagarmotha (*Cyperus scariosus* R. Br.) Essential Oil. *J. Essent. Oil-Bear. Plants,* **2016**, *19*(2), 368-373.
[http://dx.doi.org/10.1080/0972060X.2016.1148642]

[38]   Srivastava, R.K.; Singh, A.; Srivastava, G.P.; Lehri, A.; Niranjan, A.; Tewari, S.K.; Kumar, K.; Kumar, S. Chemical Constituents and Biological Activities of Promising Aromatic Plant Nagarmotha (Cyperus Scariosus R.Br.): A Review. *Proc. Indian Natl. Sci. Acad. A Phys. Sci.,* **2014**, *80*(3), 525.
[http://dx.doi.org/10.16943/ptinsa/2014/v80i3/55127]

[39]   Kasana, B.; Sharma, S.K.; Singh, L.; Mohapatra, S.; Singh, T. Cyperous Scariosis: A Potential Medicinal Herb. *Int. Res. J. Pharm.,* **2013**, *4*(6), 17-20.

[http://dx.doi.org/10.7897/2230-8407.04604]

[40]   Anonymous. Cryptocoryne spiralis (Retz.) Fisch. ex Wydler | Species. https://indiabiodiversity.org/ species/show/244496#natural-history

[41]   Wadkar, S.; Shete, C.; Inamdar, F.; Gurav, R.; Patil, K.; Ghosh, J. Phytochemical Screening and Antibacterial Activity of *Cryptocoryne Spiralis* Var. Spiralis and *Cryptocoryne Retrospiralis* (Roxb) Kunth. *Med. Aromat. Plants,* **2017**, *6*(2).
[http://dx.doi.org/10.4172/2167-0412.1000289]

[42]   Prasad, S.K.; Laloo, D.; Sahu, A.N.; Nath, G.; Hemalatha, S. *Cryptocoryne spiralis*, a substitute of *Aconitum heterophyllum* in the treatment of diarrhoea. *J. Pharm. Pharmacol.,* **2014**, *66*(12), 1808-1817.
[http://dx.doi.org/10.1111/jphp.12292] [PMID: 25130980]

[43]   John Adams, S.; Kuruvilla, G.R.; Krishnamurthy, K.V.; Nagarajan, M.; Venkatasubramanian, P. Pharmacognostic and phytochemical studies on Ayurvedic drugs Ativisha and Musta. *Rev. Bras. Farmacogn.,* **2013**, *23*(3), 398-409.
[http://dx.doi.org/10.1590/S0102-695X2013005000040]

[44]   Sharma, P. Dravyaguna-Vijnana, Part II, 4.; Choukamba orientalia: Varanasi, 2008; pp 761.

[45]   Balakrishnan, P. Amrita for Life Tinospora Cordifolia (Giloy); Balakrishnan, P., Ed.; National medicinal plat board, Ministery of AYUSH, Government of India: New delhi.

[46]   Gyanendra, P. *Dravyaguna Vijnana.,* **2005**, *Vol. 1.*

[47]   Sharma, P.; Dwivedee, B.P.; Bisht, D.; Dash, A.K.; Kumar, D. The chemical constituents and diverse pharmacological importance of *Tinospora cordifolia. Heliyon,* **2019**, *5*(9), e02437.
[http://dx.doi.org/10.1016/j.heliyon.2019.e02437] [PMID: 31701036]

[48]   Singh, D.; Chaudhuri, P.K. Chemistry and Pharmacology of *Tinospora cordifolia. Nat. Prod. Commun.,* **2017**, *12*(2), 1934578X1701200.
[http://dx.doi.org/10.1177/1934578X1701200240] [PMID: 30428235]

[49]   Alam, P.; Ali, M.; Singh, R. Madhurima; Ahmad, S.; Shakeel, F. A Validated HPLC Method for Estimation of Cordifolioside a in *Tinospora Cordifolia*, Miers and Marketed Formulations. *J. Chromatogr. Sci.,* **2009**, *47*(10), 910-913.
[http://dx.doi.org/10.1093/chromsci/47.10.910] [PMID: 19930804]

[50]   Tiwari, P.; Nayak, P.; Prusty, S.K.; Sahu, P.K. Phytochemistry and Pharmacology of *Tinospora cordifolia*: A Review. *Systematic Reviews in Pharmacy,* **2018**, *9*(1), 70-78.
[http://dx.doi.org/10.5530/srp.2018.1.14]

[51]   Balkrishna, A.; Khandrika, L.; Varshney, A. Giloy Ghanvati (*Tinospora cordifolia* (Willd.) Hook. f. and Thomson) Reversed SARS-CoV-2 Viral Spike-Protein Induced Disease Phenotype in the Xenotransplant Model of Humanized Zebrafish. *Front. Pharmacol.,* **2021**, *12*, 635510.
[http://dx.doi.org/10.3389/fphar.2021.635510] [PMID: 33953674]

[52]   Sharma, A.; Kaur, G. Tinospora Cordifolia as a Potential Neuroregenerative Candidate against Glutamate Induced Excitotoxicity: An *in Vitro* Perspective 11 Medical and Health Sciences 1109 Neurosciences. *BMC Complement. Altern. Med.,* **2018**, *18*(1), 1-17.
[PMID: 29295712]

[53]   Anonymous. Glimpses of CCRAS Contributions (50 Glorious Years) Medicinal Plants Research, III.; Central Council For Research In Ayurvedic Sciences; Ministry of AYUSH, Government of India New Delhi, 2018.

[54]   Santhosh Kumar, J. U.; Krishna, V.; Seethapathy, G. S.; Ganesan, R.; Ravikanth, G.; Shaanker, R. U. Assessment of Adulteration in Raw Herbal Trade of Important Medicinal Plants of India Using DNA Barcoding. *3 Biotech,* **2018**, *8* (3).
[http://dx.doi.org/10.1007/s13205-018-1169-3]

[55]   Hegde, S.; Jayaraj, M. A Review of the Medicinal Properties, Phytochemical and Biological Active Compounds of Tinospora Sinensis (Lour.) Merr. *J. Biol. Act. Prod. from Nat.,* **2016**, *6*(2), 84-94.
[http://dx.doi.org/10.1080/22311866.2016.1185968]

[56]   Wen, C.; Li, J.; Xu, X.; Li, Q.; Li, Y.; Chen, Y.; Yang, G. Lignans and clerodane diterpenoids from *Tinospora sinensis. RSC Advances,* **2020**, *10*(47), 28157-28163.
[http://dx.doi.org/10.1039/D0RA04917D] [PMID: 35519134]

[57]   Lam, S. H.; Chen, P. H.; Hung, H. Y.; Hwang, T. L.; Chiang, C. C.; Thang, T. D.; Kuo, P. C.; Wu, T. S. Chemical Constituents from the Stems of Tinospora Sinensis and Their Bioactivity. *Mol.* **2018**, *23* (10), 2541.
[http://dx.doi.org/10.3390/molecules23102541]

[58]   Gowthami, R.; Sharma, N.; Pandey, R.; Agrawal, A. Status and consolidated list of threatened medicinal plants of India. *Genet. Resour. Crop Evol.,* **2021**, *68*(6), 2235-2263.
[http://dx.doi.org/10.1007/s10722-021-01199-0] [PMID: 34054223]

[59]   https://indiabiodiversity.org/species/show/250719

[60]   Parveen, A.; Adams, J.S.; Raman, V.; Budel, J.M.; Zhao, J.; Babu, G.N.M.; Ali, Z.; Khan, I.A. Comparative Morpho-Anatomical and HPTLC Profiling of Tinospora Species and Dietary Supplements. *Planta Med.,* **2020**, *86*(7), 470-481.
[http://dx.doi.org/10.1055/a-1120-3711] [PMID: 32168549]

[61]   Choudhary, M.I.; Ismail, M.; Ali, Z.; Shaari, K.; Lajis, N.H. Atta-ur-Rahman Alkaloidal constituents of *Tinospora crispa. Nat. Prod. Commun.,* **2010**, *5*(11), 1934578X1000501.
[http://dx.doi.org/10.1177/1934578X1000501109] [PMID: 21213972]

[62]   Thomas, A.; Rajesh, E.K.; Kumar, D.S. The Significance of *Tinospora crispa* in Treatment of Diabetes Mellitus. *Phytother. Res.,* **2016**, *30*(3), 357-366.
[http://dx.doi.org/10.1002/ptr.5559] [PMID: 26749336]

[63]   Ahmad, W.; Jantan, I.; Bukhari, S.N.A. *Tinospora crispa* (L.) Hook. f. & Thomson: A Review of Its Ethnobotanical, Phytochemical, and Pharmacological Aspects. *Front. Pharmacol.,* **2016**, *7*(59), 59.
[http://dx.doi.org/10.3389/fphar.2016.00059] [PMID: 27047378]

[64]   Haque, M.A.; Jantan, I.; Harikrishnan, H.; Ahmad, W. Standardized ethanol extract of *Tinospora crispa* upregulates pro-inflammatory mediators release in LPS-primed U937 human macrophages through stimulation of MAPK, NF-κB and PI3K-Akt signaling networks. *BMC Complementary Medicine and Therapies,* **2020**, *20*(1), 245.
[http://dx.doi.org/10.1186/s12906-020-03039-7] [PMID: 32020859]

[65]   Parveen, A.; Wang, Y.H.; Fantoukh, O.; Alhusban, M.; Raman, V.; Ali, Z.; Khan, I.A. Development of a chemical fingerprint as a tool to distinguish closely related Tinospora species and quantitation of marker compounds. *J. Pharm. Biomed. Anal.,* **2020**, *178*, 112894.
[http://dx.doi.org/10.1016/j.jpba.2019.112894] [PMID: 31606561]

[66]   Ahmed, S.M.; Manhas, L.R.; Verma, V.; Khajuria, R.K. Quantitative determination of four constituents of Tinospora sps. by a reversed-phase HPLC-UV-DAD method. Broad-based studies revealing variation in content of four secondary metabolites in the plant from different eco-geographical regions of India. *J. Chromatogr. Sci.,* **2006**, *44*(8), 504-509.
[http://dx.doi.org/10.1093/chromsci/44.8.504] [PMID: 16959127]

[67]   Nagral, A.; Adhyaru, K.; Rudra, O.S.; Gharat, A.; Bhandare, S. Herbal Immune Booster-Induced Liver Injury in the COVID-19 Pandemic - A Case Series. *J. Clin. Exp. Hepatol.,* **2021**, *11*(6), 732-738.
[http://dx.doi.org/10.1016/j.jceh.2021.06.021] [PMID: 34230786]

[68]   Galal, A.; Raman, V.; Khan, A.; , I. *Sida Cordifolia* I. a Traditional Herb in Modern Perspective – A Review. *Curr. Tradit. Med.,* **2014**, *1*(1), 5-17.
[http://dx.doi.org/10.2174/2215083801666141226215639]

[69]   Ankit, J.; Shreya, C.; Singour, P.K.; Rajak, H. P. R. S. *Sida Cordifolia* (Linn) – An Overview. *J. Appl.*

Pharm. Sci., **2011**, *1*(2), 23-31.

[70]   Ankad, G.M.; Bhagwat, S.S.; Hegde, H.V.; Subramanya, M.D.; Upadhya, V.; Pai, S.R. Total polyphenolic contents and *in vitro* antioxidant properties of eight Sida species from Western Ghats, India. *J. Ayurveda Integr. Med.,* **2015**, *6*(1), 24-28.
[http://dx.doi.org/10.4103/0975-9476.146544] [PMID: 25878460]

[71]   Dinda, B.; Das, N.; Dinda, S.; Dinda, M.; SilSarma, I. The genus Sida L. – A traditional medicine: Its ethnopharmacological, phytochemical and pharmacological data for commercial exploitation in herbal drugs industry. *J. Ethnopharmacol.,* **2015**, *176*, 135-176.
[http://dx.doi.org/10.1016/j.jep.2015.10.027] [PMID: 26497766]

[72]   Avula, B.; Joshi, V.; Wang, Y.H.; Jadhav, A.N.; Khan, I.A. Quantitative Determination of Ecdysteroids in *Sida rhombifolia* L. and various other *Sida* Species Using LC-UV, and their Anatomical Characterization. *Nat. Prod. Commun.,* **2008**, *3*(5), 1934578X0800300.
[http://dx.doi.org/10.1177/1934578X0800300508]

[73]   Jadhav, A.N.; Pawar, R.S.; Avula, B.; Khan, I.A. Ecdysteroid Glycosides from *Sida rhombifolia* L. *Chem. Biodivers.,* **2007**, *4*(9), 2225-2230.
[http://dx.doi.org/10.1002/cbdv.200790180] [PMID: 17886841]

[74]   Mah, S.H.; Teh, S.S.; Ee, G.C.L. Anti-inflammatory, anti-cholinergic and cytotoxic effects of *Sida rhombifolia. Pharm. Biol.,* **2017**, *55*(1), 920-928.
[http://dx.doi.org/10.1080/13880209.2017.1285322] [PMID: 28152649]

[75]   Poojari, R.; Gupta, S.; Maru, G.; Khade, B.; Bhagwat, S. Sida rhombifolia ssp. retusa seed extract inhibits DEN induced murine hepatic preneoplasia and carbon tetrachloride hepatotoxicity. *Asian Pac. J. Cancer Prev.,* **2009**, *10*(6), 1107-1112.
[PMID: 20192593]

[76]   Aminah, N.S.; Laili, E.R.; Rafi, M.; Rochman, A.; Insanu, M.; Tun, K.N.W. Secondary metabolite compounds from Sida genus and their bioactivity. *Heliyon,* **2021**, *7*(4), e06682.
[http://dx.doi.org/10.1016/j.heliyon.2021.e06682] [PMID: 33912700]

[77]   Abat, J.K.; Kumar, S.; Mohanty, A.; Litscher, G.; Rocha, J. Ethnomedicinal, Phytochemical and Ethnopharmacological Aspects of Four Medicinal Plants of Malvaceae Used in Indian Traditional Medicines: A Review. *Medicines (Basel),* **2017**, *4*(4), 75.
[http://dx.doi.org/10.3390/medicines4040075] [PMID: 29057840]

[78]   Mathew, M.; Jayshree, C.; Thankachan, V.J.; Nilima, G. A phytochemical study of bala dwayam (*Sida cordifolia* & *Abutilon Indicum* linn.) And clinical evaluation of its moola churna ksheerapaka in Sandhigata vata with special reference to janu sandhi. *Int. J. Ayurveda. Med.,* **2021**, *12*(2), 292-295.
[http://dx.doi.org/10.47552/ijam.v12i3.1928]

[79]   Rajeshwari, S.; Sevarkodiyone, S. Medicinal Properties of *Abutilon Indicum. Open J. Plant Sci.,* 2018, 3 (1), 022–025.

[80]   Mei-Lin Yang, Pei-Lin Wu, Hui-Nung Shih, Tran Dinh Thang, N. X. D. Tian-S. W. Chemical Constituents from *Abutilon Indicum. J. Asian Nat. Prod. Res.,* **2008**, *10*(7), 689-693.
[http://dx.doi.org/10.1080/10286020802016545]

[81]   Guo, S.; He, M.; Liu, M.; Huang, W.; Ouyang, H.; Feng, Y.; Zhong, G.; Yang, S. Chemical Profiling of *Embelia ribes* by Ultra-High-Performance Liquid Chromatography Quadrupole Time-of-Flight Tandem Mass Spectrometry and Its Antioxidant and Anti-inflammatory Activities *In Vitro. J. Chromatogr. Sci.,* **2020**, *58*(3), 241-250.
[http://dx.doi.org/10.1093/chromsci/bmz097] [PMID: 31800022]

[82]   Kamble, V.; Attar, U.; Umdale, S.; Nimbalkar, M.; Ghane, S.; Gaikwad, N. Phytochemical analysis, antioxidant activities and optimized extraction of embelin from different genotypes of *Embelia ribes* Burm f.: a woody medicinal climber from Western Ghats of India. *Physiol. Mol. Biol. Plants,* **2020**, *26*(9), 1855-1865.
[http://dx.doi.org/10.1007/s12298-020-00859-2] [PMID: 32943821]

[83]   Souravi, K.; Rajasekharan, P. A Review on the Pharmacology of *Embelia Ribes* Burm. F.-A Threatened Medicinal Plant. *Int. J. Pharma Bio Sci.,* **2014**, *5*(2), 443-456.

[84]   Nagamani, V.; Sabitha Rani, A.; Satyakala, M. V Chandrashekar Reddy, G. N. High Performance Liquid Chromatography (HPLC) Analysis of Embelin in Different Samples of Embelis Ribes Burm. f.-a Threatened Medicinal Plant of India. *J. Med. Plants Res.,* **2013**, *7*(24), 1761-1767.

[85]   Rao, C.B.; Venkateswarlu, V. Chemical Examination of *Embelia ribes.* I. Isolation of a New Constituent, "Vilangin," Its Constitution and Synthesis. *J. Org. Chem.,* **1961**, *26*(11), 4529-4532.
        [http://dx.doi.org/10.1021/jo01069a079]

[86]   Choudhary, S.; Kaurav, H.; Chaudhary, G. Vaibidang (*Embelia ribes*): A Potential Herbal Drug in Ayurveda with Anthelmintic Property. *Int. J. Res. Appl. Sci. Biotechnol.,* **2021**, *8*(2), 237-243.
        [http://dx.doi.org/10.31033/ijrasb.8.2.31]

[87]   Khare, C.P. *Embelia Ribes* Burm. F. Indian Medicinal Plants. Springer New York; 2007. p. 1–1.

[88]   Stephan Raj, T.L.; Antoney, J.; John De Britto, A.; Abida, P. *In-vitro* Cytotoxicity Studies on Methanolic Leaf Extract of *Embelia Ribes* Burm F - an Important Traditional Medicinal Plant of Kerala. *Advances in Cytology & Pathology,* **2016**, *1*(1), 6-8.
        [http://dx.doi.org/10.15406/acp.2016.01.00002]

[89]   Hossan, M.S.; Fatima, A.; Rahmatullah, M.; Khoo, T.J.; Nissapatorn, V.; Galochkina, A.V.; Slita, A.V.; Shtro, A.A.; Nikolaeva, Y.; Zarubaev, V.V.; Wiart, C. Antiviral activity of *Embelia ribes* Burm. f. against influenza virus *in vitro. Arch. Virol.,* **2018**, *163*(8), 2121-2131.
        [http://dx.doi.org/10.1007/s00705-018-3842-6] [PMID: 29633078]

[90]   Agyare, C.; Boakye, Y.D.; Bekoe, E.O.; Hensel, A.; Dapaah, S.O.; Appiah, T. Review: African medicinal plants with wound healing properties. *J. Ethnopharmacol.,* **2016**, *177*, 85-100.
        [http://dx.doi.org/10.1016/j.jep.2015.11.008] [PMID: 26549271]

[91]   Bai, R.; Jie, X.; Yao, C.; Xie, Y. Discovery of small-molecule candidates against inflammatory bowel disease. *Eur. J. Med. Chem.,* **2020**, *185*(1), 111805.
        [http://dx.doi.org/10.1016/j.ejmech.2019.111805] [PMID: 31703817]

[92]   Akhtar, N.; Mohammed, S.A.A.; Khan, R.A.; Yusuf, M.; Singh, V.; Mohammed, H.A.; Al-Omar, M.S.; Abdellatif, A.A.H.; Naz, M.; Khadri, H. Self-Generating nano-emulsification techniques for alternatively-routed, bioavailability enhanced delivery, especially for anti-cancers, anti-diabetics, and miscellaneous drugs of natural, and synthetic origins. *J. Drug Deliv. Sci. Technol.,* **2020**, *58*(1), 101808.
        [http://dx.doi.org/10.1016/j.jddst.2020.101808]

[93]   Kumar, D.; Kumar, A.; Prakash, O. Potential antifertility agents from plants: A comprehensive review. *J. Ethnopharmacol.,* **2012**, *140*(1), 1-32.
        [http://dx.doi.org/10.1016/j.jep.2011.12.039] [PMID: 22245754]

[94]   Durg, S.; Veerapur, V.P.; Neelima, S.; Dhadde, S.B. Antidiabetic activity of *Embelia ribes,* embelin and its derivatives: A systematic review and meta-analysis. *Biomed. Pharmacother.,* **2017**, *86*, 195-204.
        [http://dx.doi.org/10.1016/j.biopha.2016.12.001] [PMID: 27984799]

[95]   Caruso, F.; Rossi, M.; Pedersen, J.Z.; Incerpi, S. Computational studies reveal mechanism by which quinone derivatives can inhibit SARS-CoV-2. Study of embelin and two therapeutic compounds of interest, methyl prednisolone and dexamethasone. *J. Infect. Public Health,* **2020**, *13*(12), 1868-1877.
        [http://dx.doi.org/10.1016/j.jiph.2020.09.015] [PMID: 33109497]

[96]   Annapurna, D.; Srivastava, A.; Rathore, T.S. Impact of Population Structure, Growth Habit and Seedling Ecology on Regeneration of *Embelia ribes* Burm. f. —Approaches toward a Quasi *in situ* Conservation Strategy. *Am. J. Plant Sci.,* **2013**, *4*(6), 28-35.
        [http://dx.doi.org/10.4236/ajps.2013.46A005]

[97]   Venkatasubramanian, P.; Godbole, A.; Vidyashankar, R.; Kuruvilla, G.R. Evaluation of Traditional

Anthelmintic Herbs as Substitutes for the Endangered *Embelia Ribes*, Using Caenorhabditis Elegans Model. *Curr. Sci.,* **2013**, *105*(11), 1593-1598.

[98]   Ved, D.; Singh, A. Identity of Vidanga- A Plant Drug in Trade. *Medicinal plants of conservation concern.* **2006**.

[99]   Pandey, A.K.; Ojha, V. Estimation of embelin in embelia tsjeriam-cottam fruits by HPLC to standardize harvesting time. *Indian J. Pharm. Sci.,* **2011**, *73*(2), 216-219.
        [http://dx.doi.org/10.4103/0250-474X.91563] [PMID: 22303066]

[100]   Gideon, A.V.; Britto, J.S. HPLC and GC-MS Analysis Of Bioactive Compounds In *Embelia Tsjeriam-Cottam* (Roem. & Schult.) A. Dc-A Threatened Species. *Int. J. Sci. Technol. Res.,* **2020**, *9*(3), 1766-1771.

[101]   Nafees, H.; Nefees, S.; Nizamudeen, S. A Comprehensive Review on *Embelia Tsjeriam-Cottam* A.DC. *Sci. Lett.,* **2020**, *1*(1), 1-3.

[102]   Poojari, D.R. Phytochemical Fingerprinting, Cytotoxic, Antimicrobial, Antitubercular, Antimycotic Potentials of *Sida Rhombifolia* Subsp. Retusa and *Embelia Tsjeriam-Cottam*. In Asia Pacific Life Sciences Compendium **2011**, 201-214.

[103]   Lall, N.; Kishore, N.; Fibrich, B.; Lambrechts, I. *In vitro* and *In vivo* activity of *Myrsine africana* on elastase inhibition and anti-wrinkle activity. *Pharmacogn. Mag.,* **2017**, *13*(52), 583-589.
        [http://dx.doi.org/10.4103/pm.pm_145_17] [PMID: 29200717]

[104]   Venkatasubramanian, P.; Balasubramani, S.P.; Nandi, S.K.; Tariq, M. Bioactive Metabolite Profiling for Identification of Elite Germplasms:A Conservation Strategy for Threatened Medicinal Plants. *Curr. Sci.,* **2018**, *114*(3), 554-561.
        [http://dx.doi.org/10.18520/cs/v114/i03/554-561]

[105]   Singh, H.B.; Bharati, K. Avinash. Enumeration of Dyes. In Handbook of Natural Dyes and Pigments; Elsevier **2014**, 33-260.

[106]   Zou, Y-P.; Tan, C.H.; Wang, B-D.; Zhu, D.Y.; Kim, S.K. Chemical Constituents from *Myrsine africana* L. *Helv. Chim. Acta,* **2008**, *91*(11), 2168-2173.
        [http://dx.doi.org/10.1002/hlca.200890234]

[107]   Kupchan, S.M.; Steyn, P.S.; Grove, M.D.; Horsfield, S.M.; Meitner, S.W. Tumor inhibitors. XXXV. Myrsine saponin, the active principle of *Myrsine africana*. *J. Med. Chem.,* **1969**, *12*(1), 167-169.
        [http://dx.doi.org/10.1021/jm00301a045] [PMID: 5763016]

[108]   Kabubii, Z.N.; Mbaria, J.; Mathiu, M. Acute toxicity studies of *Myrsine africana* aqueous seed extract in male Wistar rats on some hematological and biochemical parameters. *Clinical Phytoscience,* **2015**, *1*(1), 9.
        [http://dx.doi.org/10.1186/s40816-015-0010-3]

[109]   Fibrich, B.; Gao, X.; Puri, A.; Banga, A.K.; Lall, N. *In Vitro* Antioxidant, Anti-Inflammatory and Skin Permeation of *Myrsine africana* and Its Isolated Compound Myrsinoside B. *Front. Pharmacol.,* **2020**, *10*, 1410.
        [http://dx.doi.org/10.3389/fphar.2019.01410] [PMID: 31969815]

[110]   Azam, S.; Bashir, S.; Ahmad, B. Anti-spasmodic action of crude methanolic extract and a new compound isolated from the aerial parts of *Myrsine africana*. *BMC Complement. Altern. Med.,* **2011**, *11*(1), 55.
        [http://dx.doi.org/10.1186/1472-6882-11-55] [PMID: 21733176]

[111]   https://www.nmpb.nic.in/medicinal_list

[112]   Shanmugam, S.; Baby, J.P.; Chandran, R.; Thankarajan, S.; Thangaraj, P. *Maesa indica*: a nutritional wild berry rich in polyphenols with special attention to radical scavenging and inhibition of key enzymes, α-amylase and α-glucosidase. *J. Food Sci. Technol.,* **2016**, *53*(7), 2957-2965.
        [http://dx.doi.org/10.1007/s13197-016-2263-3] [PMID: 27765966]

[113] Maesa indica (Roxb.) A. DC. Species. India Biodiversity Portal. https://indiabiodiversity.org/species/show/32702

[114] Kuruvilla, G.R.; Neeraja, M.; Srikrishna, A.; Subba Rao, G.S.R.; Sudhakar, A.V.S.; Venkatasubramanian, P. A New Quinone from Maesa Indica (Roxb.) A. DC, (Myrsinaceae). *Indian J. Chem. - Sect. B Org. Med. Chem.,* **2010**, *49*(12), 1637-1641.

[115] Natarajan, B.; Paulsen, B.S. An ethnopharmacological study from thane district, maharashtra, India: traditional knowledge compared with modern biological science. *Pharm. Biol.,* **2000**, *38*(2), 139-151. [http://dx.doi.org/10.1076/1388-0209(200004)38:2;1-1;FT139] [PMID: 21214452]

CHAPTER 4

Synthetic and Natural Agents as Bacterial Biofilm Inhibitors

Ethiraj Kannatt Radhakrishnan[1,*] and **Anjitha Theres Benny**[1]

[1] *Department of Chemistry, School of Advanced Science, VIT, Vellore, Tamil Nadu-632014, India*

Abstract: A biofilm is a form of bacterial cluster normally seen in environmental niches. They are immobile communities that colonize and develop on medical implants like sutures, catheters and dental implants, which can be treated only by their removal, leading to unaffordable treatment. The main biofilm consequence is its increased tolerance to negative environmental conditions, which includes resistance to antibiotics and antimicrobial agents. The high resistance of bacterial biofilm towards external stress and antibiotics is due to the extracellular polymeric matrix, which provides a barrier from the external environment. The biofilm development is facilitated by the cell-to-cell communication mechanism of bacteria called quorum sensing, which promotes the bacterial community to mature. There is a huge number of naturally occurring chemical compounds that can act as antibiofilm agents. Different chemical compounds resist bacterial biofilm growth by different mechanisms depending on the chemical structure of the molecule, and the stage of biofilm formation at which we introduce the chemical compound into the biofilm system. The anti-biofilm activity of a natural or synthetic compound mainly depends on certain aspects; some of them will deal with the inhibition of the formation of the polymer matrix, some others may suppress the cell adhesion and its attachment to itself or an external surface, while others deal with the interruption of extracellular polymeric matrix generation and lessening virulence factors production, thereby hindering QS network and biofilm development.

Keywords: Antagonistic, Antibiofilm, Antimicrobial, Autoinducers, Efflux Pump, Extracellular Polymeric Natrix, Multidrug-resistant, N-acyl Homoserine Lactones, Persisters, Photodynamic Therapy, Magnetic Nanoparticles, Violacein, Virulence Factor, Quorum Sensing, Quorum Quenching.

INTRODUCTION

Today microbial control is an ever-increasing economic concern disturbing human beings and animals. There are many phases for this crisis, making it difficult to overcome; the existence of various antimicrobial resistance and

[*] **Corresponding author Ethiraj Kannatt Radhakrishnan:** Department of Chemistry, School of Advanced Science, VIT, Vellore, Tamil Nadu-632014, India; Email: ethukr@gmail.com

Shazia Anjum (Ed.)

altering regulations in the bacterial body due to the increased awareness of the bacteria to its surroundings may make the antibiotics inefficient. Antimicrobial resistance occurs naturally in a microorganism and is a dynamic threat due to its capability to evolve and express resistant genes, finally leading to the selection of resistant microbial clones. This fact pointed to the requirement for new, potent antimicrobials, which can overcome the negatives of the existing ones [1]. Recent literature review shows advancements in the field of developing potent antimicrobial compounds. Jaspreet S. Dhau *et al.*, studied the anti-bacterial efficiency of various pyridylselenium compounds like bis[3-(4-chloro-N,N-diethylpyridine-2-carboxamide)] diselenide and bis(3-bromo-2-pyridyl) diselenide against different bacterial strains, including *Bacillus pumilus* (MTCC-1607), *Escherichia coli* (MTCC-1687), *Bacillus subtilis* (MTCC-441), *Staphylococcus aureus* (MTCC-737) and *Pseudomonas oleovorans* (MTCC-617) [2 - 4] .

Biofilm formation is a significant field to study once dealing with antimicrobials and antimicrobial resistance of bacterial biofilm. Biofilms are aggregates of multicellular organisms found associated with abiotic or biotic surfaces where bacteria are found embedded in extracellular polymeric matrix [5]. They express higher resistance to antibiotics than planktonic ones due to the poor penetration of drugs into the biofilm [6]. The major reason for the increased resistance of biofilm is the presence of an extracellular polymeric matrix [7].

The extracellular matrix, composed of polysaccharides, proteins, lipids, and DNA, slows or nullifies the diffusion of antibiotics into the biofilm. The resistance of biofilm thus leads to its propagation and further development [8]. Along with the inhibition of antibiotic entry into the cells, bacteria can also resist antibiotic drugs by some other mechanisms. Any kind of variations in the microenvironment of biofilm-like, change in temperature, low availability of water, and change in availability of nutrients, oxidative stress, and starvation may activate some adaptive stress responses inherent in bacteria. This response will then further lead to the alteration of the bacterial cell by which it enters into the spore-like persister state, where they are extremely safe. The presence of persisters inside the biofilm is the reason for the high antibiotic resistance [9]. Another mechanism by which bacterial biofilm resists antibiotics is the method known as efflux pumping. The efflux system allows the expelling of antibiotics, biocides, metabolic products, organic solvents, and dyes out of the biofilm system to enhance biofilm development. Hence, in order to overcome its activity, promising modifications are required in developing new antibiotics [10].

In nature, microorganisms rarely live in plantonic form, but rather they prefer communal growth or aggregates. Bacteria achieve the self-immobilisation in aquatic or soil systems by the cell surface hydrophobicity of the organism.

Bacterial cell surface hydrophobicity promotes bacterial colonisation and hence biofilm formation [11]. The studies done by various researchers found that there is a positive correlation between cell surface hydrophobicity and virulence factors and biofilm formation [12]. Hence, drugs that are capable of reducing the thickness and cell surface hydrophobicity of the bacteria can lead to a reduction in biofilm formation.

All the known mechanisms of bacterial resistance to antibiotics make the chemists aware of developing more potent antibiotics which can overcome all the possible resistance mechanisms. The chapter deals with a few methods by which biofilm inhibition can be achieved by making use of various synthetic and natural compounds. The methods include quorum quenching, extracellular polymeric matrix formation, inhibition of biofilm formation, and efflux pump inhibition.

QUORUM QUENCHERS

Due to the overuse of antibiotics, bacteria become multidrug-resistant, and it is an immediate necessity to find an alternative method for antimicrobial therapies. The most promising strategy for that is to target the main physiological property in the biofilm, and it is quorum sensing (QS). QS is the mechanism by which bacteria communicate with each other. The mechanism is based on the constant flow of signalling molecules called autoinducers (AI) [13]. In the case of gram-negative bacteria, N-acyl homoserine lactones (AHLs) play the role of AI, and in gram positive bacteria, it is AIPs. [14].

Quorum quenching (QQ) that can disrupt the communication of bacteria can act as a driving force for the lessening or even complete inhibition of virulence factors and biofilm formation. The quorum quenching approaches include the use of structural analogues of auto-inductors which are QS receptors. The structural analogues of these can be synthesized in laboratories or can be isolated from natural sources. There are a vast number of naturally occurring compounds that can hinder the communication of microbes [15, 16]. There are different methods by which QS can be inhibited, and the mechanisms involved in quorum sensing inhibition are listed below.

- Inhibiting the synthesis of signal molecules by blocking Lux operon proteins [17].
- Enzymatic degradation [18] or inactivation of signal molecules by changing the pH to alkaline [19] or by changing temperature [19] and thereby leading to lactonolysis [20].
- The enzymatic degradation of AHL is the best method of QQ. The enzymatic degradation can be catalysed by enzymes like lactonases, acylases, reductases,

and oxidases. By competing with the signal molecules and receptor analogs [21].
• By hindering the signal transduction cascades [22].

The mechanism of blocking quorum sensing is represented in Fig. (**1**). The quorum quenching will inhibit the production of virulence factors and hence the biofilm formation. In Gram-negative bacteria, the AHLs synthesised by the LuxI enzyme play the role of autoinducers. They penetrate the cell membrane of bacteria, and once it reaches the threshold concentration, LuxR receptor protein gets activated, and the transcription of target effector genes occurs. In the case of Gram-positive bacteria, AIPs are synthesised in the form of propeptides, and they will export outside the cell through the ABC-ATP binding cassette transport system. After reaching the threshold concentration in the environment, the autoinducer molecules are bound by sensor proteins with kinase activity. Kinase is activated by phosphorylation. The phosphate group is transferred to the transcription regulator, which results in the activation of the transcription of the target genes.

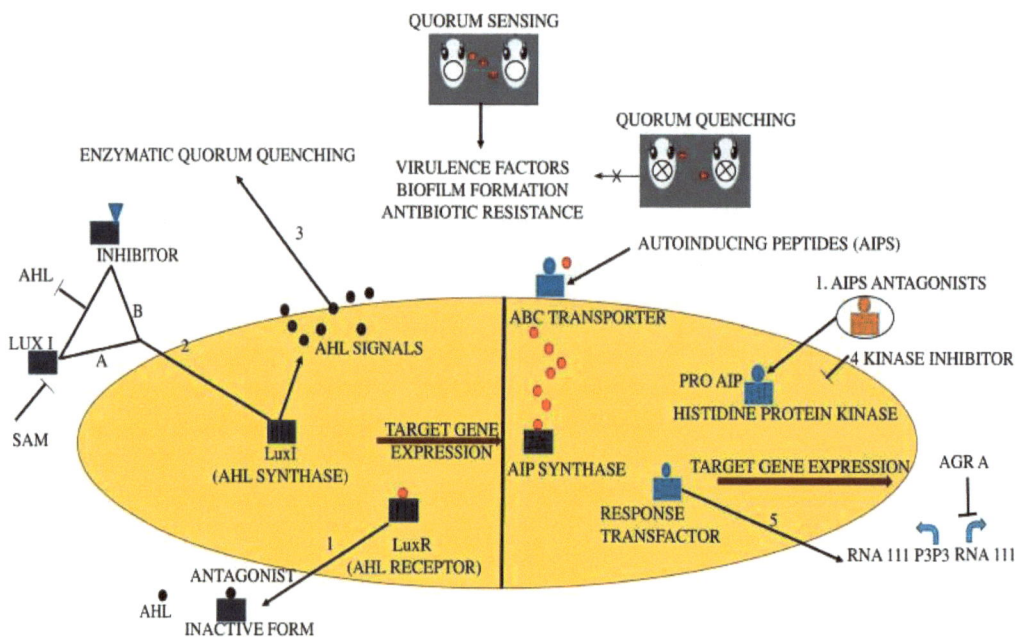

Fig. (1). Mechanisms involved in quorum quenching.

Mechanisms involved are numbered accordingly; 1-Antagonist inductor application; 2-Inhibition of the synthesis of AHL molecule; 3-AHL degradation by enzymatic methods including hydrolysis of HSL ring by lactonase, hydrolysis of an amide bond by acylase, and reduction of carbonyl or hydroxyl groups by oxidoreductase, 4- Stopage of histidine protein kinase activation by kinase inhibitor, blockage of signal transduction cascade.

Natural Products as Quorum Quenchers

Natural quorum sensing inhibitors are compounds that are extracted from natural sources like plant parts, antibodies, or enzymes. The phytochemicals and other active quorum quenchers isolated from natural products are gaining much importance as they are assumed to be nontoxic and have minimum side effects [23].

From Plant Source

Plants have been an important source of drugs to fight against various diseases since ancient times. Plant-derived medicinal products are gaining much more attention due to their potential efficiency and minimal side effects. There are numerous examples of phytochemicals that are biologically important [24]. Considering the importance of antibiofilm and quorum quenching, the compounds that have quorum quenching activities isolated from plants are Centella Asiatica and naringin, which are active against *Chromobacterium violaceum bacteria* [25] [26]. Similarly, 1, 5- dihydropyrrol-2-ones, citric acid, and fructose furoic acid ester are a few compounds that can inhibit quorum sensing in *E. coli* bacteria [27, 28]. Phytochemical compounds like coumarin, curcumin, garlic baicalin, ginseng, berberine, salicylic acid, trans cinnamaldehyde, hordenine, phillyirin, musa paradisiaca, *etc.* are effective quorum quenchers against *P. aeruginosa* [29]-[31]. *Piper nigrum* peppercorns extract were found to be quorum quenchers due to the presence of active compounds, namely piperine and trichostachine [32]. Catechins isolated from the bark of *combretum albiflorum,* which belongs to the flavonoid family found to reduce the quorum sensing expressing genes, *lasI, lasR, rhlR, rhlI,* in bacteria like *P. aeruginosa* [33]. *Achyranthes aspera* extracts with excellent pharmaceutical applications, including anti-cancer, anti-malarial and anti-peroxidative, were used as a natural brush in the southern part of India in cleaning the tooth. The stem or root parts or the burned ashes were used by them as natural brushes. Later, the *in-vitro* and *in-silico* studies done on the plant extract showed the antiquorum quenching activity of the compound against cariogenic *Streptococcus mutans* [34]. The dietary spice *Cinnamomum verum* extracted was found to have a good antibiofilm activity against *Serratia marcescenes* and *P. aeruginosa* by quorum quenching activity by reducing the swarming nature of the organism which is a good virulent factor regulated by quorum sensing [35].

Truchado, P *et al.* studied the use of phytochemicals as quorum quenchers by studying the concentration of biosensor *violacein* a response of the QS system in *Chromobacterium violaceum*. The studies revealed that compounds like cinnamaldehyde, resveratrol, pomegranate extracts, ellagic acid, and rutin can inhibit the quorum sensing by reducing the production of violacein [36]. *Syzygium aromaticum* has a potential effect on the quorum quenching activity on the violacein pigment inhibition on *C. Violaceum* and biofilm formation inhibition on clinical isolates of *P. aeruginosa* [37].

The antibiofilm and antivirulence activity screening of *Brassica oleracea var. capitata* (cabbage) and *Brassica rapa subsp. rap* a (Turnip) extracts against *P. aeruginosa* and *E. coli* clinical isolates suggest that they have a potential effect in the reduction of virulence factors, including pyocyanin and rhamnolipid production. The *in silico* studies revealed the ability of sulforaphane and iberin present in the extract to bind with the LasR regulator, which is responsible for quorum sensing in *P. aeruginosa* [38]. The antivirulence properties of *Hibiscus sabdariffa* L. (*Hs*) calyxes and two γ-lactones (hibiscus acid [HA] and its methyl ester) in *Pseudomonas aeruginosa* were analysed by Humberto Cortes-López *et al.* 2021 and found that HA is the first molecule recognised with antivirulence properties in *Hs* with the potential to prevent infections caused by *P. aeruginosa* [39]. Ahmad Fiqri Mustaqim Othman *et al.* in 2019 studied the quorum quenching activity of crude extract of *Curcuma xanthorrhiza Roxb* extract against *P. aeruginosa* ATCC35554. The studies indicate that the extract has the capability to decrease the virulence factors like pyocyanin production, swarming motility, and biofilm formation [40]. K. Marathe *et al.* in 2018 studied the antibiofilm activity of *Euphorbia trigona* extract against *Serratia marcescens* and *Proteus mirabilis*. The major part of the bioactive fraction of the extract was identified as 9,12-Octadecadienoyl chloride (Z, Z), a derivative of linoleic acid. It was then used by them for the antibiofilm activity screening. The compound decreases the prodigiosin production, swarming motility and biofilm formation in *S. marcescens*. It was also found effective in reducing urease synthesis, swarming motility, and biofilm formation in *P. mirabilis* [41]. *Eugenia uniflora* fruit is another plant part which is highly efficient against quorum sensing in *Chromobacterium violaceum*. The phenolic extract of *Eugenia uniflora* inhibited up to 96% of violacein production in *C. violaceum*, at low subinhibitory concentrations, likely due to the fruit's phenolic content [42]. Similarly, the phenolic extract of *Eugenia brasiliensis* (grumixama) also showed quorum quenching activity against *Chromobacterium violaceum* [43]. Phytochemical compounds inhibiting quorum sensing in different bacterial species are explained in the following Table **1**.

Table 1. Phytochemical compounds inhibiting quorum sensing in different bacterial species.

Phytochemical Compound	Inhibition Against	Reference
Melicopelunu-ankenda	*Escherichia coli*	[44]
Syzygium araomaticum	*Escherichia coli*	[44]
Vanila plaifolia	*Chromobacterium violaceum*	[44]
Prunus armeniaca	*Chromobacterium violaceum*	[44]
Chamaesyce hypericifolia	*Chromobacterium violaceum*	[44]
Lonicera alpigena	*Staphylococcus aureus*	[44]
Capparis spinosa	*Chromobacterium violaceum*	[44]
Moringa oleifera	*Chromobacterium violaceum*	[44]
Quercus virginiana	*Chromobacterium violaceum*	[44]
Peoonidin-3-O-galactoside	*Escherichia coli*	[45]
Coumarin derivatives	*Escherichia coli*	[46]
Sesquiterpenes	*Staphylococcus aureus*	[47]
Kaempferol, quercetin, catechin, tanninscatechin, epigallocatechin	*Staphylococcus aureus, Escherichia coli, Chromobacterium violaceum*	[48]

From Bacterial By-Products

Quorum quenching can be achieved by compounds that are obtained from prokaryotic by-products or secondary metabolites of bacteria to block their signalling molecule from reaching the receptor protein. The antagonistic action of secondary metabolites of different bacterial species acts as quorum quenchers by competing with signal molecules to bind with the receptor. Certain examples of compounds isolated from bacterial metabolites and the mechanism of action of those compounds on certain bacteria are given below Table **2**.

Synthetic Compounds as Quorum Quenchers

To compensate for all the disadvantages of naturally occurring chemical compounds, modern researchers put forward the use of synthetic molecules that are specific in their actions. By using chemical methods for quenching, one can reduce the bacterial population, which is ineffective to adapt or establish in the host cell [58]. An important virulence factor for QS which is produced by *C. violaceum* can be inhibited by derivatives of cinnamic acid like cinnamyl alchohol, and methyl cinnamate [59]. QS in *P. aeruginosa* has reported its reduction by Norspirmidine by reduction in the expression of LasI, LasR, RhLI, RhIR, MvfR genes by reducing the attachment of bacteria to the surface. Naringenin, a colourless flavourless flavanone down-regulates the expression of LasI and RhlI genes, thereby inhibiting the LuxR transcription factors leading to the decreased production of AHL. 4-Nitro-pyridine-N-oxide (4-NPO), is another chemical compound that can act as a quorum quencher by down-regulating the genes involved in virulence factor (*lasA, lasB, chiC,* and *rhlAB*) of *P. aeruginosa* [60].

Table 2. List of compounds isolated from bacterial metabolites and the mechanism of action of those compounds on certain bacteria.

Entry No	Bacterial By-Product	Name of Bacteria	Mechanism of Action and Affecting Bacteria	Reference
1	Isobutyramide and 3-methyl-N-(2-phenylethl)-butyramide	*Halobacillus salinus*	Target the Lux system of *Vibrio harveyi*	[49]
2	Phenethylamides and a cyclic dipeptide	*Bacillus cereus*	Inhibit AHL-mediated quorum sensing in *Chromobacterium violaceum*	[50]
3	Cyclic dipeptides	*Lactobacillus reuteri*	Toxin production in *Staphylococcus*	[51]
4	Yayurea A and B	*Staphylococcus delphini*	Inhibit quorum sensing mediated mechanisms such as pigment production, bio luminance and biofilm formation	[52]
5	Cis-9-octadecenoic acid	*Stenotrophomonas maltophilia*	Inhibit CviR gene	[53]
6	Tumonic acids (E, F, G and G).	*Blennothrix cantharidosmum*	Regulate bioluminescence in *Vibrio harveyi*	[54]
7	Lyngbic acid, lyngbyoic acid, Malyngolide, Pitinoic acid and peptides as microcolins	*Lyngbya majuscula*	Quorum sensing antagonistic action	[55, 56]
8	Honaucins	*Leptolyngbya crosbyana*	Inhibit quorum sensing mediated bacterial communication.	[57]

Another method by which quorum sensing can be inhibited is by synthesizing compounds that can antagonize AHL protein. As an example, compounds like metabromo-thiolactone (mBTL) can antagonize AHL in *P. aeruginosa* [61]. 2,5-Piperazinedione [62], 3-Nitro phenylacetanoyl HL (C14) [63], 4-I N-phenylacetyl-L-homoserine lactones (PHL) [64], Chloro-pyridine pharmacophore [65] and N-Decanoyl cyclopentylamid [66] are some of the synthetic compounds that can do QQ by inhibition of LasR gene. Some synthetic compounds are unrelated to AHLs in their structure but can inhibit QS by antagonistic activity, which includes thiazolidinedione type molecules with strong biofilm inhibition properties (z)-5-octylidenethiazolidine-2, 4-dione (TZD-C8 [67]. Another synthetic AHL analogues (SAHLAs) that show efficiency in quorum quenching is water-soluble macrocycles, such as cyclodextrins (CDs). They have good quorum quenching property against *P. aeruginosa* [68]. Similarly, M Molnar *et al.* in 2021 studied the quorum quenching effect of α-cyclodextrin by studying the bioluminescence response in *Aliivibrio fischeri,* which produces light based on quorum sensing. It was found that α-cyclodextrin in 10 mM at 120 min contact time caused ~64% inhibition of bioluminescence in *Aliivibrio fischeri,* which was an indication of the reduction in quorum sensing in the bacteria [69]. Derivatives of fusaric acid are also found to be active against QS in gram-negative bacteria *P. aeruginosa* [70]. The comp- ounds, namely (Z)-Ethyl 2-(1-(4-methylbenzyl)- 4-((4- methylbenzyl) amino)-5- oxopyrrolidin-2-ylidene) acetate, (Z)-Ethyl 2-(5-oxo-1-(thiophen-2-ylmethyl)-4-((thiophen-2-ylmethyl)amino)pyrrolidin-2- ylid ene) acetate, (Z)-Ethyl 2-(1-benzyl-4-(benzylamino)-5-oxopyrrolidin-2-ylidene) acetate, (Z)-Ethyl 2-(1- (furan-2-ylmethyl)-4-((furan-2- ylmethyl)amino)-5-oxopyrrolidin-2-yli dene) acetate, which are having structural similarity with HSL showed a notable ability to interfere with the green fluorescent protein fluorescence induced in the *E.coli* by 3OC6HSL [71]. Isoxazolone derivatives showed very good quorum quenching activity and also very good antibiofilm activity against both gram-negative and gram-positive bacterial human pathogens through the quorum quenching mechanism [72]. R Sathyanarayana *et al.* in 2020 studied the quorum quenching property of 1-phenyl-1*H*-2-(1-aryl-5-methyl-1*H*-1,2,3-triazol-4-yl)- 3-(*N*-aryl-carbamoylmethy- lthio)-1,2,4-triazoles against *Chromobacterium viol aceum* and *Xanthomonas campestris* pv. *Campestris* (*Xcc*). Among a set of compounds synthesised by them, compounds with an electron-withdrawing group on the *N*-phenylacetamide portion exhibited good activity with more than 80% inhibition of violacein [73].

Enzymatic Quorum Quenching

Enzymatic quorum quenching is the process by which certain enzymes degrade autoinducers which eventually stops bacterial communication and, thereby, QS and bacterial biofilm formation (Fig. **2**).

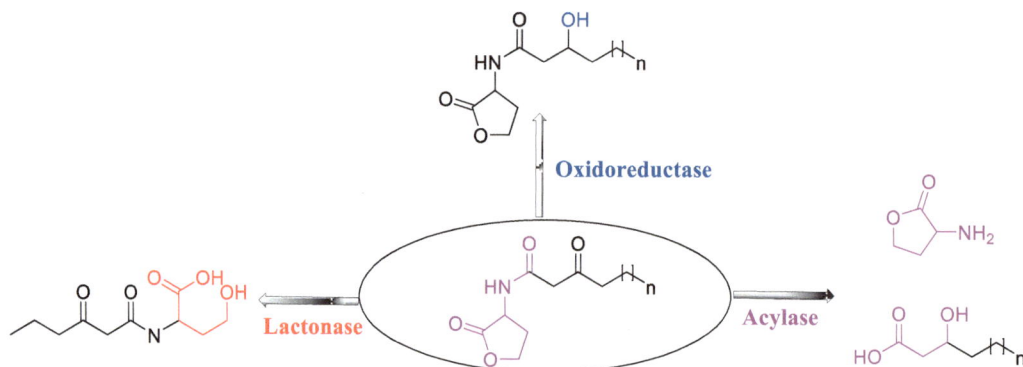

Fig. (2). Enzymatic activity of quorum quenching [58].

The hypothesis of QQ was taken into consideration from the microorganisms coexisting with QS and QQ activities [74]. The different chemical reactions taking place behind QQ bacteria are decarboxylation, deamination, deacylation, lactonolysis. Enzymes found degrading AI is characterized under the categories including lactonase enzymes, acylase enzymes, and oxidoreductase enzymes [21].

Lactonase Enzymes

Lactonase enzyme also called acyl-homoserine lactonase, is a metalloenzyme that is produced by certain bacterial species. As the name indicates, they are enzymes that can lactonase or inactivate the acyl-homoserine lactone ring [75]. Lactonase has the ability to hydrolyze the ester bond of the lactone ring of acyl-homoserine lactones and thereby prevents the signal molecule from reaching and binding to the transcriptional regulators or the receptor site.

The first enzyme recognized as a QQ lactonase is AiiA *isolated* from *Bacillus sp.* strain 240B1 [76, 77]. Other known lactonase enzymes include AhlS isolated from *Solibacillus silvestris* StLB046 [78], AhlD isolated from *Arthrobacter sp.* IBN110 [79], AttM (AiiB) from *Agrobacterium tumefaciens* [31], QsdR1 isolated from *Rhizobium sp.* NGR234 [80], AhlK from *Klebsiella pneumonia* KCTC2241 [79] are a few among them.

Acylase Enzymes

Acylase enzymes or N-Acyl homoserine lactone acylase (AHL acylase) is another enzyme responsible for disrupting quorum sensing in bacteria by hydrolysis of acylhomoserine lactone. The enzyme *Variovorax paradoxus* was identified as potent enough to use AHL as a source of nitrogen and energy. HSL produced by the degradation of AHL acts as a source of nitrogen, and the corresponding fatty acid by-product as the source of energy. AhlM isolated from *Streptomyces sp.* M664 [81], AiiD isolated from *Ralstonia sp.* XJ12B [82], Aac isolated from *Ralstonia solanacearum* GMI1000 [83], HacB (PA0305) from *P. aeruginosa* PAO1 [84], AiiO from *Ochrobactrum* sp. A44 [85] are a few examples of acylase enzymes.

Oxidoreductase Enzymes

Oxidoreductase enzymes target the acyl side chain by an oxidative or reductive activity. The oxidation or reduction that takes place on the acyl chain catalyses a modification in the chemical structure of the signal molecule without degrading it. The modification generated on the signal molecule thus affects the specificity of the signal molecule leading to the disturbance in the activation of QS mediated genes and hence hinderers the quorum sensing [86]. CYP102A1 (P450BM-3) isolated from *Bacillus megaterium* [86], n.i isolated from *Rhodococcus erythropolis* W2 [86], and BpiB09 from Soil metagenome [86] are few among many of the oxidoreductase known today.

Nanoparticles as Quorum Quenchers

Nanoparticles are also found to be good candidates in QQ [87]. Mycofabricated silver nanoparticles with QS-regulated virulence factors and selenium nanoparticles (Se-NPs) with honey phytochemicals are some of the nanosized quorum quenchers active against P. aeruginosa biofilm [88]. Gold nanoparticles also show a remarkable effect on quorum quenching [89]. Gold nanoparticles coated with acyl-homoserine lactone lactonase like AiiA, (AuNPs) were tested against proteus species [90]. The proteins coated on the nanoparticles break the lactone bond of acyl-homoserine lactone and thereby inhibit quorum sensing [91].

García-Lara B *et al.* 2015 studied the effects of ZnO nanoparticles against six clinical strains from cystic fibrosis patients. ZnO nanoparticles were found effective in reducing pyocyanin, elastase, and biofilm formation for most of the strains. The data indicate the efficiency of ZnO nanoparticles against *P. aeruginosa* recalcitrant infections [92]. Similarly, silicon dioxide nanoparticles (Si-NP) were used to target acylhomoserine lactones (HSLs) to halt bacterial communication. When Si-NP were surface functionalized with β-cyclodextrin (β-

CD) and introduced into the bacterial culture of *Vibrio fischeri* whose luminous output depends upon HSL-mediated QS, there was a dramatic reduction in bacterial communication. Reductions in luminescence were recognised through quantitative polymerase chain reaction (qPCR) analyses of luminescence genes. The results showed that with high concentrations of engineered NPs in association with quorum-quenching compounds, the chemical signals were removed from the nearby bacterial environment and thereby effectively silencing and isolating the cells [93].

EXTRACELLULAR POLYMERIC MATRIX DEGRADATION

Biofilm is a system in which microbes form a cluster by adhering to each other and itself attaching to a suitable surface [94]. The main strength of biofilm against almost all known antibiotics is its potency to show resistance to antibiotic agents, and it is due to the presence of the slimy extracellular polymeric matrix, which protects the microbes. The self-produced extracellular polymeric matrix is composed of polysaccharides, enzymes, proteins, e DNA, lipids and bio surfactants (Fig. **3**) [95].

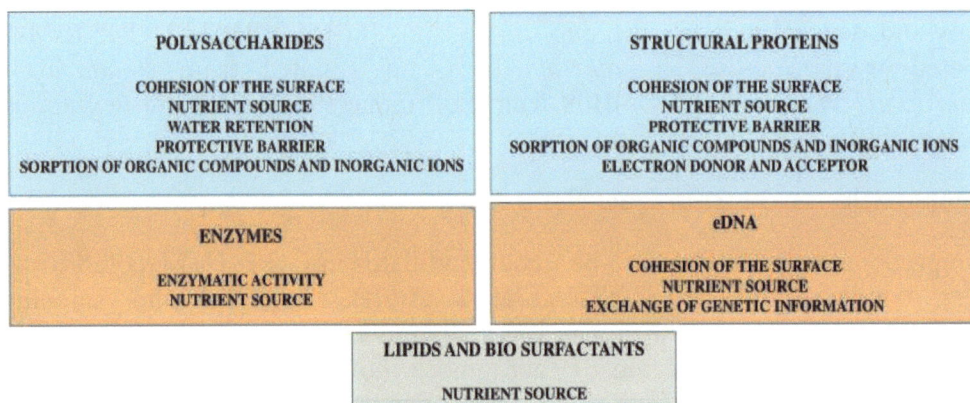

POLYSACCHARIDES

COHESION OF THE SURFACE
NUTRIENT SOURCE
WATER RETENTION
PROTECTIVE BARRIER
SORPTION OF ORGANIC COMPOUNDS AND INORGANIC IONS

STRUCTURAL PROTEINS

COHESION OF THE SURFACE
NUTRIENT SOURCE
PROTECTIVE BARRIER
SORPTION OF ORGANIC COMPOUNDS AND INORGANIC IONS
ELECTRON DONOR AND ACCEPTOR

ENZYMES

ENZYMATIC ACTIVITY
NUTRIENT SOURCE

eDNA

COHESION OF THE SURFACE
NUTRIENT SOURCE
EXCHANGE OF GENETIC INFORMATION

LIPIDS AND BIO SURFACTANTS

NUTRIENT SOURCE

Fig. (3). Extracellular polymeric matrix of biofilm.

Each constituent of the EPS matrix has its own role in biofilm maturation and growth. The cells within the matrix have the ability to mutate and survive in almost all severe environmental conditions. The matrix provides benefits including antibiotic resistance, physical barrier and protection from external stress, storage of nutrients, tolerance from desiccation, organisation of virulence factors through the processes of quorum sensing [96, 97].

The complex nature of the extracellular matrix acts as a barrier for the antimicrobial agents, as it can limit the antimicrobial from penetrating into the biofilm system [98, 99]. The antibiotics that enter the matrix interact with the components of the EPS, and the enzymes present in the matrix may degrade the antibiotics and some may form complex owing to the chelation, and this will reduce the antibiotic efficiency of the drug [100]. There are many more physical barriers in the biofilm microenvironment that prevents the antibiotics from reaching the bacteria in its full efficiency and making the bacteria multi-drug resistant [100]. In addition, the bacteria growing in the biofilm environment behaves differently than the planktonic ones [8]. The bacteria in the deeper areas of the biofilm are in an inactive state owed to decreased access to nutrients and other growth factors [100]. These bacteria have reduced susceptibility to antibiotics as they are metabolically less active [101]. Due to the complexity of composition and structure, EPS has a major role in biofilm formation, development, and resistance against antibiotics. So in order to make biofilm susceptible to antibiotics, it is important to degrade the matrix. There are different methods by which EPS degradation can be done. The different strategies include usage of enzymes, nano carries, synthetic and natural compounds, magnetic nano particles, photodynamic therapy are few of them (Fig. **4**) [102].

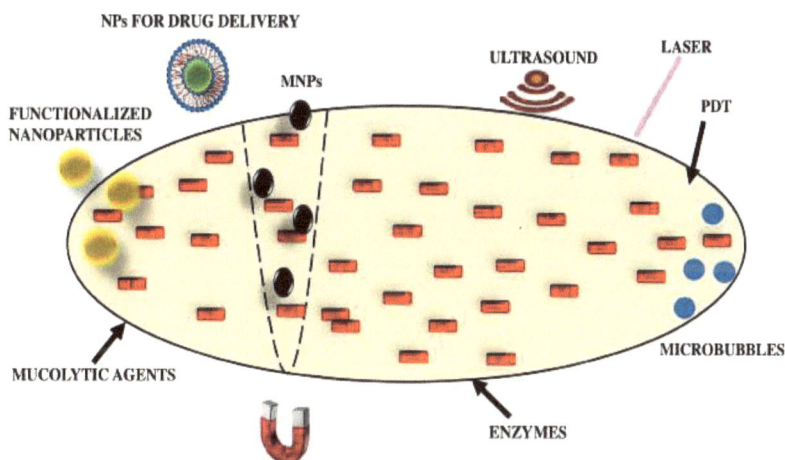

Fig. (4). Therapeutic procedures to interrupt the biofilm matrix include Functionalisd nanoparticles, NPs-nanoparticles, MNPs- magnetic nanoparticles, PDT- photodynamic therapy, Ultrasound, laser.

Enzymatic Degradation of Extracellular Polymeric Matrix

Enzymes have -increasing demand ever in medicinal chemistry as they can reduce the usage of harmful chemicals with high efficacy leading to sustainable chemistry. The enzymes such as protease, glycosidase, and DNase have potential antibiofilm activity by degrading the polymeric matrix and thereby releasing the planktonic cells [103]. The major constituent of biofilm is protein, and thus, protease enzymes are good candidates as antibiofilm agents. Proteases are well known for their ability to degrade adhesin, the membrane protein, and some other proteins which are constituents of extracellular matrix. These proteins are major ones responsible for the initial attachment of cells to each other and to solid surfaces [104]. Similarly, deoxyribonucleases or DNAse are enzymes that are capable of degrading or cleaving DNA of biofilm, making the bacteria susceptible to antibiotics [105].

Chandra Mishra *et al.* 2019 reported the antibiofilm efficiency of metalloprotease M16 isolated from *Microbacterium sp* SKS10 as a good protease enzyme. They reported that the optimum activity was shown by them at pH 12 at 60 °C, and they were more efficient than already reported enzymes like trypsin, amylase and papain. The presence of peptidase M16 improved the availability of antibiotics inside the biofilm and was reported to be noncytotoxic to epidermoid carcinoma cells (A431) [106]. Mammalian protease is another effective protease enzyme for the degradation of bacterial proteins and inhibition of bacterial growth. Human matrix metalloprotease 1 is one such mammalian protease active against *Enterococcus faecalis* biofilms by disruption of the extracellular polymeric matrix. It is a type 1 collagen that significantly inhibits *Enterococcus faecalis* biofilms, which are vancomycin-resistant [107].

Extracellular matrix degradation is a well-known and practically used method for the eradication of biofilm. However, solely targeting the matrix degradation cannot completely clear out the biofilm from the surface, whereas it triggers the release of planktonic bacteria and thereby continues the biofilm formation cycle. It is more efficient to use matrix-degrading enzymes together with antimicrobial agents by a dual targeting approach of biofilm degradation. By the advent of this dual targeting approach, one can bring the planktonic bacteria out by matrix degrading enzymes and efficiently kill the bacteria which are more exposed to antibiotics. Chen H *et al.* in 2019 reported the investigation of combining glucanohydrolase with clinically available essential oils with antimicrobial activity on cariogenic bacteria like *Streptococcus mutans*. They also showed that mutanase and dextranase synergistically breakdown the extracellular matrix and enhance bacterial killing by antimicrobial agents. They also suggest that this EPS-degrading/antimicrobial approach (EDA) effectively eliminates mixed biofilms at high risk for eradication by normal antibiofilm drugs [108].

Lungs of patients with cystic fibrosis (CF) often get infected or undergo the relapse of bacterial infection due to the formation of antibiotic-resistant biofilm of *Pseudomonas aeruginosa*. Alginate lyases are one of the best therapeutic agents for the destruction of the extracellular polymeric matrix of *Pseudomonas aeruginosa.* Hamzah H *et al.* in 2020 reported that alginate lyase enzymes (AlyP1400) of marine origin have effective antibiofilm activity against *P. aeruginosa* clinical isolate CF27. AlyP1400, in combination with clinically available antibiotics, was found to be good candidate against *P. aeruginosa* infections in CF [109].

Dental caries is one of the most prevalent infections caused by bacterial biofilms. Oral streptococci are the main group of bacteria that form early colonisation on dental surfaces. Among the streptococci, *S. mutans* is one of the major constituents. The rnc gene (SMU-1514)- ribonucleas III(RNase III), in S.mutans, is deleted, and thus, the biofilm formation is disrupted and reduces cariogenicity by making the biofilm susceptible to antimicrobial drugs. Yuxing Song YJ *et al.* in 2019 reported the synergetic effect of rnc gene deleted S. mutans with anti-bacterial aminohexadecylmethacrylate (DMAHDM) on the antibiofilm effect and protection of teeth from dental caries [110].

Lim ES *et al.* 2020 reported the antibiofilm activity of naturally available curcumin from turmeric extract. Curcumin 1% can inhibit or degrade the extracellular polymeric matrix in a catheter in 60%, and it is proved to be better than the drug nystatin and almost equivalent to the control drug chloramphenicol [111].

Papain is a proteolitic enzyme isolated from *Carica papaya* with various applications in food industries. Fulaz S *et al.* 2019 reported that the papain is an antibiofilm agent with high efficiency in breaking the extracellular matrix even if it is not an anti-bacterial agent, its efficiency in the degradation of extracellular matrix makes it a good candidate as an antibiofilm agent. They investigated the antibiofilm properties of papain against *S. aureus*, *C. jejuni* using crystal violet staining, SEM analysis and direct counting methods [112]. Patel KK *et al.,* in 2019, worked on the synergetic activity of biofilm-degrading enzymes with sodium hypochlorite. The study revealed that the combination of DNase, protease, and cellulose with sodium hypochlorite efficiently controls the biofilm of *E. coli* O157:H7 biofilms [113].

Nano Carriers in Extracellular Polymeric Matrix Degradation

Nano technology plays a dynamic part in the targeting and disruption of the extracellular polymeric matrix. The main attraction of nanoparticles as drug carriers is their ability to penetrate into the biofilm matrix and release antibiotics into the biofilm system [114]. The nanoparticles are more likely to interact with the polymeric matrix by an electrostatic force of attraction. The biofilm matrix is composed of negatively charged particles hence nanoparticles with positive charge within it can easily interact with the bacterial cell wall. The surface-attached positively charged nanoparticles will further enter the biofilm system with different mechanisms by which they are engineered.

There are different examples of nanoparticles used in the matrix disruption of biofilm. The enzyme alginate lyases immobilised on polymeric nanoparticles with ciprofloxacin loaded on it is one such example. Hwang G *et al.* 2019 reported the complete disruption of *P. aeruginosa* biofilm with no sustainable bacteria after treating it for 72 h [115].

Weldrick PJ *et al.* in 2020 used chitosan nanoparticles supported with antimicrobial cellobiose dehydrogenase and DNase 1 for the treatment of *Candida aldicans* and *S. aureus*. The cellobiose dehydrogenase acts as the antimicrobial as it has the ability to produce hydrogen peroxidase, which can generate free radicals for the promotion of oxidation of the EPS matrix [116].

The iron oxide MNPs shows characteristic antibiofilm activity by the mechanism of generation of free radicals with EPS matrix degradation and bactericidal activity [117]. Protease-functionalised nanogel carriers are another mode of treating biofilm. In this method, Manoharan A *et al.* used protease enzyme alcalae 2.4 LFG coating on carbopol nanogel to digest the EPS matrix to reach the bacteria inside the matrix and deliver antibiotics directly to their cell walls. The effectiveness of the nanocarriers against *Staphylococcus aureus, Pseudomonas aeruginosa*, Staphylococcus epidermidis, Klebsiella pneumoniae, *Escherichia coli, and Enterococcus faecalis* was carried out. The studies were also carried out with co-administration of ciprofloxacin, and there was a characteristic decrease in the biomass than the normal ciprofloxacin administration [118].

ZnO nanoparticles synthesised using extracts of *Plectranthus amboinicus* Pam-ZnO NPs were evaluated for their antibiofilm efficiency against *Staphylococcus aureus* biofilms MRSA ATCC 33591. The Pam-ZnO NPs were able to disintegrate and recalcitrant biofilm architecture by penetrating into the exopolysaccharide formed by *Staphylococcus aureus* [119]. Rajagopalan Thaya *et al.*, in 2016, studied the a*ntibiofilm activity of* chitosan-coated Ag/ZnO (CS/Ag/ZnO) nanocomposite against *B. licheniformis, B. cereus, V. parahae-molyticus* and *P. vulgaris*. The exhibited antibiofilm activity was due to the reduction in hydrophobicity index and EPS (extracellular polysaccharide) production of both Gram-positive and Gram-negative bacteria after treatment with CS/Ag/ZnO nanocomposite [120]. Simillarly, gold nanoparticles synthesised using the essential oil of Nigella sativa (NsEO-AuNPs) show antibiofilm activity against *S. aureus* and *V. harveyi* due to the inhibition of exopolysaccharide synthesis, which limits biofilm formation [121].

Synthetic Compounds in Extracellular Polymeric Matrix Degradation

In contrast to the enzymatic action on biofilm degradation, fewer reports are available for the antibiofilm activity of synthetic compounds. Mucolytic agents, including ambroxol and N-acetyl cysteine (NAC), are good candidates for antibiofilm activity [102]. NAC acts as an antibiofilm agent against quinolone-resistant *Pseudomonas aeruginosa* (QRPA) and *methicillin-resistnt Staphylococcus aureus* (MRSA) in tympanostomy tube infections was identified by Abd El-Baky RM *et al.* in 2019 [122].

NAC also shows its bacteriostatic activity when tested in planktonic bacteria. NAC 30 mM, in combination with suitable antibiotics and enzymes, shows eradication of MRSA and MSSA biofilms more than the antibiofilm activity shown by NAC alone. The maximal disruption of biofilm was a result of the intrinsic acidity of NAC. NAC enhanced the antibiotic effect of amoxicillin/clavulanate in MRSA and MSSA by the synergetic effect of the combination drug. The same effects were observed when NAC was administered with teicoplanin or oxacillin [123].

INHIBITION OF BIOFILM FORMATION

Pathogenic microorganisms have gained resistance to antibiotics currently in use, including penicillins, aminoglycosides, fluoroquinolones, and cephalosporins, by various mechanisms. The emergence of multi-drug resistance in bacteria makes them resistant to antibiotics when subjected to antibiotics with the same dosage for a prolonged time. The bacteria, upon treatment with antibiotics, start mutating and gain resistance, making them a multi-drug resistant strain. In this scenario, it is urgent to discover new compounds with potential higher than existing ones [124].

Natural Products in Inhibition of Biofilm Formation

The ethanolic extract of *Artemisia princeps* can inhibit the cariogenic property of *Streptococcus mutans* at concentrations 0.4-3.2 mg/mL asreported by Yong-Ouk You *et al.* in 2019 [125]. The antibiofilm efficacy of baicalindue to the inhibition of efflux generation was studied by Caldeira M *et al.* in 2019 [126]. Akihiko Terada *et al.*, in 2019, developed a polymer-based zwitterionic sheet with acylase I immobilised on it to provide antibiofilm activity to *Agrobacterium tumefaciens*. The quorum quenching enzyme acylase I was immobilised on a polyethylene membrane sheet grafted by glycidyl methacrylate (GMA) using radiation-induced graft polymerisation. The hydrophobicity of GMA was increased by converting the epoxy group of GMA to dimethylamino-γ-butyric acid (DMGABA). The acylase-immobilised zwitterionic membrane sheet can inhibit *Agrobacterium tumefaciens* biofilm formation [124].

Synthetic Compounds in Inhibition of Biofilm Formation

Biofilm growth on dental implants is a serious issue to be studied. The research by Shruti Vidhawan Agarwalla *et al.* in 2021 introduced the method of using graphene coating on titanium dental implants to ensure the inhibition of biofilm formation. Though there were many surface coating methods to inhibit the biofilm formations on titanium, they found that the use of graphene was more effective against it. The mechanism of action of graphene is unknown, and its effectiveness is still being studied [127].

The effect of phenyl lactic acid (PLA) against *Enterococcus faecalis* biofilm formation was done by Daoying Wang *et al.* in 2019. The inhibition of biofilm formation in *Enterococcus faecalis* at PLA concentrations of 1.25 and 2.50 mg/mL was studied by crystal violet assay, biofilm biomass assay, scanning electron microscopy, and confocal laser scanning microscopy. The inhibition of biofilm formation was identified to be obtained by the inhibition of EPS production and cell motility [128].

Helal F Hetta *et al.* in 2019 reported the effect of ketoconazole on efflux pump inhibition and thereby, biofilm formation inhibition. Docking studies revealed the effect of ketoconazole on the diminishing of NorA expression for the efflux generation. Ketoconazole itself is an antifungal drug with no anti-bacterial activity but the synergetic effect of ketoconazole with ciprofloxacin, norfloxacin, levofloxacin, and ethidium bromide shows a dramatic change in the antibiofilm activity of the drug. It can accelerate the activity of fluoroquinolones against multi-drug resistant *S. aureus* by inhibiting the efflux pump, which is one of the major reasons for biofilm formation [119].

Nanocarriers in Inhibition of Biofilm Formation

Humberto H. Lara *et al.* in 2020 reported the antibiofilm activity of silver nanoparticles against *Candida auris* biofilm by biofilm formation inhibition mechanism with half maximal inhibitory concentration (IC_{50}) of 0.06 ppm [129]. Raghvendra A. Mahamuni *et al.*, in 2019, studied the inhibition of biofilm formation by ZnO nanoparticles. ZnO possesses bactericidal activity by inducing reactive oxygen species generation, Zn^{2+} release, easy internalisation in bacterial cells, and hydrogen peroxide accumulation. These activities of ZnO get enhanced once they transform to its nano composites, and the effect of nanoparticles of ZnO on inhibition of biofilm formation was studied by the group and suggests that it is an effective compound in inhibition of multi-drug resistant biofilm formation

[130]. *Momordica* charantia silver nano particles show antibiofilm activity against *E. faecalis* and *A. hydrophila*. The decreased biofilm activity of *Mc*-Ag NPs is decreasing their hydrophobicity index [131].

EFFLUX PUMP INHIBITORS

Efflux pumps are a type of proteins present in bacteria that can expel harmful substances like secondary metabolites, quorum sensing molecules, dyes, biocides, and antimicrobials from the bacterial cells making the bacteria multi-drug resistant. The major efflux systems comprise of ATP-binding cassette (ABC), Major facilitator superfamily (MFS), resistance-nodulation-division (RND multi-drug and toxic compound extrusion (MATE) family/superfamily small multiantibiotic resistance (SMR) and [132]. Efflux pumps play a vital role in the development of drug resistance in microorganisms by decreasing antibiotic concentration inside the cell [133].

Various studies conducted in the field of biofilm formation and development suggest the role of efflux pump in increasing the anti-bacterial resistance of bacteria. The deceleration of antibiotic resistance can be achieved by increasing the potential of Efflux Pump Inhibitors (EPI). For an efflux pump inhibitor to be clinically approved, it should show less toxicity to tissues and attain the required therapeutic activity. It can function in combination with antibiotics to achieve greater effectiveness than that of individual agents alone. The studies in the field show that the emergence of a potent efflux inhibitory drug is a herculean task, and a majority of the EPIs were discovered serendipitously [134].

Many EPIs potentiating the activity of antibiotics are known to date, among which few of them attain greater interest, and they are presented in Fig. (**5**). Even if there is extensive research going on in this field, only a few EPIs have reached the clinical trials due to the toxic effects even at the concentration required for their activity. Literature reviews suggest that the only EPI that has conducted clinical development is bis (pyrimidine) sulfonamide MP-601, 205 bis (pyrimidine) sulfonamide MP-601,205 in combination with ciprofloxacin in treatment of cystic fibrosis and ventilator associated pneumonia caused by *P. aeruginosa* [132].

Natural Products as Efflux Pump Inhibitors

The method of combining antibiotic drugs with efflux inhibitors is an efficient method for increasing the activity of antibiotic drugs. Various natural products are used in this method. Maria *et al.* in 2019 combined Norfloxacin with isolated or extracted products from *Arrabidaea brachypoda* to study antibiotic effect against *Staphylococcus aureus*, *Escherchia coli* and *Candida albicans*. BR-B isolated from dichloromethane extract of plant parts showed significant antibiotic activity upon the combination with Norfloxacin by accumulating more antibiotics in the cell. The increased efficiency was achieved by inhibiting the NorA efflux [135]. α-Bisabolol is another naturally occurring sesquiterpene isolated from *matricaria chamomilla L.* plant part with NorA efflux inhibition. α-Bisabololin complexation with β-Cyclodextrin improved the physicochemical characteristics of α-Bisabololin. The complex synergism with antibiotics like tetracycline and norfloxacin increased the activity of the antibiotics by the inhibition of NorA efflux in *Staphylococcus aureus* strains [136]. Flavonoids are another set of biologically active compounds isolated from plant parts. 5, 2'-dihydroxy- 6,7,8,6'-tetramethoxyflavone in combination with rifampicin shows antimicrobial activity against *Mycobacterial aurum* and *Mycobacterial bovis BCG*. It increased the susceptibility of *Mycobacterial smegmatis* to the antibiotic rifampicin. Another flavonoid 5,6,7,8,3',4'-hexamethoxyflavone acts as one of the most potent efflux inhibitors in *Mycobacterial aurum* and *Mycobacterial smegmatis* [137].

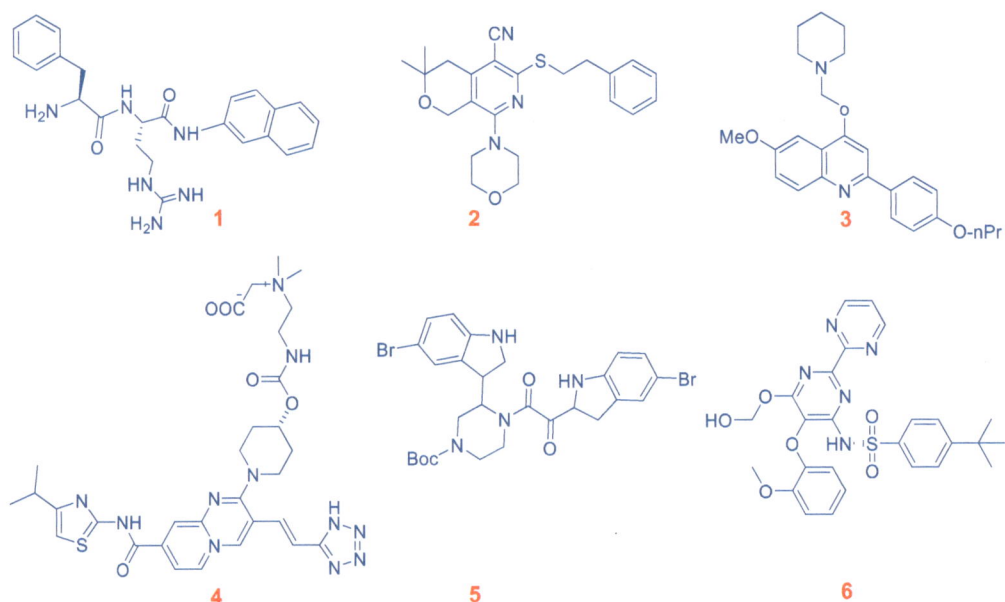

Fig. (5). Structure of 1. peptidomimetic PaβN, 2. pyranopyridine MBX2319, 3.representatives of the quinolone, 4.pyridopyrimidinone D13-9001 and 5. indole derivatives, 6.bis (pyrimidine)sulfonamide MP-601,205.

Similar to the role of phytochemical compounds, seaweeds are an important source of biologically active compounds. Lu WJ *et al.* in 2019 studied the potential of brown seaweeds *Sargassum horneri and Laminaria japonica* and the red seaweeds *Porphyra dentate*, *Gracilaria sp.* in inhibiting efflux pumping in *E.*

coli. All of these compounds show antibiotic activity in synergism with clarithromycin but to a different extent. The presence of alkaloids, indoles, phenolic compounds, pyrrole derivatives, terpenes, terpenoids and halogenated aromatic moieties in the structures incorporate them with these activities [138].

Synthetic Compounds as Efflux Pump Inhibitors

Although the use of efflux inhibitors can reduce the biofilm formation by bacteria, these molecules are harmful to human beings. Hence to decrease the quantity and, thereby the toxicity, Raquel Ferrer-Espada *et al.* in 2019 reported the use of permeability-increasing antimicrobial peptides (AMP) in combination with efflux pump inhibitors. They used polymyxin B nonpeptide (PMBN) with antibiotics in the presence of EPI and tested against *Pseudomonas aeruginosa* strains to the efflux system MexAB-OprM. The reports suggest that AMP synergizes with EPI to reduce the amount of inhibitor needed for antibiotic sensitization [139]. Multidrug-resistant *Escherichia coli* biofilm formation was reduced by using the synergism between benzylisothiocyanate in combination with metal chelators like ethylene diaminetetraacetic acid (EDTA) and efflux inhibitor phenylalanine-arginine b-naphthylamide (PAbN). The availability of efflux inhibitors will increase the antibiotic accumulation in bacterial cells and the metal chelator like EDTA will help in the release of outer membrane polysaccharides of tested *Escherichia coli* bacteria there by triggering the bactericidal activity of the antibiotic [140]. Hellewell *et al.* studied the biofilm inhibition and, thereby, the antibiofilm activity of natural products like chalcones. The studies show the significant activity of 2-phenylacetophenone against the efflux pump generation, and *trans* chalcones for its gram-negative and mycobacterial efflux pumps inhibition higher than verapamil and chloropromazine [141]. Another efflux pump protein NorA belonging to *Staphylococcus aureus,* shows resistance towards many of the antibiotics. Zimmermann *et al.* in 2019 studied the identification of an efficient efflux inhibitor, as none of the drugs known then were efficient enough for use in clinical trials due to their toxic effect of them. Finally, they found that the antibiotic ciprofloxacin, in combination with nilotinib, a tyrosine kinase inhibitor showed effectiveness in inhibiting efflux pump inhibition and thereby antibiofilm activity [142]. Cordeiro RDA *et al.* in 2019 worked on the study of anti-efflux activity of promethazine (PMZ) on Fusarium solani species complex (FSSC). PMZ shows reduction in rhodamineG efflux, cell adhesion and disruption of mature biofilms. The study reveals that the FSSC's efflux pumping is related to the antifungal tolerance of the species and the inhibition of efflux pumping triggers the susceptibility of the species to antifungals [143]. In order to achieve efflux inhibition in antimicrobial-resistant Salmonella enterica serovar Typhimurium and *Escherichia coli* species Elizabeth M. Grimsey *et al.* in 2020 conducted studies on Chlorpromazine and amitriptyline on its efflux inhibitory activity on *acrB* mediated efflux. The results revealed the antibiofilm activity of Chlorpromazine and amitriptyline species [144].

Nanoparticles as Efflux Pump Inhibitors

Silver nanoparticles with spherical nanostructure having a mean size of 38.89 nm were synthesised biologically-. Its anti-bacterial effect was determined by its ability to inhibit efflux pump in multi-drug resistant *Acinetobacter baumannii*. The real-time polymerase chain reaction results suggest that there was a significant decrease in the efflux pump gens by the action of silver nanoparticles [132]. Abdulaziz Anas *et al.* 2019 studied the sensitivity and resistance of a few bacterial pathogens, including *Vibrio alginolyticus, Escherichia coli, Staphylococcus aureus*, and Bacillus subtilis, towards silver-silica hybrid nanoparticles. The complete mortality of even highly resistant *S. aureus* was observed upon combining nanoparticles with an efflux pump inhibiting Verapamil [145]. It is a well-known fact that nano silver has bactericidal activity. Samir A. Anuj *et al.,* in 2019, studied the synergetic activity of the nano silver particles with linezolid for the enhancement of bactericidal activity. Linezolid is normally not active towards gram-negative bacteria like *E. coli* due to its rapid efflux mechanism. Hence in order to increase the efficiency and to reduce the drug dosage, the group studied the potential of biologically synthesised nano silver in the bactericidal efficiency of linezolid against *E.coli* MTCC443 [146].

CONCLUSION

To date, ample studies have been done pertaining to bacterial biofilm formation. The prior studies have not exhausted the relevance of research in this area due to the constant emergence of variant and severe biofilm infections. The multi-drug resistance of bacterial biofilm has constantly challenged the existing anti-bacterial drugs. Hence, further research in the field of biofilm is essential in addressing the critical concerns of the time that challenges life. The adequate antibiotics to combat the emerging genetically mutated bacterial biofilms ought to be researched, developed, and constantly updated. This chapter deals with a few methods by which biofilm inhibition can be achieved by making use of various synthetic and natural compounds. The methods include quorum quenching, extracellular polymeric matrix formation, inhibition of biofilm formation, efflux pump inhibition. Due to the multi-drug resistance and high tolerance of biofilm, the generation of efficient drugs to inhibit the complete growth and maturation of biofilm is a big challenge.

CONSENT FOR PUBLICATION

Not applicable.

CONFLICT OF INTEREST

The authors declare no conflict of interest, financial or otherwise.

ACKNOWLEDGEMENTS

The authors are thankful to VIT, and Vellore management.

REFERENCES

[1]   Sharma, D.; Misba, L.; Khan, A.U. Antibiotics *versus* biofilm: an emerging battleground in microbial communities. *Antimicrob. Resist. Infect. Control,* **2019**, *8*(1), 76.
      [http://dx.doi.org/10.1186/s13756-019-0533-3] [PMID: 31131107]

[2]   Dhau, J.S.; Singh, A.; Brandão, P.; Felix, V. Synthesis, characterization, X-ray crystal structure and antibacterial activity of bis[3-(4-chloro-N,N-diethylpyridine-2-carboxamide)] diselenide. *Inorg. Chem. Commun.,* **2021**, *133*, 108942.
      [http://dx.doi.org/10.1016/j.inoche.2021.108942]

[3]   Dhau, J.S.; Singh, A.; Singh, A.; Sooch, B.S.; Brandão, P.; Félix, V. Synthesis and antibacterial activity of pyridylselenium compounds: Self-assembly of bis(3-bromo-2-pyridyl)diselenide *via* intermolecular secondary and π-π stacking interactions. *J. Organomet. Chem.,* **2014**, *766*, 57-66.
      [http://dx.doi.org/10.1016/j.jorganchem.2014.05.009]

[4]   Singh, A.; Kaushik, A.; Dhau, J.S.; Kumar, R. Exploring coordination preferences and biological applications of pyridyl-based organochalcogen (Se, Te) ligands. *Coord. Chem. Rev.,* **2022**, *450*, 214254.
      [http://dx.doi.org/10.1016/j.ccr.2021.214254]

[5]   Flemming, H.C.; Wingender, J. Relevance of microbial extracellular polymeric substances (EPSs) - Part I: Structural and ecological aspects. *Water Sci. Technol.,* **2001**, *43*(6), 1-8.
      [http://dx.doi.org/10.2166/wst.2001.0326] [PMID: 11381954]

[6]   Dincer, S.; Uslu, F.M.; Delik, A. *Antibiotic Resistance in Biofilm*; Bact Biofilms, **2020**, pp. 135-148.

[7]   Mah, T.F.C.; O'Toole, G.A. Mechanisms of biofilm resistance to antimicrobial agents. *Trends Microbiol.,* **2001**, *9*(1), 34-39.
      [http://dx.doi.org/10.1016/S0966-842X(00)01913-2] [PMID: 11166241]

[8]   Pinto, R.M.; Soares, F.A.; Reis, S.; Nunes, C.; Van Dijck, P. Innovative strategies toward the disassembly of the EPS matrix in bacterial biofilms. *Front. Microbiol.,* **2020**, *11*, 952.
      [http://dx.doi.org/10.3389/fmicb.2020.00952] [PMID: 32528433]

[9]   Wood, T.K.; Knabel, S.J.; Kwan, B.W. Bacterial persister cell formation and dormancy. *Appl. Environ. Microbiol.,* **2013**, *79*(23), 7116-7121.
      [http://dx.doi.org/10.1128/AEM.02636-13] [PMID: 24038684]

[10] Aybey, A.; Usta, A.; Demirkan, E. Effects of psychotropic drugs as bacterial efflux pump inhibitors on quorum sensing regulated behaviors. *J. Microbiol. Biotechnol. Food Sci.,* **2014**, *4*(2), 128-131.
      [http://dx.doi.org/10.15414/jmbfs.2014.4.2.128-131]

[11] Miller, M.B.; Bassler, B.L. Quorum sensing in bacteria. *Annu. Rev. Microbiol.,* **2001**, *55*(1), 165-199.
      [http://dx.doi.org/10.1146/annurev.micro.55.1.165] [PMID: 11544353]

[12] Lade, H.; Paul, D.; Kweon, J.H. N-acyl homoserine lactone-mediated quorum sensing with special reference to use of quorum quenching bacteria in membrane biofouling control. *BioMed Res. Int.,* **2014**, *2014*, 1-25.
      [http://dx.doi.org/10.1155/2014/162584] [PMID: 25147787]

[13] Rehman, Z.U.; Leiknes, T. Quorum-quenching bacteria isolated from red sea sediments reduce biofilm

formation by *Pseudomonas aeruginosa*. *Front. Microbiol.*, **2018**, *9*, 1354.
[http://dx.doi.org/10.3389/fmicb.2018.01354] [PMID: 30065702]

[14]   Krasowska, A.; Sigler, K. How microorganisms use hydrophobicity and what does this mean for human needs? *Front. Cell. Infect. Microbiol.*, **2014**, *4*, 112-119.
[http://dx.doi.org/10.3389/fcimb.2014.00112] [PMID: 25191645]

[15]   Danchik, C.; Casadevall, A. Role of cell surface hydrophobicity in the pathogenesis of medically-significant fungi. *Front. Cell. Infect. Microbiol.*, **2021**, *10*, 594973.
[http://dx.doi.org/10.3389/fcimb.2020.594973] [PMID: 33569354]

[16]   Kalia, V.C. Quorum sensing inhibitors: An overview. *Biotechnol. Adv.*, **2013**, *31*(2), 224-245.
[http://dx.doi.org/10.1016/j.biotechadv.2012.10.004] [PMID: 23142623]

[17]   Lade, H.; Paul, D.; Kweon, J.H. Quorum quenching mediated approaches for control of membrane biofouling. *Int. J. Biol. Sci.*, **2014**, *10*(5), 550-565.
[http://dx.doi.org/10.7150/ijbs.9028] [PMID: 24910534]

[18]   Brackman, G.; Coenye, T. Quorum sensing inhibitors as anti-biofilm agents. *Int. J. Curr. Pharm. Res.*, **2015**, *21*(1), 5-11.
[PMID: 25189863]

[19]   Yates, E.A.; Philipp, B.; Buckley, C.; Atkinson, S.; Chhabra, S.R.; Sockett, R.E.; Goldner, M.; Dessaux, Y.; Cámara, M.; Smith, H.; Williams, P. N-acylhomoserine lactones undergo lactonolysis in a pH-, temperature-, and acyl chain length-dependent manner during growth of Yersinia pseudotuberculosis and *Pseudomonas aeruginosa*. *Infect. Immun.*, **2002**, *70*(10), 5635-5646.
[http://dx.doi.org/10.1128/IAI.70.10.5635-5646.2002] [PMID: 12228292]

[20]   Rasmussen, T.B.; Givskov, M. Quorum sensing inhibitors: a bargain of effects. *Microbiology (Reading)*, **2006**, *152*(4), 895-904.
[http://dx.doi.org/10.1099/mic.0.28601-0] [PMID: 16549654]

[21]   Vadakkan, K.; Choudhury, A.A.; Gunasekaran, R.; Hemapriya, J.; Vijayanand, S. Quorum sensing intervened bacterial signaling: Pursuit of its cognizance and repression. *J. Genet. Eng. Biotechnol.*, **2018**, *16*(2), 239-252.
[http://dx.doi.org/10.1016/j.jgeb.2018.07.001] [PMID: 30733731]

[22]   Rampioni, G.; Leoni, L.; Williams, P. The art of antibacterial warfare: Deception through interference with quorum sensing–mediated communication. *Bioorg. Chem.*, **2014**, *55*, 60-68.
[http://dx.doi.org/10.1016/j.bioorg.2014.04.005] [PMID: 24823895]

[23]   Muñoz-Cazares, N.; García-Contreras, R.; Soto-Hernández, M.; Martínez-Vázquez, M.; Castillo-Juárez, I. Natural products with quorum quenching-independent antivirulence properties. *Studies in Natural Products Chemistry*, **2018**, *57*, 327-351.
[http://dx.doi.org/10.1016/B978-0-444-64057-4.00010-7]

[24]   Katiyar, C.; Kanjilal, S.; Gupta, A.; Katiyar, S. Drug discovery from plant sources: An integrated approach. *Ayu*, **2012**, *33*(1), 10-19.
[http://dx.doi.org/10.4103/0974-8520.100295] [PMID: 23049178]

[25]   Vasavi, H.S.; Arun, A.B.; Rekha, P.D. Anti-quorum sensing activity of flavonoid-rich fraction from *Centella asiatica* L. against *Pseudomonas aeruginosa* PAO1. *J. Microbiol. Immunol. Infect.*, **2016**, *49*(1), 8-15.
[http://dx.doi.org/10.1016/j.jmii.2014.03.012] [PMID: 24856426]

[26]   Tapia-Rodriguez, M.R.; Bernal-Mercado, A.T.; Gutierrez-Pacheco, M.M.; Vazquez-Armenta, F.J.; Hernandez-Mendoza, A.; Gonzalez-Aguilar, G.A.; Martinez-Tellez, M.A.; Nazzaro, F.; Ayala-Zavala, J.F. Virulence of *Pseudomonas aeruginosa* exposed to carvacrol: alterations of the Quorum sensing at enzymatic and gene levels. *J. Cell Commun. Signal.*, **2019**, *13*(4), 531-537.
[http://dx.doi.org/10.1007/s12079-019-00516-8] [PMID: 30903602]

[27]   Amrutha, B.; Sundar, K.; Shetty, P.H. Effect of organic acids on biofilm formation and quorum

signaling of pathogens from fresh fruits and vegetables. *Microb. Pathog.,* **2017**, *111*, 156-162.
[http://dx.doi.org/10.1016/j.micpath.2017.08.042] [PMID: 28867627]

[28]   Vinothkannan, R.; Muthu Tamizh, M.; David Raj, C.; Adline Princy, S. Fructose furoic acid ester: An effective quorum sensing inhibitor against uropathogenic *Escherichia coli. Bioorg. Chem.,* **2018**, *79*, 310-318.
[http://dx.doi.org/10.1016/j.bioorg.2018.05.009] [PMID: 29800818]

[29]   Hemmati, F.; Salehi, R.; Ghotaslou, R.; Samadi Kafil, H.; Hasani, A.; Gholizadeh, P.; Nouri, R.; Ahangarzadeh Rezaee, M. Quorum Quenching: A potential target for antipseudomonal therapy. *Infect. Drug Resist.,* **2020**, *13*, 2989-3005.
[http://dx.doi.org/10.2147/IDR.S263196] [PMID: 32922047]

[30]   Bahari, S.; Zeighami, H.; Mirshahabi, H.; Roudashti, S.; Haghi, F. Inhibition of *Pseudomonas aeruginosa* quorum sensing by subinhibitory concentrations of curcumin with gentamicin and azithromycin. *J. Glob. Antimicrob. Resist.,* **2017**, *10*, 21-28.
[http://dx.doi.org/10.1016/j.jgar.2017.03.006] [PMID: 28591665]

[31]   McCarthy, R.R.; O'Gara, F. The impact of phytochemicals present in the diet on microbial signalling in the human gut. *J. Funct. Foods,* **2015**, *14*, 684-691.
[http://dx.doi.org/10.1016/j.jff.2015.02.032]

[32]   Juan, V.; Ramírez-ch, E.; Gutierrez-villagomez, J.M.; García-gonz, J.P.; Molina-torres, J. Heliyon Bioautography and GC-MS based identi fi cation of piperine and trichostachine as the active quorum quenching compounds in black pepper. *Helion,* **2020**, *6*, e031370.

[33]   Vandeputte, O.M.; Kiendrebeogo, M.; Rajaonson, S.; Diallo, B.; Mol, A.; El Jaziri, M.; Baucher, M. Identification of catechin as one of the flavonoids from Combretum albiflorum bark extract that reduces the production of quorum-sensing-controlled virulence factors in *Pseudomonas aeruginosa* PAO1. *Appl. Environ. Microbiol.,* **2010**, *76*(1), 243-253.
[http://dx.doi.org/10.1128/AEM.01059-09] [PMID: 19854927]

[34]   Yadav, R.; Rai, R.; Yadav, A.; Pahuja, M.; Solanki, S.; Yadav, H. Evaluation of antibacterial activity of *Achyranthes aspera* extract against *Streptococcus mutans*: An *in vitro* study. *J. Adv. Pharm. Technol. Res.,* **2016**, *7*(4), 149-152.
[http://dx.doi.org/10.4103/2231-4040.191426] [PMID: 27833895]

[35]   Yamarthi, A.; Jonnalgadda, S. Quorum quenching ability of dietary spice Cinnamomum verum on pathogenic bacteria quorum quenching ability of dietary spice cinnamomum verum on pathogenic bacteria introduction : Quorum sensing is a bacterial cell communication mechanism which is mediated. *Int. J. Pharm. Sci. Res.,* **2014**, *5*, 5216-5223.

[36]   Truchado, P.; Tomás-Barberán, F.A.; Allende, A.; Ponce, A. Selected phytochemical bioactive compounds as quorum sensing inhibitors. *Acta Hortic.,* **2012**, *939*(939), 93-97.
[http://dx.doi.org/10.17660/ActaHortic.2012.939.11]

[37]   Mutungwa, W.; Alluri, N.; Majumdar, M. Anti-quorum sensing activity of some commonly used traditional indian spices. *Int. J. Pharm. Pharm. Sci.,* **2015**, *7*, 80-83.

[38]   Sakr, M.; Ibrahim, N.; Ali, S.; Alzahaby, N.; Omar, A.; Khairy, W.; Zohdy, B.; Qassem, O.; Saleh, S. Identification of potential quorum quenching compounds in Brassica oleracea var. capitata against MDR *Pseudomonas aeruginosa* and *Escherichia coli* clinical isolates. *Archives of Pharmaceutical Sciences Ain Shams University,* **2021**, *5*(1), 128-142.
[http://dx.doi.org/10.21608/aps.2021.76856.1062]

[39]   Cortes-López, H.; Castro-Rosas, J.; García-Contreras, R.; Rodríguez-Zavala, J.S.; González-Pedrajo, B.; Díaz-Guerrero, M.; Hernández-Morales, J.; Muñoz-Cazares, N.; Soto-Hernández, M.; Ruíz-Posadas, L.M.; Castillo-Juárez, I. Antivirulence Activity of a Dietary Phytochemical: Hibiscus Acid Isolated from *Hibiscus sabdariffa* L. Reduces the Virulence of *Pseudomonas aeruginosa* in a Mouse Infection Model. *J. Med. Food,* **2021**, *24*(9), 934-943.
[http://dx.doi.org/10.1089/jmf.2020.0135] [PMID: 33751918]

[40]   Othman, A.F.M.; Rukayadi, Y.; Radu, S. Inhibition of *pseudomonas aeruginosa* quorum sensing by curcuma xanthorrhiza roxb. extract. *J. Pure Appl. Microbiol.,* **2019**, *13*(3), 1335-1347.
[http://dx.doi.org/10.22207/JPAM.13.3.05]

[41]   Marathe, K.; Nashikkar, N.; Bundale, S.; Upadhyay, A. Analysis of quorum quenching potential of euphorbia trigona mill. *Artic Int J Pharm Sci Res,* **2019**, *10*, 1372-1386.
[http://dx.doi.org/10.13040/IJPSR.0975-8232.10(3).1372-86]

[42]   Rodrigues, A.C.; Zola, F.G.; Ávila Oliveira, B.D.; Sacramento, N.T.B.; da Silva, E.R.; Bertoldi, M.C.; Taylor, J.G.; Pinto, U.M. Quorum quenching and microbial control through phenolic extract of Eugenia uniflora fruits. *J. Food Sci.,* **2016**, *81*(10), M2538-M2544.
[http://dx.doi.org/10.1111/1750-3841.13431] [PMID: 27603708]

[43]   Rodrigues, A.C.; Rodrigues, B.D; silva, E.R.; Bertoldi, M.C.; Pinto, U.M. Anti-quorum sensing activity of phenolic extract from *Eugenia brasiliensis. Food Sci. Technol,* **2016**, *36*, 337-343.
[http://dx.doi.org/10.1590/1678-457X.0089]

[44]   John, N.; Ramesh, S. Anti-quorum sensing properties of medicinal plants–A review. *In AIP Conference Proceedings,* **2020**, *2263*, p. 030011.
[http://dx.doi.org/10.1063/5.0016830]

[45]   Cătunescu, G.M.; Rotar, A.M.; Pop, C.R.; Diaconeasa, Z.; Bunghez, F.; Socaciu, M.I.; Semeniuc, C.A. Influence of extraction pre-treatments on some phytochemicals and biological activity of Transylvanian cranberries (Vaccinium vitis-idea L.). *Lebensm. Wiss. Technol.,* **2019**, *102*, 385-392.
[http://dx.doi.org/10.1016/j.lwt.2018.12.062]

[46]   Kowalczyk, P.; Madej, A.; Paprocki, D.; Szymczak, M.; Ostaszewski, R. Coumarin derivatives as new toxic compounds to selected K12, R1–R4 E. coli Strains. *Materials (Basel),* **2020**, *13*(11), 2499-2506.
[http://dx.doi.org/10.3390/ma13112499] [PMID: 32486298]

[47]   Elmasri, W.A.; Hegazy, M.E.F.; Aziz, M.; Koksal, E.; Amor, W.; Mechref, Y.; Hamood, A.N.; Cordes, D.B.; Paré, P.W. Biofilm blocking sesquiterpenes from Teucrium polium. *Phytochemistry,* **2014**, *103*, 107-113.
[http://dx.doi.org/10.1016/j.phytochem.2014.03.029] [PMID: 24735824]

[48]   Zhang, J.; Rui, X.; Wang, L.; Guan, Y.; Sun, X.; Dong, M. Polyphenolic extract from Rosa rugosa tea inhibits bacterial quorum sensing and biofilm formation. *Food Control,* **2014**, *42*, 125-131.
[http://dx.doi.org/10.1016/j.foodcont.2014.02.001]

[49]   Teasdale, M.E.; Liu, J.; Wallace, J.; Akhlaghi, F.; Rowley, D.C. Secondary metabolites produced by the marine bacterium *Halobacillus salinus* that inhibit quorum sensing-controlled phenotypes in gram-negative bacteria. *Appl. Environ. Microbiol.,* **2009**, *75*(3), 567-572.
[http://dx.doi.org/10.1128/AEM.00632-08] [PMID: 19060172]

[50]   Teasdale, M.E.; Donovan, K.A.; Forschner-Dancause, S.R.; Rowley, D.C. Gram-positive marine bacteria as a potential resource for the discovery of quorum sensing inhibitors. *Mar. Biotechnol. (NY),* **2011**, *13*(4), 722-732.
[http://dx.doi.org/10.1007/s10126-010-9334-7] [PMID: 21152942]

[51]   Li, J.; Wang, W.; Xu, S.X.; Magarvey, N.A.; McCormick, J.K. *Lactobacillus reuteri* -produced cyclic dipeptides quench *agr* -mediated expression of toxic shock syndrome toxin-1 in staphylococci. *Proc. Natl. Acad. Sci. USA,* **2011**, *108*(8), 3360-3365.
[http://dx.doi.org/10.1073/pnas.1017431108] [PMID: 21282650]

[52]   Chu, Y.Y.; Nega, M.; Wölfle, M.; Plener, L.; Grond, S.; Jung, K.; Götz, F. A new class of quorum quenching molecules from Staphylococcus species affects communication and growth of gram-negative bacteria. *PLoS Pathog.,* **2013**, *9*(9), e1003654.
[http://dx.doi.org/10.1371/journal.ppat.1003654] [PMID: 24098134]

[53]   Singh, V.K.; Kavita, K.; Prabhakaran, R.; Jha, B. *Cis* -9-octadecenoic acid from the rhizospheric bacterium *Stenotrophomonas maltophilia* BJ01 shows quorum quenching and anti-biofilm activities.

Biofouling, **2013**, *29*(7), 855-867.
[http://dx.doi.org/10.1080/08927014.2013.807914] [PMID: 23844805]

[54] Clark, B.R.; Engene, N.; Teasdale, M.E.; Rowley, D.C.; Matainaho, T.; Valeriote, F.A.; Gerwick, W.H. Natural products chemistry and taxonomy of the marine cyanobacterium *Blennothrix cantharidosmum. J. Nat. Prod.,* **2008**, *71*(9), 1530-1537.
[http://dx.doi.org/10.1021/np800088a] [PMID: 18698821]

[55] Dobretsov, S.; Teplitski, M.; Alagely, A.; Gunasekera, S.P.; Paul, V.J. Malyngolide from the cyanobacterium *Lyngbya majuscula* interferes with quorum sensing circuitry. *Environ. Microbiol. Rep.,* **2010**, *2*(6), 739-744.
[http://dx.doi.org/10.1111/j.1758-2229.2010.00169.x] [PMID: 23766278]

[56] Kwan, J.C.; Meickle, T.; Ladwa, D.; Teplitski, M.; Paul, V.; Luesch, H. Lyngbyoic acid, a "tagged" fatty acid from a marine cyanobacterium, disrupts quorum sensing in *Pseudomonas aeruginosa. Mol. Biosyst.,* **2011**, *7*(4), 1205-1216.
[http://dx.doi.org/10.1039/c0mb00180e] [PMID: 21258753]

[57] Choi, H.; Mascuch, S.J.; Villa, F.A.; Byrum, T.; Teasdale, M.E.; Smith, J.E.; Preskitt, L.B.; Rowley, D.C.; Gerwick, L.; Gerwick, W.H. Honaucins A-C, potent inhibitors of inflammation and bacterial quorum sensing: synthetic derivatives and structure-activity relationships. *Chem. Biol.,* **2012**, *19*(5), 589-598.
[http://dx.doi.org/10.1016/j.chembiol.2012.03.014] [PMID: 22633410]

[58] Gupta, K.; Daroch, P.; Harjai, K.; Chhibber, S. Parallels among natural and synthetically modified quorum-quenching strategies as convoy to future therapy. *Microbiology (Reading),* **2019**, *165*(12), 1265-1281.
[http://dx.doi.org/10.1099/mic.0.000826] [PMID: 31264956]

[59] Malheiro, J.F.; Maillard, J.Y.; Borges, F.; Simões, M. Evaluation of cinnamaldehyde and cinnamic acid derivatives in microbial growth control. *Int. Biodeterior. Biodegradation,* **2019**, *141*, 71-78.
[http://dx.doi.org/10.1016/j.ibiod.2018.06.003]

[60] Paluch, E.; Rewak-Soroczyńska, J.; Jędrusik, I.; Mazurkiewicz, E.; Jermakow, K. Prevention of biofilm formation by quorum quenching. *Appl. Microbiol. Biotechnol.,* **2020**, *104*(5), 1871-1881.
[http://dx.doi.org/10.1007/s00253-020-10349-w] [PMID: 31927762]

[61] O'Loughlin, C.T.; Miller, L.C.; Siryaporn, A.; Drescher, K.; Semmelhack, M.F.; Bassler, B.L. A quorum-sensing inhibitor blocks *Pseudomonas aeruginosa* virulence and biofilm formation. *Proc. Natl. Acad. Sci. USA,* **2013**, *110*(44), 17981-17986.
[http://dx.doi.org/10.1073/pnas.1316981110] [PMID: 24143808]

[62] Musthafa, K.S.; Balamurugan, K.; Pandian, S.K.; Ravi, A.V. 2,5-Piperazinedione inhibits quorum sensing-dependent factor production in *Pseudomonas aeruginosa* PAO1. *J. Basic Microbiol.,* **2012**, *52*(6), 679-686.
[http://dx.doi.org/10.1002/jobm.201100292] [PMID: 22359266]

[63] Geske, G.D.; Mattmann, M.E.; Blackwell, H.E. Evaluation of a focused library of N-aryl l-homoserine lactones reveals a new set of potent quorum sensing modulators. *Bioorg. Med. Chem. Lett.,* **2008**, *18*(22), 5978-5981.
[http://dx.doi.org/10.1016/j.bmcl.2008.07.089] [PMID: 18760602]

[64] Geske, G.D.; O'Neill, J.C.; Miller, D.M.; Mattmann, M.E.; Blackwell, H.E. Modulation of bacterial quorum sensing with synthetic ligands: systematic evaluation of N-acylated homoserine lactones in multiple species and new insights into their mechanisms of action. *J. Am. Chem. Soc.,* **2007**, *129*(44), 13613-13625.
[http://dx.doi.org/10.1021/ja074135h] [PMID: 17927181]

[65] Nandi, S. Recent advances in ligand and structure based screening of potent quorum sensing inhibitors against antibiotic resistance induced bacterial virulence. *Recent Pat. Biotechnol.,* **2016**, *10*(2), 195-216.

[http://dx.doi.org/10.2174/1872208310666160728104450] [PMID: 27468815]

[66]　Ishida, T.; Ikeda, T.; Takiguchi, N.; Kuroda, A.; Ohtake, H.; Kato, J. Inhibition of quorum sensing in *Pseudomonas aeruginosa* by N-acyl cyclopentylamides. *Appl. Environ. Microbiol.,* **2007**, *73*(10), 3183-3188.
　　　　[http://dx.doi.org/10.1128/AEM.02233-06] [PMID: 17369333]

[67]　Lidor, O.; Al-Quntar, A.; Pesci, E.C.; Steinberg, D. Mechanistic analysis of a synthetic inhibitor of the *Pseudomonas aeruginosa* LasI quorum-sensing signal synthase. *Sci. Rep.,* **2015**, *5*(1), 16569.
　　　　[http://dx.doi.org/10.1038/srep16569] [PMID: 26593271]

[68]　Ziegler, E.W.; Brown, A.B.; Nesnas, N.; Chouinard, C.D.; Mehta, A.K.; Palmer, A.G. β-Cyclodextrin encapsulation of synthetic AHLs: Drug delivery implications and quorum-quenching exploits. *ChemBioChem,* **2021**, *22*(7), 1292-1301.
　　　　[http://dx.doi.org/10.1002/cbic.202000773] [PMID: 33238068]

[69]　Molnár, M.; Fenyvesi, É.; Berkl, Z.; Németh, I.; Fekete-Kertész, I.; Márton, R.; Vaszita, E.; Varga, E.; Ujj, D.; Szente, L. Cyclodextrin-mediated quorum quenching in the Aliivibrio fischeri bioluminescence model system – Modulation of bacterial communication. *Int. J. Pharm.,* **2021**, *594*, 120150.
　　　　[http://dx.doi.org/10.1016/j.ijpharm.2020.120150] [PMID: 33321169]

[70]　Tung, T.T.; Jakobsen, T.H.; Dao, T.T.; Fuglsang, A.T.; Givskov, M.; Christensen, S.B.; Nielsen, J. Fusaric acid and analogues as Gram-negative bacterial quorum sensing inhibitors. *Eur. J. Med. Chem.,* **2017**, *126*, 1011-1020.
　　　　[http://dx.doi.org/10.1016/j.ejmech.2016.11.044] [PMID: 28033578]

[71]　Qin, X.; Thota, G.K.; Singh, R.; Balamurugan, R.; Goycoolea, F.M. Synthetic homoserine lactone analogues as antagonists of bacterial quorum sensing. *Bioorg. Chem.,* **2020**, *98*, 103698.
　　　　[http://dx.doi.org/10.1016/j.bioorg.2020.103698] [PMID: 32217369]

[72]　Kadam, H.K.; Salkar, K.; Naik, A.P.; Naik, M.M.; Salgaonkar, L.N.; Charya, L.; Pinto, K.C.; Mandrekar, V.K.; Vaz, T. Silica Supported Synthesis and Quorum Quenching Ability of Isoxazolones Against Both Gram Positive and Gram Negative Bacterial Pathogens. *ChemistrySelect,* **2021**, *6*(42), 11718-11728.
　　　　[http://dx.doi.org/10.1002/slct.202101798]

[73]　Sathyanarayana, R.; Bajire, S.K.; Poojary, B.; Shastry, R.P.; Kumar, V.; Chandrashekarappa, R.B. Design, synthesis, antibacterial and quorum quenching studies of 1,2,5-trisubstituted 1,2,4-triazoles. *J. Indian Chem. Soc.,* **2021**, *18*(5), 1051-1066.
　　　　[http://dx.doi.org/10.1007/s13738-020-02093-9]

[74]　Sikdar, R.; Elias, M. Quorum quenching enzymes and their effects on virulence, biofilm, and microbiomes: a review of recent advances. *Expert Rev. Anti Infect. Ther.,* **2020**, *18*(12), 1221-1233.
　　　　[http://dx.doi.org/10.1080/14787210.2020.1794815] [PMID: 32749905]

[75]　d'Angelo-Picard, C.; Faure, D.; Penot, I.; Dessaux, Y. Diversity of N-acyl homoserine lactone-producing and -degrading bacteria in soil and tobacco rhizosphere. *Environ. Microbiol.,* **2005**, *7*(11), 1796-1808.
　　　　[http://dx.doi.org/10.1111/j.1462-2920.2005.00886.x] [PMID: 16232294]

[76]　Thomas, P.W.; Stone, E.M.; Costello, A.L.; Tierney, D.L.; Fast, W. The quorum-quenching lactonase from *Bacillus thuringiensis* is a metalloprotein. *Biochemistry,* **2005**, *44*(20), 7559-7569.
　　　　[http://dx.doi.org/10.1021/bi050050m] [PMID: 15895999]

[77]　Fetzner, S. Quorum quenching enzymes. *J. Biotechnol.,* **2015**, *201*, 2-14.
　　　　[http://dx.doi.org/10.1016/j.jbiotec.2014.09.001] [PMID: 25220028]

[78]　Morohoshi, T.; Tominaga, Y.; Someya, N.; Ikeda, T. Complete genome sequence and characterization of the N-acylhomoserine lactone-degrading gene of the potato leaf-associated Solibacillus silvestris. *J. Biosci. Bioeng.,* **2012**, *113*(1), 20-25.
　　　　[http://dx.doi.org/10.1016/j.jbiosc.2011.09.006] [PMID: 22019407]

[79] Park, S; Lee, SJ; Oh, T; Oh, J; Koo, B; Yum, D AhlD, an N-acylhomoserine lactonase in Arthrobacter sp., and predicted homologues in other bacteria. *Microbiology (Reading).*, **2003**, *149*(Pt 6), 1541-1550.

[80] Krysciak, D.; Schmeisser, C.; Preuß, S.; Riethausen, J.; Quitschau, M.; Grond, S.; Streit, W.R. Involvement of multiple loci in quorum quenching of autoinducer I molecules in the nitrogen-fixing symbiont Rhizobium (Sinorhizobium) sp. strain NGR234. *Appl. Environ. Microbiol.*, **2011**, *77*(15), 5089-5099.
[http://dx.doi.org/10.1128/AEM.00112-11] [PMID: 21642401]

[81] Park, S.Y.; Kang, H.O.; Jang, H.S.; Lee, J.K.; Koo, B.T.; Yum, D.Y. Identification of extracellular N-acylhomoserine lactone acylase from a Streptomyces sp. and its application to quorum quenching. *Appl. Environ. Microbiol.*, **2005**, *71*(5), 2632-2641.
[http://dx.doi.org/10.1128/AEM.71.5.2632-2641.2005] [PMID: 15870355]

[82] Lin, Y.H.; Xu, J.L.; Hu, J.; Wang, L.H.; Ong, S.L.; Leadbetter, J.R.; Zhang, L.H. Acyl-homoserine lactone acylase from Ralstonia strain XJ12B represents a novel and potent class of quorum-quenching enzymes. *Mol. Microbiol.*, **2003**, *47*(3), 849-860.
[http://dx.doi.org/10.1046/j.1365-2958.2003.03351.x] [PMID: 12535081]

[83] Chen, C.N.; Chen, C.J.; Liao, C.T.; Lee, C.Y. A probable aculeacin A acylase from the Ralstonia solanacearum GMI1000 is N-acyl-homoserine lactone acylase with quorum-quenching activity. *BMC Microbiol.*, **2009**, *9*(1), 89.
[http://dx.doi.org/10.1186/1471-2180-9-89] [PMID: 19426552]

[84] Wahjudi, M.; Papaioannou, E.; Hendrawati, O.; van Assen, A.H.G.; van Merkerk, R.; Cool, R.H.; Poelarends, G.J.; Quax, W.J. PA0305 of *Pseudomonas aeruginosa* is a quorum quenching acylhomoserine lactone acylase belonging to the Ntn hydrolase superfamily. *Microbiology (Reading)*, **2011**, *157*(7), 2042-2055.
[http://dx.doi.org/10.1099/mic.0.043935-0] [PMID: 21372094]

[85] Czajkowski, R.; Krzyżanowska, D.; Karczewska, J.; Atkinson, S.; Przysowa, J.; Lojkowska, E.; Williams, P.; Jafra, S. Inactivation of AHLs by Ochrobactrum sp. A44 depends on the activity of a novel class of AHL acylase. *Environ. Microbiol. Rep.*, **2011**, *3*(1), 59-68.
[http://dx.doi.org/10.1111/j.1758-2229.2010.00188.x] [PMID: 23761232]

[86] Chen, F.; Gao, Y.; Chen, X.; Yu, Z.; Li, X. Quorum quenching enzymes and their application in degrading signal molecules to block quorum sensing-dependent infection. *Int. J. Mol. Sci.*, **2013**, *14*(9), 17477-17500.
[http://dx.doi.org/10.3390/ijms140917477] [PMID: 24065091]

[87] Gökalsın, B.; Berber, D.; Sesal, N.C. *Pseudomonas aeruginosa* quorum sensing and biofilm inhibition. *Quorum Sensing*, **2019**, 227-256.
[http://dx.doi.org/10.1016/B978-0-12-814905-8.00009-5]

[88] Velázquez-Velázquez, J.L.; Santos-Flores, A.; Araujo-Meléndez, J.; Sánchez-Sánchez, R.; Velasquillo, C.; González, C.; Martínez-Castañon, G.; Martinez-Gutierrez, F. Anti-biofilm and cytotoxicity activity of impregnated dressings with silver nanoparticles. *Mater. Sci. Eng. C*, **2015**, *49*, 604-611.
[http://dx.doi.org/10.1016/j.msec.2014.12.084] [PMID: 25686989]

[89] Hayat, S.; Muzammil, S.; Shabana, ; Aslam, B.; Siddique, M.H.; Saqalein, M.; Nisar, M.A. Quorum quenching: role of nanoparticles as signal jammers in Gram-negative bacteria. *Future Microbiol.*, **2019**, *14*(1), 61-72.
[http://dx.doi.org/10.2217/fmb-2018-0257] [PMID: 30539663]

[90] Vinoj, G.; Pati, R.; Sonawane, A.; Vaseeharan, B. *In vitro* cytotoxic effects of gold nanoparticles coated with functional acyl homoserine lactone lactonase protein from *Bacillus licheniformis* and their antibiofilm activity against Proteus species. *Antimicrob. Agents Chemother.*, **2015**, *59*(2), 763-771.
[http://dx.doi.org/10.1128/AAC.03047-14] [PMID: 25403677]

[91] Kaufmann, G.F.; Sartorio, R.; Lee, S.H.; Rogers, C.J.; Meijler, M.M.; Moss, J.A.; Clapham, B.;

Brogan, A.P.; Dickerson, T.J.; Janda, K.D. Revisiting quorum sensing: Discovery of additional chemical and biological functions for 3-oxo- *N* -acylhomoserine lactones. *Proc. Natl. Acad. Sci. USA,* **2005**, *102*(2), 309-314.
[http://dx.doi.org/10.1073/pnas.0408639102] [PMID: 15623555]

[92]   García-Lara, B.; Saucedo-Mora, M.Á.; Roldán-Sánchez, J.A.; Pérez-Eretza, B.; Ramasamy, M.; Lee, J.; Coria-Jimenez, R.; Tapia, M.; Varela-Guerrero, V.; García-Contreras, R. Inhibition of quorum-sensing-dependent virulence factors and biofilm formation of clinical and environmental *Pseudomonas aeruginosa* strains by ZnO nanoparticles. *Lett. Appl. Microbiol.,* **2015**, *61*(3), 299-305.
[http://dx.doi.org/10.1111/lam.12456] [PMID: 26084709]

[93]   Miller, K.P.; Wang, L.; Chen, Y.P.; Pellechia, P.J.; Benicewicz, B.C.; Decho, A.W. Engineering nanoparticles to silence bacterial communication. *Front. Microbiol.,* **2015**, *6*, 189-196.
[http://dx.doi.org/10.3389/fmicb.2015.00189] [PMID: 25806030]

[94]   Watnick, P.; Kolter, R. Biofilm, city of microbes. *J. Bacteriol.,* **2000**, *182*(10), 2675-2679.
[http://dx.doi.org/10.1128/JB.182.10.2675-2679.2000] [PMID: 10781532]

[95]   Donelli G, editor. Microbial biofilms: methods and protocols. Humana press 2014; 1147: 33-41.
[http://dx.doi.org/10.1007/978-1-4939-0467-9]

[96]   Hu, X.; Kang, F.; Yang, B.; Zhang, W.; Qin, C.; Gao, Y. Extracellular polymeric substances acting as a permeable barrier hinder the lateral transfer of antibiotic resistance genes. *Front. Microbiol.,* **2019**, *10*, 736.
[http://dx.doi.org/10.3389/fmicb.2019.00736] [PMID: 31057498]

[97]   Flemming, H.C.; Wingender, J. The biofilm matrix. *Nat. Rev. Microbiol.,* **2010**, *8*(9), 623-633.
[http://dx.doi.org/10.1038/nrmicro2415] [PMID: 20676145]

[98]   Stone, W.; Wolfaardt, G. Measuring microbial metabolism in atypical environments. *Methods Microbiol.,* **2018**, *45*, 123-144.
[http://dx.doi.org/10.1016/bs.mim.2018.07.004]

[99]   Di Martino, P. Extracellular polymeric substances, a key element in understanding biofilm phenotype. *AIMS Microbiol.,* **2018**, *4*(2), 274-288.
[http://dx.doi.org/10.3934/microbiol.2018.2.274] [PMID: 31294215]

[100]   Flemming, H.C.; Wingender, J.; Szewzyk, U.; Steinberg, P.; Rice, S.A.; Kjelleberg, S. Biofilms: an emergent form of bacterial life. *Nat. Rev. Microbiol.,* **2016**, *14*(9), 563-575.
[http://dx.doi.org/10.1038/nrmicro.2016.94] [PMID: 27510863]

[101]   Algburi, A.; Comito, N.; Kashtanov, D.; Dicks, L.M.T.; Chikindas, M.L. Control of biofilm formation: antibiotics and beyond. *Appl. Environ. Microbiol.,* **2017**, *83*(3), e02508-16.
[http://dx.doi.org/10.1128/AEM.02508-16] [PMID: 27864170]

[102]   Leroy, C.; Delbarre, C.; Ghillebaert, F.; Compere, C.; Combes, D. Effects of commercial enzymes on the adhesion of a marine biofilm-forming bacterium. *Biofouling,* **2008**, *24*(1), 11-22.
[http://dx.doi.org/10.1080/08927010701784912] [PMID: 18058451]

[103]   Ganesh, A.; Nagendrababu, V.; John, A.; Deivanayagam, K. The effect of addition of an eps degrading enzyme with and without detergent to 2% chlorhexidine on disruption of *enterococcus faecalis* biofilm: A confocal laser scanning microscopic study. *J. Clin. Diagn. Res.,* **2015**, *9*(11), ZC61-ZC65.
[http://dx.doi.org/10.7860/JCDR/2015/14602.6829] [PMID: 26675655]

[104]   Lister, J.L.; Horswill, A.R. *Staphylococcus aureus* biofilms: recent developments in biofilm dispersal. *Front. Cell. Infect. Microbiol.,* **2014**, *4*, 178-187.
[http://dx.doi.org/10.3389/fcimb.2014.00178] [PMID: 25566513]

[105]   Kumar, L.; Cox, C.R.; Sarkar, S.K. Matrix metalloprotease-1 inhibits and disrupts *Enterococcus faecalis* biofilms. *PLoS One,* **2019**, *14*(1), e0210218.
[http://dx.doi.org/10.1371/journal.pone.0210218] [PMID: 30633757]

[106]   Saggu, S.K.; Jha, G.; Mishra, P.C. Enzymatic Degradation of Biofilm by Metalloprotease From

Microbacterium sp. SKS10. *Front. Bioeng. Biotechnol.,* **2019**, *7*, 192-205.
[http://dx.doi.org/10.3389/fbioe.2019.00192] [PMID: 31448272]

[107] Daboor, S.M.; Rohde, J.R.; Cheng, Z. Disruption of the extracellular polymeric network of *Pseudomonas aeruginosa* biofilms by alginate lyase enhances pathogen eradication by antibiotics. *J. Cyst. Fibros.,* **2021**, *20*(2), 264-270.
[http://dx.doi.org/10.1016/j.jcf.2020.04.006] [PMID: 32482592]

[108] Chen, H.; Zhang, B.; Weir, M.D.; Homayounfar, N.; Fay, G.G.; Martinho, F.; Lei, L.; Bai, Y.; Hu, T.; Xu, H.H.K. S. mutans gene-modification and antibacterial resin composite as dual strategy to suppress biofilm acid production and inhibit caries. *J. Dent.,* **2020**, *93*, 103278.
[http://dx.doi.org/10.1016/j.jdent.2020.103278] [PMID: 31945398]

[109] Hamzah, H; Hertiani, T; Pratiwi, SU; Nuryastuti, T Inhibitory activity and degradation of curcumin as anti-biofilm polymicrobial on catheters. *Int. J. Res.,* **2020**, *11*, 830-5.

[110] Song, Y.J.; Yu, H.H.; Kim, Y.J.; Lee, N.K.; Paik, H.D. The use of papain for the removal of biofilms formed by pathogenic *Staphylococcus aureus* and *Campylobacter jejuni. Lebensm. Wiss. Technol.,* **2020**, *127*, 109383.
[http://dx.doi.org/10.1016/j.lwt.2020.109383]

[111] Lim, E.S.; Koo, O.K.; Kim, M.J.; Kim, J.S. Bio-enzymes for inhibition and elimination of *Escherichia coli* O157:H7 biofilm and their synergistic effect with sodium hypochlorite. *Sci. Rep.,* **2019**, *9*(1), 9920.
[http://dx.doi.org/10.1038/s41598-019-46363-w] [PMID: 31289312]

[112] Fulaz, S.; Vitale, S.; Quinn, L.; Casey, E. Nanoparticle–Biofilm Interactions: The role of the EPS matrix. *Trends Microbiol.,* **2019**, *27*(11), 915-926.
[http://dx.doi.org/10.1016/j.tim.2019.07.004] [PMID: 31420126]

[113] Patel, K.K.; Tripathi, M.; Pandey, N.; Agrawal, A.K.; Gade, S.; Anjum, M.M.; Tilak, R.; Singh, S. Alginate lyase immobilized chitosan nanoparticles of ciprofloxacin for the improved antimicrobial activity against the biofilm associated mucoid *P. aeruginosa* infection in cystic fibrosis. *Int. J. Pharm.,* **2019**, *563*, 30-42.
[http://dx.doi.org/10.1016/j.ijpharm.2019.03.051] [PMID: 30926526]

[114] Tan, Y.; Ma, S.; Liu, C.; Yu, W.; Han, F. Enhancing the stability and antibiofilm activity of DspB by immobilization on carboxymethyl chitosan nanoparticles. *Microbiol. Res.,* **2015**, *178*, 35-41.
[http://dx.doi.org/10.1016/j.micres.2015.06.001] [PMID: 26302845]

[115] Hwang, G.; Paula, A.J.; Hunter, E.E.; Liu, Y.; Babeer, A.; Karabucak, B.; Stebe, K.; Kumar, V.; Steager, E.; Koo, H. Catalytic antimicrobial robots for biofilm eradication. *Sci. Robot.,* **2019**, *4*(29), eaaw2388.
[http://dx.doi.org/10.1126/scirobotics.aaw2388] [PMID: 31531409]

[116] Weldrick, P.J.; Hardman, M.J.; Paunov, V.N. Enhanced clearing of wound-related pathogenic bacterial biofilms using protease-functionalized antibiotic nanocarriers. *ACS Appl. Mater. Interfaces,* **2019**, *11*(47), 43902-43919.
[http://dx.doi.org/10.1021/acsami.9b16119] [PMID: 31718141]

[117] Subbiahdoss, G.; Sharifi, S.; Grijpma, D.W.; Laurent, S.; van der Mei, H.C.; Mahmoudi, M.; Busscher, H.J. Magnetic targeting of surface-modified superparamagnetic iron oxide nanoparticles yields antibacterial efficacy against biofilms of gentamicin-resistant staphylococci. *Acta Biomater.,* **2012**, *8*(6), 2047-2055.
[http://dx.doi.org/10.1016/j.actbio.2012.03.002] [PMID: 22406508]

[118] Manoharan, A.; Das, T.; Whiteley, G.S.; Glasbey, T.; Kriel, F.H.; Manos, J. The effect of N-acetylcysteine in a combined antibiofilm treatment against antibiotic-resistant *Staphylococcus aureus. J. Antimicrob. Chemother.,* **2020**, *75*(7), 1787-1798.
[http://dx.doi.org/10.1093/jac/dkaa093] [PMID: 32363384]

[119] Abd El-Baky, R.M.; Sandle, T.; John, J.; Abuo-Rahma, G.E.D.A.A.; Hetta, H.F. A novel mechanism

of action of ketoconazole: inhibition of the *NorA* efflux pump system and biofilm formation in multidrug-resistant *Staphylococcus aureus. Infect. Drug Resist.,* **2019**, *12*, 1703-1718.
[http://dx.doi.org/10.2147/IDR.S201124] [PMID: 31354319]

[120] Yang, Y.; Hwang, E.; Park, B.I.; Choi, N.Y.; Kim, K.J.; You, Y.O. *Artemisia princeps* Inhibits Growth, Biofilm Formation, and Virulence Factor Expression of *Streptococcus mutans. J. Med. Food,* **2019**, *22*(6), 623-630.
[http://dx.doi.org/10.1089/jmf.2018.4304] [PMID: 31021282]

[121] Bhattacharyya, P.; Gurung, J.; Khyriem, A.B.; Banik, A.; Lyngdoh, W.V.; Choudhury, B. Association of biofilm production with multidrug resistance among clinical isolates of Acinetobacter baumannii and *Pseudomonas aeruginosa* from intensive care unit. *Indian J. Crit. Care Med.,* **2013**, *17*(4), 214-218.
[http://dx.doi.org/10.4103/0972-5229.118416] [PMID: 24133328]

[122] Bao, Q.; Xie, L.; Ohashi, H.; Hosomi, M.; Terada, A. Inhibition of Agrobacterium tumefaciens biofilm formation by acylase I-immobilized polymer surface grafting of a zwitterionic group-containing polymer brush. *Biochem. Eng. J.,* **2019**, *152*, 107372-107379.
[http://dx.doi.org/10.1016/j.bej.2019.107372]

[123] Agarwalla, S.V.; Ellepola, K.; Costa, M.C.F.; Fechine, G.J.M.; Morin, J.L.P.; Castro Neto, A.H.; Seneviratne, C.J.; Rosa, V. Hydrophobicity of graphene as a driving force for inhibiting biofilm formation of pathogenic bacteria and fungi. *Dent. Mater.,* **2019**, *35*(3), 403-413.
[http://dx.doi.org/10.1016/j.dental.2018.09.016] [PMID: 30679015]

[124] Vijayakumar, S.; Vinoj, G.; Malaikozhundan, B.; Shanthi, S.; Vaseeharan, B. Plectranthus amboinicus leaf extract mediated synthesis of zinc oxide nanoparticles and its control of methicillin resistant *Staphylococcus aureus* biofilm and blood sucking mosquito larvae. *Spectrochim. Acta A Mol. Biomol. Spectrosc.,* **2015**, *137*, 886-891.
[http://dx.doi.org/10.1016/j.saa.2014.08.064] [PMID: 25280336]

[125] Thaya, R.; Malaikozhundan, B.; Vijayakumar, S.; Sivakamavalli, J.; Jeyasekar, R.; Shanthi, S.; Vaseeharan, B.; Ramasamy, P.; Sonawane, A. Chitosan coated Ag/ZnO nanocomposite and their antibiofilm, antifungal and cytotoxic effects on murine macrophages. *Microb. Pathog.,* **2016**, *100*, 124-132.
[http://dx.doi.org/10.1016/j.micpath.2016.09.010] [PMID: 27622344]

[126] Manju, S.; Malaikozhundan, B.; Vijayakumar, S.; Shanthi, S.; Jaishabanu, A.; Ekambaram, P.; Vaseeharan, B. Antibacterial, antibiofilm and cytotoxic effects of Nigella sativa essential oil coated gold nanoparticles. *Microb. Pathog.,* **2016**, *91*, 129-135.
[http://dx.doi.org/10.1016/j.micpath.2015.11.021] [PMID: 26703114]

[127] Agarwalla, S.V.; Ellepola, K.; Silikas, N.; Castro Neto, A.H.; Seneviratne, C.J.; Rosa, V. Persistent inhibition of Candida albicans biofilm and hyphae growth on titanium by graphene nanocoating. *Dent. Mater.,* **2021**, *37*(2), 370-377.
[http://dx.doi.org/10.1016/j.dental.2020.11.028] [PMID: 33358443]

[128] Liu, F.; Sun, Z.; Wang, F.; Liu, Y.; Zhu, Y.; Du, L.; Wang, D.; Xu, W. Inhibition of biofilm formation and exopolysaccharide synthesis of *Enterococcus faecalis* by phenyllactic acid. *Food Microbiol.,* **2020**, *86*, 103344.
[http://dx.doi.org/10.1016/j.fm.2019.103344] [PMID: 31703877]

[129] Lara, H.H.; Ixtepan-Turrent, L.; Jose Yacaman, M.; Lopez-Ribot, J. Inhibition of Candida auris biofilm formation on medical and environmental surfaces by silver nanoparticles. *ACS Appl. Mater. Interfaces,* **2020**, *12*(19), 21183-21191.
[http://dx.doi.org/10.1021/acsami.9b20708] [PMID: 31944650]

[130] Mahamuni-Badiger, P.P.; Patil, P.M.; Badiger, M.V.; Patel, P.R.; Thorat- Gadgil, B.S.; Pandit, A.; Bohara, R.A. Biofilm formation to inhibition: Role of zinc oxide-based nanoparticles. *Mater. Sci. Eng. C,* **2020**, *108*, 110319.
[http://dx.doi.org/10.1016/j.msec.2019.110319] [PMID: 31923962]

[131]   Blanco, P.; Hernando-Amado, S.; Reales-Calderon, J.; Corona, F.; Lira, F.; Alcalde-Rico, M.; Bernardini, A.; Sanchez, M.; Martinez, J. Bacterial multidrug efflux pumps: much more than antibiotic resistance determinants. *Microorganisms,* **2016**, *4*(1), 14-33.
[http://dx.doi.org/10.3390/microorganisms4010014] [PMID: 27681908]

[132]   de Sousa Andrade, L.M.; de Oliveira, A.B.M.; Leal, A.L.A.B.; de Alcântara Oliveira, F.A.; Portela, A.L.; de Sousa Lima Neto, J.; de Siqueira-Júnior, J.P.; Kaatz, G.W.; da Rocha, C.Q.; Barreto, H.M. Antimicrobial activity and inhibition of the NorA efflux pump of *Staphylococcus aureus* by extract and isolated compounds from Arrabidaea brachypoda. *Microb. Pathog.,* **2020**, *140*, 103935.
[http://dx.doi.org/10.1016/j.micpath.2019.103935] [PMID: 31857236]

[133]   Reza, A.; Sutton, J.M.; Rahman, K.M. Effectiveness of efflux pump inhibitors as biofilm disruptors and resistance breakers in gram-negative (ESKAPEE) bacteria. *Antibiotics (Basel),* **2019**, *8*(4), 229-248.
[http://dx.doi.org/10.3390/antibiotics8040229] [PMID: 31752382]

[134]   Lamut, A.; Peterlin Mašič, L.; Kikelj, D.; Tomašič, T. Efflux pump inhibitors of clinically relevant multidrug resistant bacteria. *Med. Res. Rev.,* **2019**, *39*(6), 2460-2504.
[http://dx.doi.org/10.1002/med.21591] [PMID: 31004360]

[135]   Pereira da Cruz, R.; Sampaio de Freitas, T.; do Socorro Costa, M.; Lucas dos Santos, A.T.; Ferreira Campina, F.; Pereira, R.L.S.; Bezerra, J.W.A.; Quintans-Júnior, L.J.; De Souza Araújo, A.A.; De Siqueira Júnior, J.P.; Iriti, M.; Varoni, E.M.; De Menezes, I.R.A.; Melo Coutinho, H.D.; Bezerra Morais-Braga, M.F. Effect of α-Bisabolol and Its β-Cyclodextrin Complex as TetK and NorA Efflux Pump Inhibitors in *Staphylococcus aureus* Strains. *Antibiotics (Basel),* **2020**, *9*(1), 28-36.
[http://dx.doi.org/10.3390/antibiotics9010028] [PMID: 31947642]

[136]   Solnier, J.; Martin, L.; Bhakta, S.; Bucar, F. Flavonoids as novel efflux pump inhibitors and antimicrobials against both environmental and pathogenic intracellular mycobacterial species. *Molecules,* **2020**, *25*(3), 734-746.
[http://dx.doi.org/10.3390/molecules25030734] [PMID: 32046221]

[137]   Lu, W.J.; Lin, H.J.; Hsu, P.H.; Lai, M.; Chiu, J.Y.; Lin, H.T.V. Brown and red seaweeds serve as potential efflux pump inhibitors for drug-resistant *Escherichia coli. Evid. Based Complement. Alternat. Med.,* **2019**, *2019*, 1-12.
[http://dx.doi.org/10.1155/2019/1836982] [PMID: 30713568]

[138]   Malaikozhundan, B.; Vaseeharan, B.; Vijayakumar, S.; Sudhakaran, R.; Gobi, N.; Shanthini, G. Antibacterial and antibiofilm assessment of Momordica charantia fruit extract coated silver nanoparticle. *Biocatal. Agric. Biotechnol.,* **2016**, *8*, 189-196.
[http://dx.doi.org/10.1016/j.bcab.2016.09.007]

[139]   Ferrer-Espada, R.; Shahrour, H.; Pitts, B.; Stewart, P.S.; Sánchez-Gómez, S.; Martínez-de-Tejada, G. A permeability-increasing drug synergizes with bacterial efflux pump inhibitors and restores susceptibility to antibiotics in multi-drug resistant *Pseudomonas aeruginosa* strains. *Sci. Rep.,* **2019**, *9*(1), 3452.
[http://dx.doi.org/10.1038/s41598-019-39659-4] [PMID: 30837499]

[140]   Lin, K.H.; Lo, C.C.; Chou, M.C.; Yeh, T.H.; Chen, K.L.; Liao, W.Y.; Lo, H.R. Synergistic actions of benzyl isothiocyanate with ethylenediaminetetraacetic acid and efflux pump inhibitor phenylalanine-arginine β-naphthylamide against multidrug-resistant *escherichia coli. Microb. Drug Resist.,* **2020**, *26*(5), 468-474.
[http://dx.doi.org/10.1089/mdr.2019.0118] [PMID: 31755808]

[141]   Hellewell, L.; Bhakta, S. Chalcones, stilbenes and ketones have anti-infective properties *via* inhibition of bacterial drug-efflux and consequential synergism with antimicrobial agents. *Access Microbiol.,* **2020**, *2*(4), acmi000105.
[http://dx.doi.org/10.1099/acmi.0.000105] [PMID: 33005869]

[142]   Zimmermann, S.; Klinger-Strobel, M.; Bohnert, J.A.; Wendler, S.; Rödel, J.; Pletz, M.W.; Löffler, B.;

Tuchscherr, L. Clinically approved drugs inhibit the *Staphylococcus aureus* multidrug NorA efflux pump and reduce biofilm formation. *Front. Microbiol.,* **2019**, *10*, 2762-2775.
[http://dx.doi.org/10.3389/fmicb.2019.02762] [PMID: 31849901]

[143] A Cordeiro, R.; Portela, F.V.M.; Pereira, L.M.G.; de Andrade, A.R.C.; de Sousa, J.K.; Aguiar, A.L.R.; Pergentino, M.L.M.; de Sales, G.S.; de Oliveira, J.S.; Medrano, D.J.A.; Brilhante, R.S.N.; Rocha, M.F.G.; SCM Castelo-Branco, D.; Sidrim, J.J.C. Efflux pump inhibition controls growth and enhances antifungal susceptibility of *Fusarium solani* species complex. *Future Microbiol.,* **2020**, *15*(1), 9-20.
[http://dx.doi.org/10.2217/fmb-2019-0186] [PMID: 32043371]

[144] Grimsey, E.M.; Fais, C.; Marshall, R.L.; Ricci, V.; Ciusa, M.L.; Stone, J.W.; Ivens, A.; Malloci, G.; Ruggerone, P.; Vargiu, A.V.; Piddock, L.J.V. Chlorpromazine and amitriptyline are substrates and inhibitors of the AcrB multidrug efflux pump. *MBio,* **2020**, *11*(3), e00465-20.
[http://dx.doi.org/10.1128/mBio.00465-20] [PMID: 32487753]

[145] Jose, J.; Anas, A.; Jose, B.; Puthirath, A.B.; Athiyanathil, S.; Jasmin, C.; Anantharaman, M.R.; Nair, S.; Subrahmanyam, C.; Biju, V. Extinction of antimicrobial resistant pathogens using silver embedded silica nanoparticles and an efflux pump blocker. *ACS Appl. Bio Mater.,* **2019**, *2*(11), 4681-4686.
[http://dx.doi.org/10.1021/acsabm.9b00614] [PMID: 35021465]

[146] Anuj, S.A.; Gajera, H.P.; Hirpara, D.G.; Golakiya, B.A. Bacterial membrane destabilization with cationic particles of nano-silver to combat efflux-mediated antibiotic resistance in Gram-negative bacteria. *Life Sci.,* **2019**, *230*, 178-187.
[http://dx.doi.org/10.1016/j.lfs.2019.05.072] [PMID: 31152810]

CHAPTER 5

Quercetin Chemistry, Structural Modifications, Sar Studies and Therapeutic Applications: An Update

Nazia Banday[1], Prince Ahad Mir[2], Mudasir Maqbool[3], Rafia Jan[4], Nyira Shafi[5], Roohi Mohi-ud-din[1,6,*] and Reyaz Hassan Mir[7,8,*]

[1] *Pharmacognosy and Phytochemistry Lab, Department of Pharmaceutical Sciences, University of Kashmir, Hazratbal, Srinagar-190006, Kashmir, India*

[2] *Khalsa College of Pharmacy, G.T. Road, Amritsar, 143002 Punjab, India*

[3] *Pharmacy Practice Division, Department of Pharmaceutical Sciences, University of Kashmir, Hazratbal, Srinagar, 190006, Kashmir, India*

[4] *Defence Research and Development Organization (DRDO), Hospital, Khonmoh, Srinagar 190001, Jammu & Kashmir, India*

[5] *Pharmacology Division, Department of Pharmaceutical Sciences, University of Kashmir, Hazratbal, Srinagar, 190006, Kashmir, India*

[6] *Sher-I-Kashmir Institute of Medical Sciences, Soura, Srinagar, Jammu, and Kashmir, India*

[7] *Pharmaceutical Chemistry Division, Chandigarh College of Pharmacy, Landran, Punjab-140301, India*

[8] *Pharmaceutical Chemistry Division, Department of Pharmaceutical Sciences, University of Kashmir, Hazratbal, Srinagar-190006, Kashmir, India*

Abstract: Natural products are investigated for their remunerative effects on health. Quercetin, a flavonoid, is commonly distributed in vegetables and fruits. Quercetin is used as a supplement in food and as a phytochemical remedy against several diseases, including circulatory dysfunction, neurodegeneration, diabetes, cancer, and inflammation. The most prominent property of quercetin is its antioxidant activity, enabling it to douse free radicals. Derivatives of quercetin are essential metabolites, and even various conjugates are being advocated by the Food and Drug Administration (FDA) for use in humans. So, the biosynthesis of quercetin derivatives is a predominant field of research. Methylation and glycosylation are two essential strategies used to synthesize various metabolites of quercetin that do not exist in nature. This review

---

* **Corresponding authors Roohi Mohi-ud-din and Reyaz Hassan Mir:** Pharmacognosy and Phytochemistry Lab, Department of Pharmaceutical Sciences, University of Kashmir, Hazratbal, Srinagar-190006, Kashmir, India; Tel: +917006320884; and Pharmaceutical Chemistry Division, Chandigarh College of Pharmacy, Landran, Punjab-140301, India; Tel: +917051433380; E-mails: roohisofi@gmail.com; reyazhassan249@gmail.com

Shazia Anjum (Ed.)

summmarizes quercetin chemistry, structural modifications, Structure-Activity Relationship (SAR) studies, and therapeutic applications of quercetin.

Keywords: Flavonoids, Quercetin Derivatives, Quercetin, SAR Studies, Therapeutic Applications.

1. INTRODUCTION TO FLAVONOIDS

Flavonoids are a group of plant-derived substances with a similar flavone structure. The basic skeleton comprises two aromatic rings (A and B) attached to a heterocyclic ring (C) that integrates the aromatic rings [1, 2] (Fig. **1**). Flavonoids are available in glycoside-bound and free aglycone [3, 4]. There are over 4,000 different types of flavonoids in nature, which are classified as anthocyanidins, flavones, chalcones, flavonols, and isoflavones. Flavonoids exhibit various pharmacological effects, such as antimicrobial, antioxidant, anti-inflammatory, and hepatoprotective [5 - 13].

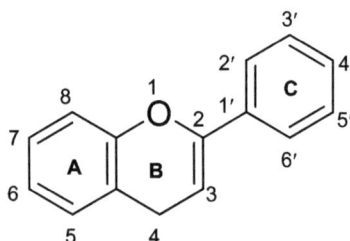

Fig. (1). Fundamental arrangement of flavonoid.

1.1. Quercetin Chemistry and Source

The chemical name for quercetin is (2-(3,4-dihydroxy phenyl)-3,5,7-trihydroxy-4-H chromen-4-one) Fig. (**2**) [14, 15]. The word Quercetin is derived from the Latin word Quercetum, which means oak forest. It has a yellow color to it. It is insoluble in cold water, slightly soluble in hot water, and entirely soluble in lipids and alcohol [16, 17]. It's one of the most potent antioxidants, usually found in edible plants [18 - 21]. Quercetin possesses many beneficial qualities, including anti-inflammatory, central nervous system stimulant, anticancer, and anti-infection [22]. Quercetin can also affect blood clotting *via* thrombin inhibition [23]. Quercetin has been shown to have neuroprotective properties in both *in-vivo* and *in-vitro* investigations [24]. Additionally, quercetin is used for ischemia [25], Huntington's disorder [26], and Parkinson's disorder [27].

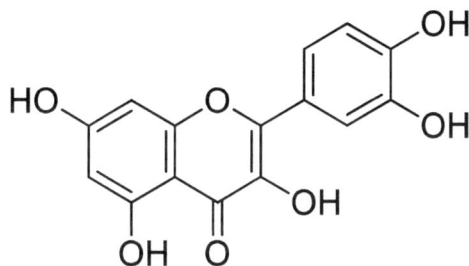

Fig. (2). Chemical structure of quercetin [14, 15].

Quercetin is a di-phenyl propane molecule with 15 carbon atoms in its structure. It is made up of two benzene rings and a pyran ring. 4-oxo-flavonoid is a flavonoid with a carbonyl group at the C-4 position in its 'C' ring. Flavonoids are divided into sub-classes based on pyran ring oxidation and substitutions, flavones, flavonols, flavanones, flavan-3-ols, flavonols, and isoflavones [28, 29]. With a chemical formula of $C_{15}H_{10}O_7$, quercetin belongs to the flavone subclass of flavonoids. According to IUPAC nomenclature, it is also known as 2-(3,--Dihydroxyphenyl)-5,7-dihydroxy-4H-1-benzopyran-4-one. Five hydroxyl groups can be found in quercetin at positions 3, 5, 7, 3', and 4'. It is an aglycone because quercetin lacks an associated sugar moiety. The production of glycosidic quercetin occurs when at position 3 hydroxyl group is replaced by glucose, galactose, rhamnose, or rutinose. Quercetin is water-insoluble or nearly insoluble. The addition of (glucose, rhamnose, or rutinose) to quercetin enhances its solubility in water thus, unlike quercetin, glycosidic quercetin is water-soluble [22, 30]. Due to numerous hydroxyl groups, it has been attributed to the cause of its photo-degradation, in addition to being responsible for its antioxidant capabilities. It has been claimed that the 3,3' and 4' positions hydroxyl groups are principally accountable for their photo-labile feature, while the hydroxyl groups at the 5 and 7 locations play no role [31]. Quercetin is well-known for its anti-inflammatory properties. In addition, glycosylated quercetin has been found to have lower anti-inflammatory properties than quercetin [32]. When quercetin is glycosylated at position 3, it loses its capacity to neutralize free radicals and inhibit Acetylcholine levels [33]. When quercetin is methylated at the 4' and 7' sites, its anticancer capabilities enhance. The metabolic stability of quercetin can be improved by replacing the hydroxyl group with an O-methylated group [34]. The presence of a double bond across carbon 2 and 3 in quercetin, as well as the hydroxyl group in the 'B' ring, is critical for thrombin inhibition. When hydroxyl groups in the 'B' and 'C' rings are replaced with methoxy groups, the inhibiting activity of thrombin is reduced, but replacing hydroxyl groups in the 'A' ring with methoxy groups increases the inhibitory activity of thrombin [35]. Due to the catechol group in the 'B' ring, a 2,3 double bond in the 'C' ring, and a hydroxyl group at C-3 position, quercetin leads to oxidative stress by increasing Reactive oxygen species (ROS) generation and reactive metabolites [36]. *In-vitro* investigations have shown that substituting hydroxyl groups at positions 3, 5, and 7, substituting methoxy groups or hydrogen atoms at position 3', and substituting hydroxyl or methoxy groups at the 4' position can boost quercetin's neuroprotective activity [37, 38].

The glycosides isoquercetin, rutin, and hyperin are the most abundant forms of quercetin found in vascular plants. It was isolated in its natural state from various plant components, including leaves, buds, and fruits. Compositae, Solanaceae, Rhamnaceae, and Passiflora are just a few of the families that contain a significant quantity of quercetin (Table **1**) [39]. Apples, asparagus, berries, capers, red-leaf lettuce, and onion contain a significantly higher concentration of quercetin [19, 38, 40]. It has been shown that when quercetin is held at elevated temperatures, the amount of quercetin is significantly reduced. For example, onions stored at a temperature of 100°C lost approximately 25% to 33% of their quercetin concentration. On the other hand, strawberries were found to contain more quercetin after being stored at 20°C for nine months. It was discovered to have increased by approximately 32%. Additionally, it was observed that plants exposed to UV light had a higher quercetin concentration than plants grown in greenhouses [41]. Tomatoes cultivated conventionally contain less quercetin than those grown organically [23].

Table 1. Various plant sources of quercetin.

S.No.	Common Name	Botanical Name	Active Parts and Family	Quercetin Content (mg/100g)	Ref.
1.	Apple	*Malus domestica*	Fruits, Rosaceae	4.42	[42]
2.	Blueberries	*Vaccinium angustifolium*	Fruits, Ericaceae	2.70	[43, 44]
3.	Buckthorn	*Rhamnus alaternus*	Bark, Rhamnaceae	19.37	[45]
4.	Chicory	*Cichorium intybus*	Leaves, Compositae	-	[46]
5.	Cranberries, raw	*Vaccinium subg. Oxycoccus*	Fruits	15.09	[47]]
6.	Drumstick tree	*Moringa oleifera*	Leaves, Moringaceae	-	[48, 49]
7.	Goldenrod	*Solidago canadensis*	Flowering parts, Compositae	-	[50]
8.	Grapevines	*Vitis vinifera*	Fruits, Vitaceae	2.32	[45, 51]
9.	Green tea	*Camellia sinensis*	Leaves, Theaceae	2.69	[52, 53]
10.	Mahkotadewa	*Phaleria macrocarpa*	Seeds, Thymelaceae	-	[54]
11.	Maidenhair tree	*Ginkgo biloba*	Leaves, Ginkgoaceae	-	[55]
12.	Mango	*Mangifera indica*	Fruits, Anacardiaceae	-	[56]

(Table 1) cont.....

S.No.	Common Name	Botanical Name	Active Parts and Family	Quercetin Content (mg/100g)	Ref.
13.	Pepper weed	*Lepidium latifolium*	Roots and leaves, Brassicaceae	-	[57, 58]
14.	Passionflower	*Passiflora incarnate*	Leaves, Passifloraceae	-	[59]
15.	Pomegranate	*Punica granatum*	Fruits, Lythraceae	0.77	[60]
16.	Quince	*Cydonia oblonga*	Fruits and leaves, Rosaceae	-	[61]
17.	Red onion	*Allium cepa*	Fruits, Amaryllidaceae	13.27	[62, 63]
18.	Rue	*Ruta graveolens*	Leaves, Rutaceae	-	[60]
19.	Sapodilla	*Achras sapota)*	Fruits, Sapotaceae	-	[58]
20.	Spinach	*Spinacia oleracea*	Leaves	27.2	[64]
21.	Tomato	*Solanum lycopersicum*	Fruits, Solanaceae	0.5	[65]
22.	Yarrow	*Achillea millefolium*	Flowering tops, Compositae	5.67	[66]
23.	Fennel leaves	*Foeniculum vulgare*	Leaves	46.8	[67]

1.2. Structure of Quercetin and Its Derivatives

Nobel Prize winner Albert Szent Gyorgyi first revealed nutritional flavonoids in 1936 and were extensively documented for their latent effects on humans. Quercetin, a top class of flavonoids, is mainly present in vegetables and fruits and is one of the most effective antioxidants of polyphenols [68]. Quercetin has also been reported to possess potent antibacterial, antiviral, and anti-carcinogenic potency [69]. Numerous quercetin conjugates are synthesized by glycosylating these OH groups. Isoquercetin structurally contains glucose bonded at position 3 of quercetin, while as in hyperoside (quercetin 3-O-galactoside), the same position is substituted by galactose. Similarly, quercetin 7-O-rhamnoside and quercetin 3-O-rhamnoside can be synthesized by substituting rhamnosyl at 3-OH or 7-OH, respectively.

Various quercetin conjugates have disaccharides, like rutinose, a combination of glucose and rhamnose, and are labeled as α-L-rhamnopyranosyl-(1 → 6)- β---glucopyranose. When rutinose is substituted at 3-OH in quercetin leads to the synthesis of the vital compound rutin. Similarly, avicularin a quercetin conjugate has arabinofuranose at 3-OH position. Some quercetin conjugates contain more than two sugar molecules, *e.g.*, enzymatically modified isoquercitrin (EMIQ), possess 10 glucose molecules substituted at 3-OH in quercetin structure and oligoglucosylated rutin, that have 5 glucose molecules bonded with glucose residue of rutin.

Various quercetin conjugates are also methyl-substituted, *e.g.*, quercetin 4$'$-methyl ether, tamrixetin, substituted with an additional methyl moiety at the 4th position. Similarly, rhamnetin (7$'$-*O*-methoxy quercetin possesses a methyl group at position 7-OH. Furthermore, rhamnazin, and dimethylated quercetin were substituted with two methyl moieties at positions 3$'$ and 7-OH. Isorhamnetin, a methyl-substituted flavonol, can be converted into isorhamnetin 3-O-rutinosi-e-4'-O-glucoside, isorhamnetin 3-O-rutinoside-7-O-glucoside, and isorhamnetin 3-O-rutinoside by glycosylation process. Several other quercetin conjugates have methyl and glycosyl substituted at OH groups in quercetin structure, *e.g.*, tamarixetin 3-O-β-D-glucoside that possesses glucose at 3rd position while methyl at 4$'$ position. Structures of certain specified quercetin derivatives are given in Fig. (**3**) [70].

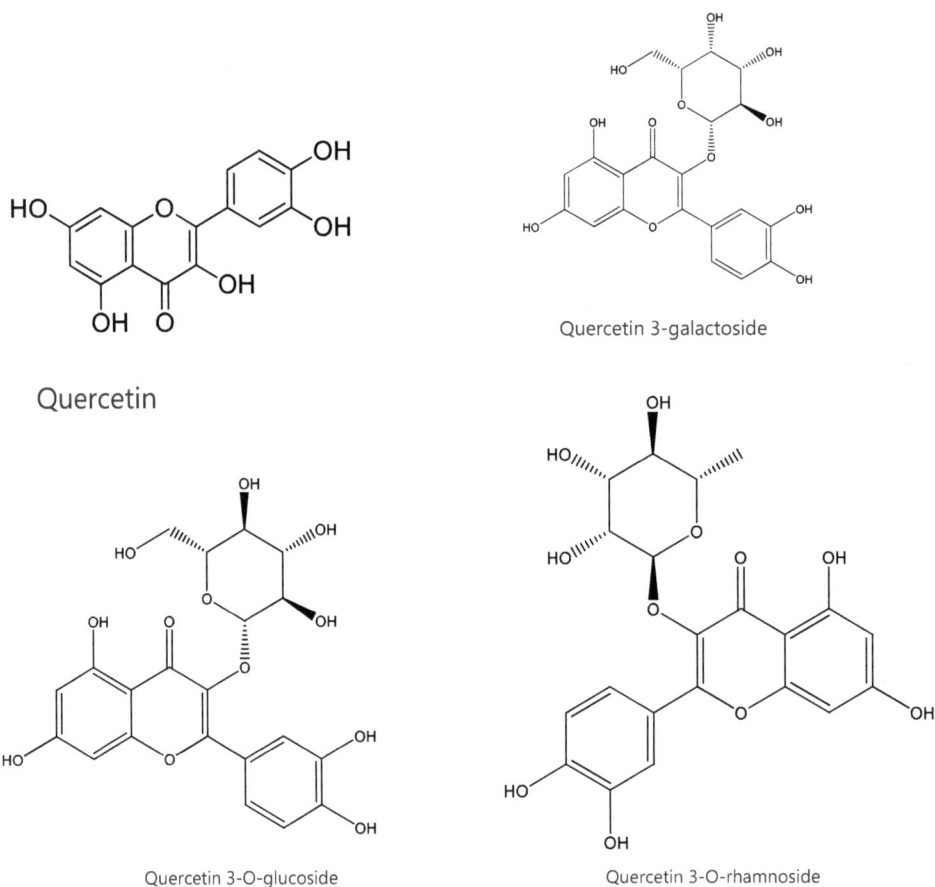

Quercetin

Quercetin 3-galactoside

Quercetin 3-O-glucoside

Quercetin 3-O-rhamnoside

(Fig. 3) contd.....

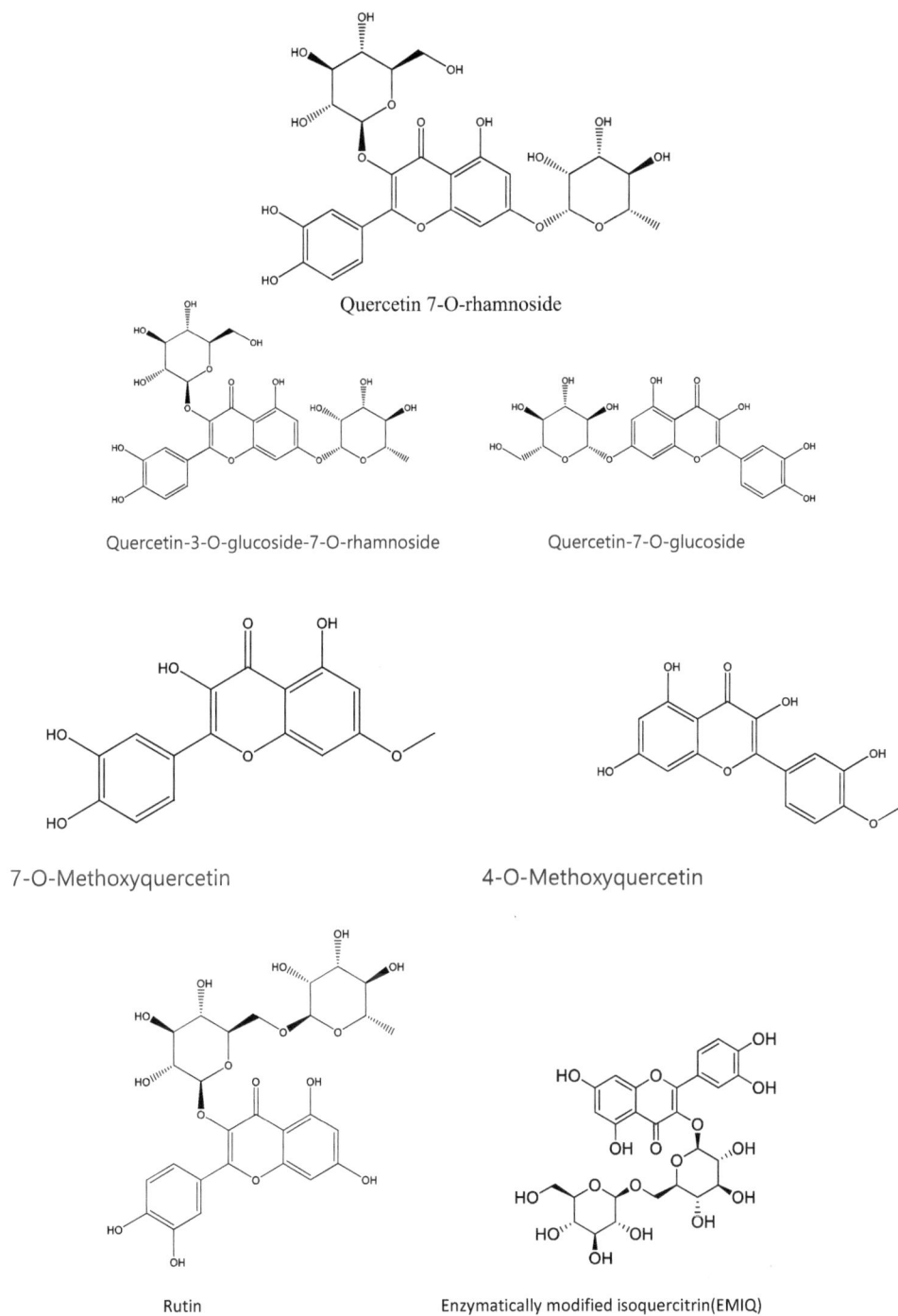

Quercetin 7-O-rhamnoside

Quercetin-3-O-glucoside-7-O-rhamnoside

Quercetin-7-O-glucoside

7-O-Methoxyquercetin

4-O-Methoxyquercetin

Rutin

Enzymatically modified isoquercitrin(EMIQ)

Fig. (3). Structure of quercetin and some of its derivatives.

2. SAR OF QUERCETIN AND ITS DERIVATIVES

Quercetin and its derivatives have revealed various health-related issues, predominantly due to variations at the vital locations of quercetin structure. Typically, the OH groups at positions number 3 and 7 in the quercetin structure are modified with glycosides. However, at positions 3′, 4′ and position 7, methylation is commonly preferred. Lesjak *et al.* demonstrated the structure-activity relationship between quercetin and its six conjugates and evaluated their anti-inflammatory and antioxidant potency. They revealed that chemically changing OH groups in quercetin decreased its antioxidant potency and reported that the OH group at position 3 is vital for antioxidant potency. On the other hand, no direct connection was found between the extent of quercetin-free hydroxyl groups and inflammatory mediator's inhibition potency. They also reported that tamarixetin, a monomethylated quercetin has potent anti-inflammatory potency compared to quercetin and its other conjugates [71, 72]. Santos *et al.* studied the lipid peroxidation inhibition potency and mitochondrial membrane permeability transition (MMPT) of eight chemically correlated flavonoids in rat liver mitochondria. They reported that substituting multiple methyl groups with hydroxyl groups enhances the lipid peroxidation inhibition potency and decreases the effect on mitochondrial respiration [73]. Similarly, Lee *et al.* studied the anti-obesity potential of quercetin aglycon (Quer) and quercetin 3-*O*-glycoside (Q3G) and reported that Q3G possesses a more potent anti-obesity effect than Quercetin, which is facilitated through lipogenesis and adipocyte differentiation inhibition, reducing serum lipids and decreasing body weight gain [74].

Briefly, quercetin and its conjugates are essential substances having different activities and potencies. In addition, an individual component can be used pharmacologically due to extraordinary biological potency. Therefore, for the synthesis of dynamic conjugates, alteration in quercetin structure is necessary and for which hydroxylation, glycosylation, and methylation are some vital reactions. These reactions yield various quercetin conjugates that are not only new but are also potent and have a wide range of pharmacological activity. Similarly, the structural activity relationship study of quercetin and its conjugates gives essential knowledge about the increased potency of the conjugates with the least side effects. Still, a lot of work has to be done to discover various techniques by which a parent molecule is modified to new conjugates and to understand the efficacy of conjugates with the modification in structure. This can also provide a new field of research to numerous investigators.

3. QUERCETIN: THERAPEUTIC APPLICATIONS

3.1. Alzheimer's Disease

Quercetin (Qu) was found to abolish the pathological hallmarks of (AD) and improve cognitive function in a transgenic mouse model. Reduction in β-amyloidosis and tauopathy was observed as depicted by a decrease in the levels of amyloid β [75]. Quercetin prevented the hyperphosphorylation of tau proteins induced by (OA) in HT22 cells by altering MAPKs and PI3K/Akt/GSK signaling cascade [76]. Quercetin (Qu) improved the cognitive function in the PPswe/PS1dE9 transgenic mouse model of AD by decreasing the plaque burden and preventing mitochondrial dysfunction by activating the AMPK pathway [77].

3.2. Cancer

3.2.1. Colorectal Cancer

Yang *et al.* evaluated the anticancer activity of quercetin in the HT-29 colon cancer cell line and reported the decrease in viability in these cell lines. The apoptosis mediated by quercetin was observed due to the inhibitory effect on the Akt-CSN6-Myc signaling cascade [78]. Quercetin exerts significant anticancer potential against colon cancer cell lines, CACO-2, and SW-620 cells. The apoptosis was due to a suppressive effect on the NF-κB pathway and reduction in the level of Bcl2 and upregulated Bax expression [79]. Further quercetin increased TRIAL-mediated apoptosis by redistributing DR4 and DR5 into lipid rafts [80].

3.2.2. Gastric Cancer

Quercetin restricted the growth of (GCSCs) by triggering the intrinsic apoptotic pathway and inhibiting the PI3K/Akt cascade. Molecular analysis revealed the increased expression of caspase-3 and -9, Bax, and cytochrome c and a reduction in Bcl-2 expression and Akt [81]. The antimetastatic potential of quercetin in gastric cancer cells was observed by modulating the expression of NF-κb, PKC-δ, ERK1/2, and AMPKα [82]. Moreover, the study by wang *et al.* also showed the anticancer potential of quercetin in AGS and MKN28 cell lines through alteration of Akt-mTOR signaling and hypoxia-induced factor 1α (HIF-1α) signaling [83].

3.2.3. Prostate Cancer

The subjection of PCa cells to varying concentrations of quercetin revealed the decrease in cell viability in a dose and time-dependent manner relative to the control groups. However, no effect was observed on normal prostate cells. Quercetin induces apoptosis and necrosis in PCa cells by influencing the mitochondrial structural integrity and impairment in ROS homeostasis, ultimately leading to PCa cell death [84]. Quercetin exhibits anticancer potential in the LNCaP prostate cancer cell line by suppressing the expression of androgen receptors apart from their activity in these cells. The androgen receptors are key players responsible for the growth and progression of prostate cancer [85].

3.2.4. Lung Cancer

Quercetin has been proven to possess a suppressive effect on lung cancer cells in both *in-vivo* and *in-vitro* through an inhibitory effect on the expression of aurora B. Aurora B is a serine-threonine kinase, overexpression of which is observed in certain cancers including lung cancer and it facilitates tumorigenesis and progression of cancer cells [86]. Yang *et al.* further authenticated the anticancer activity of quercetin glucuronides in NCI-H209. Quercetin suppressed the proliferation of NCI-H209 cells through the arrest of the cell cycle at the G2/M phase and apoptosis by triggering the release of apoptotic proteins such as caspases [87].

3.2.5. Breast Cancer

Quercetin attacks and demolishes breast cancer stem cells by decreasing the expression of (ALDH1A1), (CXCR4), Mucin 1 (MUC1), and (EpCAM) [88]. Chein *et al.* evaluated the activity of quercetin in the MDA-MB-231 breast cancer cell line. They concluded apoptotic mediated cancer cell death is depicted by an increase in the expression of caspases (caspase 3, 8, and 9). Further, increase in the expression of pro-apoptotic proteins (Bax) and a reduced expression of antiapoptotic proteins (Bcl-2) [89]. Moreover, it was observed that quercetin enhances the cytotoxic efficiency of Topotecan by about 1.3 fold in the MDA-MB-231 cell line and 1.4 fold in the MCF-7 cell line [90].

3.2.6. Pancreatic Cancer

Quercetin induces apoptotic cell death in pancreatic cancer cell growth both *in-vitro* and *in-vivo*. Quercetin negatively impacts pancreatic cancer stem cells through inhibition of proliferation, invasion, and self-renewal ability of these cells stem cells, which were mainly attributed to the changes in the levels of β-catenin [91].

3.3. Cardiovascular Disease

A study by Nickel *et al.* concluded that the immunoregulatory activity of quercetin is responsible for the anti-atherosclerotic activity of quercetin [92]. Quercetin revealed a protective effect against myocardial ischemic and reperfusion injury in a rat model through an inhibitory effect on the expression of IL-10, TNF-α, and other inflammatory cytokines [93]. Another study also concluded that quercetin's role in managing acute myocardial damage is attributed to its antioxidant, antiapoptotic, and anti-inflammatory properties. The decreased expression of inflammatory markers such as TNF-α and IL-1β and oxidative markers such as SOD and CAT were significantly reduced in the quercetin treatment group [94]. Moreover, quercetin alone or in combination with atorvastatin was identified as an encouraging cardioprotective agent in the treatment of myocardial ischemia [95]. Quercetin revealed the cardioprotective effect in cardiac fibrosis caused by isoproterenol in a rat model. The effect was more pronounced than its glycosidic derivative rutin [96]. The doxorubicin-induced cytotoxic effect in H9C2 cells was decreased by quercetin, and enhancement in the repair system in these cardiomyocytes was also observed [97].

3.4. Anti-inflammatory Activity

Quercetin is a flavonoid with unusual biological properties which can enhance cognitive and emotional efficiency and also prevent infection [22, 98]. Quercetin has been described as a strong anti-inflammatory agent with a high propensity to counter inflammation [22, 99, 100]. It has anti-inflammatory properties, which could be displayed in various cell types within both human as well as animal models [22]. Various laboratory studies have elucidated that quercetin inhibits the production of various factors such as lipopolysaccharide (LPS)- induced tumor necrosis factor α within macrophagic cells and the development of LPS in the lung cells (A549) induced by IL-8 [22, 101]. Quercetin can prevent Interleukin (IL)-1α levels of LPS-mediated mRNA and TNF-alpha, leading to decreased apoptotic neuronal injury due to microglial activation [101, 102]. Quercetin prevents the production of enzymes that produce inflammation (lipoxygenase (LOX) and cyclooxygenase (COX)) [22, 103, 104]. By inhibiting the production of Syk-and Src-induced (PI3K)-(p85) tyrosine phosphorylation and the resulting Toll-Like Receptor 4 (TLR4)/MyD88/PI3K cluster, it limits LPS-induced inflammatory response, which inhibits signaling pathway stimulation related with RAW 264.7 cells [22, 105]. The assessment of the inflammatory response caused by quercetin *versus* H_2O_2 showed the potential benefits of quercetin in human endothelial vein umbilical cells (HUVECs) on inflammatory response [22, 106].

In conjunction with pretreatment with quercetin, apoptotic cell death was significantly exacerbated as calculated by the immunoblotting of caspase 3 and cleaved caspase 3 activity. In addition, Quercetin suppresses the phosphorylation of 2 kinases (LPS-induced), such as p38 MAP and (JNK/SAPK) kinase, enzymes involved in cell growth inhibition, analogous to apoptosis activation [107, 108]. The research concluded that by increasing cytokine secretion, quercetin exerted a defensive role against irradiation-induced inflammation in rodents [22, 109]. Quercetin reduced histopathological clinical manifestations of inflammation of acute nature in animals treated by blocking the mobilization of leukocytes, reducing the levels of chemokines and lipid peroxidation of the end-product malondialdehyde and antioxidative action in the experimental rat model [22, 110]. Quercetin has improved allergic encephalomyelitis (EAE) by the suppression of Th 1 differentiation and IL-12 signaling [22, 111] and In Dark Agouti rats, experimental autoimmune myocarditis (EAM) interferes with the development of anti-inflammatory (IL-10) cytokines and/or proinflammatory (IL-17 and TNF-alpha) [22, 112]. The accumulation and activation of immune cells, including anti-inflammatory cells, is most certainly reliably blocked by Quercetin, whereas genetic appearance correlated with mitochondrial oxidative phosphorylation in experimental mice on a specific diet is explicitly enhanced. Reduction in oxidative stress and κB-NF function may have been attributed to the avoidance of immune cell aggregation and induction in experimental mice which were on a specific diet and chronic epididymal adipose tissue inflammation [22, 113]. The anti-inflammatory function of quercetin is consistent with its free radical-scavenging and antioxidant effects in several studies [114 - 116]. In addition, the development of TNF-α cytokines could be induced by NF-κB [116, 117]. Elimination of reactive species of oxygen could thus prevent oxidation and simultaneously prevent inflammation [116]. In summary, these results indicate that, at most in coronary inflammatory diseases, quercetin may function as an important protective agent [107, 108].

3.5. Anti-Diabetic Activity

Quercetin is implicated in many biological processes, including glucose homeostasis, utilizing glucose in peripheral tissues, sensitizing and secreting insulin, and inhibiting the absorption of intestinal glucose [118, 119]. The latest detailed meta-analysis and review of animal research found that at doses of 10 mg/kg, 25mg/kg, and 50 mg/kg body weight, quercetin reduces serum glucose levels [119, 120]. Quercetin is derived from berries, which slows down the oxygen intake of adenosine diphosphate by activating GLUT 4 efflux and development in isolated mitochondria, stimulating (AMPK) cascade. This pathway has a metformin-like effect [119, 121]. The antihyperglycemic function of quercetin includes GLUT2 glucose absorption, phosphoinositide 3-kinase activation (PI3K) suppression, and the reduction of insulin-based lipid peroxidation [122]. Glucokinase development, GLUT 4-stimulating hyperglycemia, glycogenolysis, and hepatic gluconeogenesis are decreased by the treatment of streptozotocin (STZ)-induced diabetic rats using quercetin, thereby increasing liver glucose metabolism [119, 123]. Quercetin supplementation reduced blood glucose levels for two weeks, improved gene expression associated with cell survival and liver proliferation, as well as elevated serum insulin in diabetic STZ-induced mice [119, 124]. Intraperitoneal infusion of quercetin into diabetic STZ-induced rats showed a decline in high blood sugar, triglycerides and plasma cholesterol, increased glucose resistance and hepatic glucokinase action [119, 125]. Co-treating with sitagliptin (a selective inhibitor of dipeptidyl peptidase-IV) and quercetin has shown improved performance in oxidative and inflammatory conditions, metabolic activity, blood glucose control, the activity of pancreatic cells, and islet framework in STZ-mediated diabetes mellitus in experimental rats [119, 126]. Quercetin prevents the activity of an inhibitor of tyrosine kinase, which has shown an influence on diabetes [119, 127]. The hypolipidemic, hypoglycemic, and antioxidant implications of supplementation quercetin have recently been explored in the type 2 diabetes mellitus animal model. Quercetin can also be effective in growing type 2 diabetes mellitus hyperglycemia, metabolic syndrome, and oxidative stress [108, 128]. However, quercetin's antidiabetic function is stated to be achieved from a cellular perspective by enhancing the metabolism of glucose by an insulin-independent process that involves (AMPK) whose stimulation in the muscle tissues ends in the translocation of the GLUT4 glucose transporter to the surface of the cell while AMPK decreases in the liver cell [108, 125].

3.6. Antioxidant Activity of Quercetin

Fascinatingly, Quercetin's health advantages are a result of its antioxidant action since it has been demonstrated to decrease oxidative stress [129]. Quercetin has been described as a powerful antioxidant due to its ability to neutralize oxidizing agents such as $ONOO^-$, O_2, and NO [130]. To avoid the toxicity of quercetin metabolic products, it should be taken in combination with other antioxidants, including glutathione and ascorbate [131]. The signaling mechanism involved in protection against oxidative stress is the interaction of Nrf2 with antioxidant response elements. According to Dong *et al.*, Quercetin is believed to activate the Nrf2-ARE pathway, resulting in the upregulation of antioxidant enzymes including catalase, glutathione reductase (RS), (HO-1), (GST), thioredoxin reductase (TrxR) and superoxide dismutase (SOD) [132, 133]. Quercetin's anti-oncogenic effect has been demonstrated because it is a good iron chelator, avoiding cell damage caused by iron overload [134]. Quercetin lowers plasma LDL levels by avoiding lipid peroxidation and boosting the production of glutathione, reducing the likelihood of atherosclerotic plaque development and, as a result, lowering the risk of coronary heart disease [135, 136]. Quercetin protects cells from cellular damage caused by radiation and other carcinogens by acting as a free radical scavenger and increasing endogenous antioxidant levels. Quercetin has a strong anti-carcinogenic impact on colon, lung, prostate, cervical, liver, and breast carcinomas. This *in-vivo* investigation on Quercetin-treated rats revealed a significant reduction in lipid peroxidation and hydrogen peroxide levels, as well as an increase in glutathione levels, indicating Quercetin's anticancer action [137]. Quercetin is beneficial in the treatment of neurodegenerative diseases such as Parkinson's and Alzheimer's disease by reducing lipid membrane damage in the brain [101, 138]. Concurrent investigations established that Quercetin protects rats' brains and diabetic neuropathy retinas from oxidative stress produced by acrylamide and cadmium fluoride [139]. Quercetin functions as a nephropro-tective and hepatoprotective agent against kidney and Liver damage caused by sodium fluoride and tertiary butyl hydrogen peroxide in rats, as evidenced by *in-vivo* investigations [140, 141]. Glutathione regulates calcium absorption in the intestines. However, owing to oxidative stress, the amount of glutathione in the gut decreases, inhibiting calcium absorption, whereas Quercetin also keeps redox balance in the gut and improves absorption of calcium from the intestines, according to research [142]. Moreover, Quercetin generates an antioxidant defence mechanism that protects the body from oxidative damage caused by smoking and exercise [141, 143]. In the enterocytes and the liver, quercetin undergoes substantial metabolization, resulting in the formation of many metabolites. With these modifications, quercetin can be glucuronidated, sulfated, and methylated. Furthermore, quercetin undergoes *in-vivo* oxidation, resulting in the formation of quercetin-quinone and quercetin-quinone methide [144, 145].

3.7. ANTIOBESITY

Obesity is a pathophysiological condition of the body characterized by oxidative stress induced by an excess of (ROS) such as peroxyl and hydrogen peroxide [146]. The antioxidant property of quercetin has been proven to have anti-obesity properties. According to reports, quercetin works as an anti-obesity drug by suppressing the gene expression of various enzymes and receptors, such as PPAR-γ and FAS, as well as the activity of Acetyl-CoA carboxylase (ACC), causing lipogenesis and adipogenesis to be disrupted [147]. Data revealed that Quercetin greatly increases the AMPK signal pathway while concurrently reducing phosphorylation of JNK and ERK, resulting in apoptosis and antilipogenesis activities [148 - 150]. Results reveal a marked decline in glucose absorption and cell proliferation in Quercetin-treated rat adipocytes and 3T3 L1 preadipocytes *in-vitro* [151, 152]. Additionally, studies have shown that Quercetin increases (NF-kB) regulation and decreases proinflammatory factors and cytokines, making it an excellent treatment for hyperlipidemia [153, 154]. According to researchers, the molecular mechanism underlying Quercetin's anti-obesity action is that it regulates hepatic gene expression associated with fat metabolism [155]. *In-vivo* experiments on mice, Quercetin administration significantly reduced obesity generated by a high-fat diet, body weight, and liver weight and also significantly decreased the HFD-induced increase in serum lipid profile and TBARS [156]. Additional research on HFD mice indicated that Quercetin inhibits lipogenesis by activating the AMPK/PPAR-γ pathway and thereby targeting the few proteins UCP1 in white/brown adipose tissues [157, 158].

CONCLUSION

From the past few years, naturally occurring bioactive molecules have gotten wider attention due to their potential health benefits, and Quercetin is one such example having immense therapeutic potential present in various food products that exhibit tremendous biological activities, including anti-inflammatory, anti-obesity, antioxidant, anti-diabetic, anticancer, and CVD. Quercetin has also been reported for its neuroprotective action against various neurodegenerative diseases. Moreover, quercetin derivatives are important metabolites that have high biological activity. So the generation of these active metabolites by modification of quercetin with reactions like methylations, glycosylation, and hydroxylations is essential. Glycosylation produces quercetin derivatives having sugar units at various hydroxyl groups that create novel metabolites and increased activity. Furthermore, SAR studies of quercetin and its derivatives also provide information for increasing the efficacy of the metabolites with reduced toxicity. So more work needs to be done in the future in order to understand the change in the activity of metabolites with the change in structure.

CONSENT FOR PUBLICATION

Not applicable.

CONFLICT OF INTEREST

The authors declare no conflict of interest, financial or otherwise.

ACKNOWLEDGEMENTS

The Authors acknowledge Chandigarh College of Pharmacy for providing the necessary facilities to carry out this work.

REFERENCES

[1]   Haddad, P.; Eid, H. The Antidiabetic Potential of Quercetin: Underlying Mechanisms. *Curr. Med. Chem.,* **2017**, *24*(4), 355-364.
        [http://dx.doi.org/10.2174/0929867323666160909153707] [PMID: 27633685]

[2]   Mir, R.H.; Masoodi, M.H.J.C.B.C. Anti-inflammatory plant polyphenolics and cellular action mechanisms **2020**, *16*(6), 809-817.
        [http://dx.doi.org/10.2174/1573407215666190419205317]

[3]   Ross, J.A.; Kasum, C.M. Dietary flavonoids: bioavailability, metabolic effects, and safety. *Annu. Rev. Nutr.,* **2002**, *22*(1), 19-34.
        [http://dx.doi.org/10.1146/annurev.nutr.22.111401.144957] [PMID: 12055336]

[4]   Ulusoy, H.G.; Sanlier, N. A minireview of quercetin: from its metabolism to possible mechanisms of its biological activities. *Crit. Rev. Food Sci. Nutr.,* **2020**, *60*(19), 3290-3303.
        [http://dx.doi.org/10.1080/10408398.2019.1683810] [PMID: 31680558]

[5]   Kandaswami, C.; Lee, L.T.; Lee, P.P.; Hwang, J.J.; Ke, F.C.; Huang, Y.T.; Lee, M.T. The antitumor activities of flavonoids. *in vivo.,* **2005**, *19*(5), 895-909.
        [PMID: 16097445]

[6]   Rauf, A.; Imran, M.; Khan, I.A.; ur-Rehman, M.; Gilani, S.A.; Mehmood, Z.; Mubarak, M.S. Anticancer potential of quercetin: A comprehensive review. *Phytother. Res.,* **2018**, *32*(11), 2109-2130.
        [http://dx.doi.org/10.1002/ptr.6155] [PMID: 30039547]

[7]   Mir, P. A. Anticancer Potential of Thymoquinone: A Novel Bioactive Natural Compound from *Nigella sativa* L *Anti-Can. Agents. Med. Chem.,* **2022**, *22*(20).
        [http://dx.doi.org/10.2174/1871520622666220511233314]

[8]   Mir, R.H. Resveratrol: a potential drug candidate with multispectrum therapeutic application. *Studies. Nat. Products. Chem.,* **2022**, *Vol. 73*, 99-137.

[9]   Mir, R.H. Curcumin as a privileged scaffold molecule for various biological targets in drug development. *Stud. Nat. Prod. Chem.,* **2022**, *73*, 405-434.
        [http://dx.doi.org/10.1016/B978-0-323-91097-2.00010-8]

[10]   Mir, R.H. Isoflavones of Soy: Chemistry and Health Benefits. In: *Edible Plants in Health and Diseases*; Springer, **2022**; pp. 303-324.
        [http://dx.doi.org/10.1007/978-981-16-4880-9_13]

[11]   Mir, R.H. *Nigella sativa* as a therapeutic candidate for arthritis and related disorders. In: *Black Seeds (Nigella Sativa)*; Elsevier, **2022**; pp. 295-312.

[12]   Mohi-Ud-Din, R.; Mir, R. H.; Sabreen, S.; Jan, R.; Pottoo, F. H.; Singh, I. P. Recent Insights into Therapeutic Potential of Plant-Derived Flavonoids against Cancer. *Anticancer. AgentS. Med. Chem.,* **2022**, *22*(20), 3343-3369.
        [http://dx.doi.org/10.2174/1871520622666220421094055]

[13]   Mohi-Ud-Din, R. Berberine in the Treatment of Neurodegenerative Diseases and Nanotechnology Enabled Targeted Delivery. *Comb. Chem. High. Throughput. Screen.,* **2022**, *25*(4), 616-633.
        [http://dx.doi.org/10.2174/1386207324666210804122539]

[14]   Parasuraman, S.; Anand David, A.V.; Arulmoli, R. Overviews of biological importance of quercetin: A bioactive flavonoid. *Pharmacogn. Rev.,* **2016**, *10*(20), 84-89.
        [http://dx.doi.org/10.4103/0973-7847.194044] [PMID: 28082789]

[15] D'Andrea, G. Quercetin: A flavonol with multifaceted therapeutic applications? *Fitoterapia.,* **2015**, *106*, 256-271.
[http://dx.doi.org/10.1016/j.fitote.2015.09.018] [PMID: 26393898]

[16] Lakhanpal, P. Quercetin: A Versatile Flavonoid. *Int. J. Med. Update.,* **2007**, *2*(11), 01.
[http://dx.doi.org/10.4314/ijmu.v2i2.39851]

[17] Batiha, G.E.S.; Beshbishy, A.M.; Ikram, M.; Mulla, Z.S.; El-Hack, M.E.A.; Taha, A.E.; Algammal, A.M.; Elewa, Y.H.A. The Pharmacological Activity, Biochemical Properties, and Pharmacokinetics of the Major Natural Polyphenolic Flavonoid: Quercetin. *Foods.,* **2020**, *9*(3), 374.
[http://dx.doi.org/10.3390/foods9030374] [PMID: 32210182]

[18] Brüll, V.; Burak, C.; Stoffel-Wagner, B.; Wolffram, S.; Nickenig, G.; Müller, C.; Langguth, P.; Alteheld, B.; Fimmers, R.; Naaf, S.; Zimmermann, B.F.; Stehle, P.; Egert, S. Effects of a quercetin-rich onion skin extract on 24 h ambulatory blood pressure and endothelial function in overweight-t--obese patients with (pre-)hypertension: a randomised double-blinded placebo-controlled cross-over trial. *Br. J. Nutr.,* **2015**, *114*(8), 1263-1277.
[http://dx.doi.org/10.1017/S0007114515002950] [PMID: 26328470]

[19] Kim, D. H. MicroRNA targeting by quercetin in cancer treatment and chemoprotection. *Pharmacolog. Res.,* **2019**, 147.
[http://dx.doi.org/10.1016/j.phrs.2019.104346]

[20] Kawabata, K.; Mukai, R.; Ishisaka, A. Quercetin and related polyphenols: new insights and implications for their bioactivity and bioavailability. *Food Funct.,* **2015**, *6*(5), 1399-1417.
[http://dx.doi.org/10.1039/C4FO01178C] [PMID: 25761771]

[21] Harwood, M.; Danielewska-Nikiel, B.; Borzelleca, J.F.; Flamm, G.W.; Williams, G.M.; Lines, T.C. A critical review of the data related to the safety of quercetin and lack of evidence of *in vivo* toxicity, including lack of genotoxic/carcinogenic properties. *Food Chem. Toxicol.,* **2007**, *45*(11), 2179-2205.
[http://dx.doi.org/10.1016/j.fct.2007.05.015] [PMID: 17698276]

[22] Li, Y.; Yao, J.; Han, C.; Yang, J.; Chaudhry, M.; Wang, S.; Liu, H.; Yin, Y. Quercetin, inflammation and immunity. *Nutrients.,* **2016**, *8*(3), 167.
[http://dx.doi.org/10.3390/nu8030167] [PMID: 26999194]

[23] Kaneider, N.C.; Mosheimer, B.; Reinisch, N.; Patsch, J.R.; Wiedermann, C.J. Inhibition of thrombin-induced signaling by resveratrol and quercetin: effects on adenosine nucleotide metabolism in endothelial cells and platelet–neutrophil interactions. *Thromb Res.,* **2004**, *vol. 114*(3), 185-194.

[24] Rishitha, N.; Muthuraman, A. Therapeutic evaluation of solid lipid nanoparticle of quercetin in pentylenetetrazole induced cognitive impairment of zebrafish. *Life Sci.,* **2018**, *199*, 80-87.
[http://dx.doi.org/10.1016/j.lfs.2018.03.010] [PMID: 29522770]

[25] Li, X.; Wang, H.; Gao, Y.; Li, L.; Tang, C.; Wen, G.; Zhou, Y.; Zhou, M.; Mao, L.; Fan, Y. Protective Effects of Quercetin on Mitochondrial Biogenesis in Experimental Traumatic Brain Injury *via* the Nrf2 Signaling Pathway. *PLoS One.,* **2016**, *11*(10), e0164237.
[http://dx.doi.org/10.1371/journal.pone.0164237] [PMID: 27780244]

[26] Sandhir, R.; Mehrotra, A. Quercetin supplementation is effective in improving mitochondrial dysfunctions induced by 3-nitropropionic acid: Implications in Huntington's disease. *Biochim. Biophys. Acta Mol. Basis Dis.,* **2013**, *1832*(3), 421-430.
[http://dx.doi.org/10.1016/j.bbadis.2012.11.018] [PMID: 23220257]

[27] El-Horany, H. E.; El-latif, R. N. A.; ElBatsh, M. M.; Emam, M. N. Ameliorative Effect of Quercetin on Neurochemical and Behavioral Deficits in Rotenone Rat Model of Parkinson's Disease: Modulating Autophagy (Quercetin on Experimental Parkinson's Disease). *Parkinsons Dis.,* **2016**, *30*(7), 360-369.

[28] Rosa, L.A.l.; Alvarez-Parrilla, E.; González-Aguilar, G.A. Fruit and vegetable phytochemicals: hemistry, nutritional value, and stability 2010. http://site.ebrary.com/id/10342780
[http://dx.doi.org/10.1002/jbt.21821]

[29]   Aherne, S. A.; O'Brien, N. M. Dietary flavonols: chemistry, food content, and metabolism. *Nutrition.,* **2002**, *18*(1), 75-81.
[http://dx.doi.org/10.1016/S0899-9007(01)00695-5]

[30]   Kumar, S.; Sharma, H.; Yadav, K. Quercetin and metabolic syndrome. *EJPMR.,* **2016**, *3*(5), 701-709.

[31]   Dall'Acqua, S.; Miolo, G.; Innocenti, G.; Caffieri, S. The photodegradation of quercetin: relation to oxidation. *Molecules.,* **2012**, *17*(8), 8898-8907.
[http://dx.doi.org/10.3390/molecules17088898] [PMID: 22836209]

[32]   Kim, H.P.; Son, K.H.; Chang, H.W.; Kang, S.S. Anti-inflammatory plant flavonoids and cellular action mechanisms. *J. Pharmacol. Sci.,* **2004**, *96*(3), 229-245.
[http://dx.doi.org/10.1254/jphs.CRJ04003X] [PMID: 15539763]

[33]   Ganeshpurkar, A.; Saluja, A.K. The Pharmacological Potential of Rutin. *Saudi Pharm. J.,* **2017**, *25*(2), 149-164.
[http://dx.doi.org/10.1016/j.jsps.2016.04.025] [PMID: 28344465]

[34]   Shi, Z.H.; Li, N.G.; Tang, Y.P.; Shi, Q.P.; Tang, H.; Li, W.; Zhang, X.; Fu, H.A.; Duan, J.A. Biological evaluation and SAR analysis of O-methylated analogs of quercetin as inhibitors of cancer cell proliferation. *Drug Dev. Res.,* **2014**, *75*(7).
[http://dx.doi.org/10.1002/ddr.21181] [PMID: 24976071]

[35]   Shi, Z.H.; Li, N.G.; Tang, Y.P.; Wei-Li, ; Lian-Yin, ; Yang, J.P.; Hao-Tang, ; Duan, J.A. Metabolism-based synthesis, biologic evaluation and SARs analysis of O-methylated analogs of quercetin as thrombin inhibitors. *Eur. J. Med. Chem.,* **2012**, *54*, 210-222.
[http://dx.doi.org/10.1016/j.ejmech.2012.04.044] [PMID: 22647223]

[36]   Gliszczyńska-Świgło, A.; van der Woude, H.; de Haan, L.; Tyrakowska, B.; Aarts, J. M. M. J. G.; Rietjens, I. M. C. M. The role of quinone reductase (NQO1) and quinone chemistry in quercetin cytotoxicity. *Toxicology in vitro.,* **2003**, *17*(4), 423-431.
[http://dx.doi.org/10.1016/S0887-2333(03)00047-X]

[37]   Echeverry, C. Pretreatment with Natural Flavones and Neuronal Cell Survival after Oxidative Stress: A Structure–Activity Relationship Study. *J. Agricul. Food. Chem.,* **2010**, *58*(4), 2111-2115.
[http://dx.doi.org/10.1021/jf902951v]

[38]   Khan, H.; Ullah, H.; Aschner, M.; Cheang, W.S.; Akkol, E.K. Neuroprotective Effects of Quercetin in Alzheimer's Disease. *Biomolecules.,* **2019**, *10*(1), 59.
[http://dx.doi.org/10.3390/biom10010059]

[39]   Alok, S.; Jain, S. K.; Verma, A.; Kumar, M.; Mahor, A.; Sabharwal, M. Herbal antioxidant in clinical practice: A review. *Asian Pac. J. Trop. Biomed.,* **2014**, *4*(1), 78-84.
[http://dx.doi.org/10.1016/S2221-1691(14)60213-6]

[40]   Costa, L.G.; Garrick, J.M.; Roquè, P.J.; Pellacani, C. Mechanisms of Neuroprotection by Quercetin: Counteracting Oxidative Stress and More. *Oxid. Med. Cell. Longev.,* **2016**, *2016*, 1-10.
[http://dx.doi.org/10.1155/2016/2986796] [PMID: 26904161]

[41]   Suganthy, N.; Devi, K.P.; Nabavi, S.F.; Braidy, N.; Nabavi, S.M. Bioactive effects of quercetin in the central nervous system: Focusing on the mechanisms of actions. *Biomed. Pharmacother.,* **2016**, *84*, 892-908.
[http://dx.doi.org/10.1016/j.biopha.2016.10.011] [PMID: 27756054]

[42]   Newcomb, R.D.; Crowhurst, R.N.; Gleave, A.P.; Rikkerink, E.H.A.; Allan, A.C.; Beuning, L.L.; Bowen, J.H.; Gera, E.; Jamieson, K.R.; Janssen, B.J.; Laing, W.A.; McArtney, S.; Nain, B.; Ross, G.S.; Snowden, K.C.; Souleyre, E.J.F.; Walton, E.F.; Yauk, Y.K. Analyses of expressed sequence tags from apple. *Plant Physiol.,* **2006**, *141*(1), 147-166.
[http://dx.doi.org/10.1104/pp.105.076208] [PMID: 16531485]

[43]   Huang, W.-y.; Zhang, H.-c.; Liu, W.-x.; Li, C.-y. Survey of antioxidant capacity and phenolic composition of blueberry, blackberry, and strawberry in Nanjing. *J. Zhejiang Univ. Sci. B.,* **2012**, *vol.*

13(2), 94-102.
[http://dx.doi.org/10.1631/jzus.B1100137]

[44] Roopchand, D.E.; Kuhn, P.; Rojo, L.E.; Lila, M.A.; Raskin, I. Blueberry polyphenol-enriched soybean flour reduces hyperglycemia, body weight gain and serum cholesterol in mice. *Pharmacol. Res.,* **2013**, *68*(1), 59-67.
[http://dx.doi.org/10.1016/j.phrs.2012.11.008] [PMID: 23220243]

[45] Boussahel, S. Flavonoid profile, antioxidant and cytotoxic activity of different extracts from *Algerian Rhamnus alaternus* L. bark. *(in eng), Pharmacogn Mag.,* **2015**, *11*(1), 102-109.
[http://dx.doi.org/10.4103/0973-1296.157707]

[46] Street, R.A.; Sidana, J.; Prinsloo, G. Cichorium intybus: Traditional Uses, Phytochemistry, Pharmacology, and Toxicology. *Evid. Based Complementary Altern. Med.,* **2013**, *2013*(579319).
[http://dx.doi.org/10.1155/2013/579319]

[47] Neto, C. C.; Amoroso, J. W.; Liberty, A. M. Anticancer activities of cranberry phytochemicals: an update. *Mol. Nutr. Food. Res.,* **2008**, *52*(1), 18-27.
[http://dx.doi.org/10.1002/mnfr.200700433]

[48] Leone, A.; Spada, A.; Battezzati, A.; Schiraldi, A.; Aristil, J.; Bertoli, S. Cultivation, Genetic, Ethnopharmacology, Phytochemistry and Pharmacology of *Moringa oleifera* Leaves: An Overview. *Int. J. Mol. Sci.,* **2015**, *16*(12), 12791-12835.
[http://dx.doi.org/10.3390/ijms160612791] [PMID: 26057747]

[49] Saini, R. K.; Sivanesan, I.; Keum, Y.-S. Phytochemicals of *Moringa oleifera*: a review of their nutritional, therapeutic and industrial significance. *3 Biotech.,* **2016**, *6*(2), 203.
[http://dx.doi.org/10.1007/s13205-016-0526-3]

[50] Apati, P. HPLC Analysis of the flavonoids in pharmaceutical preparations from canadian goldenrod (*Solidago canadensis*). *Chromatographia.,* **2002**, *56*(1), 65-68.
[http://dx.doi.org/10.1007/BF02494115]

[51] Manela, N. Phenylalanine and tyrosine levels are rate-limiting factors in production of health promoting metabolites in Vitis vinifera cv. Gamay Red cell suspension. *Front. Plant. Sci.,* **2015**, *6*(538).
[http://dx.doi.org/10.3389/fpls.2015.00538]

[52] Zhou, X.-Q.; Zeng, X.-N.; Kong, H.; Sun, X.-L. Neuroprotective effects of berberine on stroke models *in vitro* and *in vivo. Neuroscience Letters.,* **2008**, *447*(1), 31-36.
[http://dx.doi.org/10.1016/j.neulet.2008.09.064]

[53] Thakur, D.; Das, S. C.; Sabhapondit, S.; Tamuly, P.; Deka, D. K. Antimicrobial Activities of Tocklai Vegetative Tea Clones. *Ind. J. Microbiol.,* **2011**, *51*, 450-455.
[http://dx.doi.org/10.1007/s12088-011-0190-6]

[54] Altaf, R.; Asmawi, M.B.; Dewa, A.; Sadikun, A.; Umar, M. Phytochemistry and medicinal properties of Phaleria macrocarpa (Scheff.) Boerl. extracts. *Pharmacogn. Rev.,* **2013**, *7*(1), 73-80.
[http://dx.doi.org/10.4103/0973-7847.112853] [PMID: 23922460]

[55] Chan, P.C.; Xia, Q.; Fu, P.P. Ginkgo biloba leave extract: biological, medicinal, and toxicological effects. *J. Environ. Sci. Health Part C Environ. Carcinog. Ecotoxicol. Rev.,* **2007**, *25*(3), 211-244.
[http://dx.doi.org/10.1080/10590500701569414] [PMID: 17763047]

[56] Gondi, M.; Prasada Rao, U.J.S. Ethanol extract of mango (*Mangifera indica* L.) peel inhibits α-amylase and α-glucosidase activities, and ameliorates diabetes related biochemical parameters in streptozotocin (STZ)-induced diabetic rats. *J. Food Sci. Technol.,* **2015**, *52*(12), 7883-7893.
[http://dx.doi.org/10.1007/s13197-015-1963-4] [PMID: 26604360]

[57] Kaur, T.; Hussain, K.; Koul, S.; Vishwakarma, R.; Vyas, D. Evaluation of nutritional and antioxidant status of *Lepidium latifolium* Linn.: a novel phytofood from Ladakh. *PLoS One.,* **2013**, *8*(8), e69112.
[http://dx.doi.org/10.1371/journal.pone.0069112] [PMID: 23936316]

[58]   Srivastava, M.; Hegde, M.; Chiruvella, K.K.; Koroth, J.; Bhattacharya, S.; Choudhary, B.; Raghavan, S.C. Sapodilla plum (Achras sapota) induces apoptosis in cancer cell lines and inhibits tumor progression in mice. *Sci. Rep.,* **2015**, *4*(1), 6147.
        [http://dx.doi.org/10.1038/srep06147] [PMID: 25142835]

[59]   Aman, U.; Subhan, F.; Shahid, M.; Akbar, S.; Ahmad, N.; Ali, G.; Fawad, K.; Sewell, R.D.E. Passiflora incarnata attenuation of neuropathic allodynia and vulvodynia apropos GABA-ergic and opioidergic antinociceptive and behavioural mechanisms. *BMC Complement. Altern. Med.,* **2016**, *16*(1), 77.
        [http://dx.doi.org/10.1186/s12906-016-1048-6] [PMID: 26912265]

[60]   Choudhary, M.; Kumar, V.; Malhotra, H.; Singh, S. Medicinal plants with potential anti-arthritic activity. *J. Intercult. Ethnopharmacol.,* **2015**, *4*(2), 147-179.
        [http://dx.doi.org/10.5455/jice.20150313021918] [PMID: 26401403]

[61]   Oliveira, A. P. Targeted metabolites and biological activities of Cydonia oblonga Miller leaves. *Food. Res. Int.,* **2012**, *46*(2), 496-504.
        [http://dx.doi.org/10.1016/j.foodres.2010.10.021]

[62]   Henagan, T. M. *in vivo* effects of dietary quercetin and quercetin-rich red onion extract on skeletal muscle mitochondria, metabolism, and insulin sensitivity. *Genes & Nutrition.,* **2014**, *10*(1), 2.

[63]   Oliveira, T.T.; Campos, K.M.; Cerqueira-Lima, A.T.; Cana Brasil Carneiro, T.; da Silva Velozo, E.; Ribeiro Melo, I.C.A.; Figueiredo, E.A.; de Jesus Oliveira, E.; de Vasconcelos, D.F.S.A.; Pontes-d--Carvalho, L.C.; Alcântara-Neves, N.M.; Figueiredo, C.A. Potential therapeutic effect of *Allium cepa* L. and quercetin in a murine model of Blomia tropicalis induced asthma. *Daru.,* **2015**, *23*(1), 18.
        [http://dx.doi.org/10.1186/s40199-015-0098-5] [PMID: 25890178]

[64]   Bozack, A. Effect of Organic and Conventional Farming Practices on Quercetin Content in Spinach, *Spinacia oleracea* **2006**, *5*(8), 1-15.

[65]   Bovy, A.; Schijlen, E.; Hall, R.D. Metabolic engineering of flavonoids in tomato (*Solanum lycopersicum*): the potential for metabolomics. *Metabolomics.,* **2007**, *3*(3), 399-412.
        [http://dx.doi.org/10.1007/s11306-007-0074-2] [PMID: 25653576]

[66]   Benedek, B.; Kopp, B. Achillea millefolium L. s.l. revisited: Recent findings confirm the traditional use. *Wiener Medizinische Wochenschrift.,* **2007**, *157*(13), 312-314.

[67]   Y. Teimoori-Boghsani, M. B. Bagherieh-Najjar, M. J. Mianabadi, and By-product, Investigation of phytochemical and antioxidant capacity of Fennel (*Foeniculum vulgare* Mill.) against gout. vol. 7, no. 1, pp. 59-65, 2018.

[68]   Prior, R.L. Fruits and vegetables in the prevention of cellular oxidative damage. *Am. J. Clin. Nutr.,* **2003**, *78*(3) Suppl., 570S-578S.
        [http://dx.doi.org/10.1093/ajcn/78.3.570S] [PMID: 12936951]

[69]   Harborne, J.B.; Williams, C.A. Advances in flavonoid research since 1992. *Phytochem.,* **2000**, *55*(6), 481-504.
        [http://dx.doi.org/10.1016/S0031-9422(00)00235-1] [PMID: 11130659]

[70]   Magar, R. T.; Sohng, J. K. A review on structure, modifications and structure-activity relation of quercetin and its derivatives. *J Microbiol Biotechnol.,* **2020**, *30*(1).
        [http://dx.doi.org/10.4014/jmb.1907.07003]

[71]   Lesjak, M.; Beara, I.; Simin, N.; Pintać, D.; Majkić, T.; Bekvalac, K.; Orčić, D.; Mimica-Dukić, N. Antioxidant and anti-inflammatory activities of quercetin and its derivatives. *J. Funct. Foods.,* **2018**, *40*, 68-75.
        [http://dx.doi.org/10.1016/j.jff.2017.10.047]

[72]   Rice-Evans, C.A.; Miller, N.J.; Paganga, G. Structure-antioxidant activity relationships of flavonoids and phenolic acids. *Free Radic. Biol. Med.,* **1996**, *20*(7), 933-956.
        [http://dx.doi.org/10.1016/0891-5849(95)02227-9] [PMID: 8743980]

[73] Santos, A.C.; Uyemura, S.A.; Lopes, J.L.C.; Bazon, J.N.; Mingatto, F.E.; Curti, C. Effect of naturally occurring flavonoids on lipid peroxidation and membrane permeability transition in mitochondria. *Free Radic. Biol. Med.,* **1998**, *24*(9), 1455-1461.
[http://dx.doi.org/10.1016/S0891-5849(98)00003-3] [PMID: 9641263]

[74] Lee, C.W.; Seo, J.Y.; Lee, J.; Choi, J.W.; Cho, S.; Bae, J.Y.; Sohng, J.K.; Kim, S.O.; Kim, J.; Park, Y.I. 3-O-Glucosylation of quercetin enhances inhibitory effects on the adipocyte differentiation and lipogenesis. *Biomed. Pharmacother.,* **2017**, *95*, 589-598.
[http://dx.doi.org/10.1016/j.biopha.2017.08.002] [PMID: 28869898]

[75] Sabogal-Guáqueta, A. M.; Muñoz-Manco, J. I.; Ramírez-Pineda, J. R.; Lamprea-Rodriguez, M.; Osorio, E.; Cardona-Gómez, G. P. The flavonoid quercetin ameliorates Alzheimer's disease pathology and protects cognitive and emotional function in aged triple transgenic Alzheimer's disease model mice. *Neuropharmacology.,* **2015**, *93*, 134-145.
[http://dx.doi.org/10.1016/j.neuropharm.2015.01.027]

[76] Jiang, W.; Luo, T.; Li, S.; Zhou, Y.; Shen, X.Y.; He, F.; Xu, J.; Wang, H.Q. Quercetin Protects against Okadaic Acid-Induced Injury *via* MAPK and PI3K/Akt/GSK3β Signaling Pathways in HT22 Hippocampal Neurons. *PLoS One.,* **2016**, *11*(4), e0152371.
[http://dx.doi.org/10.1371/journal.pone.0152371] [PMID: 27050422]

[77] Wang, D-M.; Li, S-Q.; Wu, W-L.; Zhu, X-Y.; Wang, Y.; Yuan, H-Y. Effects of Long-Term Treatment with Quercetin on Cognition and Mitochondrial Function in a Mouse Model of Alzheimer's Disease. In: *Neurochemi. Res*; , **2014**; 39, pp. (8)1533-1543.

[78] Yang, L.; Liu, Y.; Wang, M.; Qian, Y.; Dong, X.; Gu, H.; Wang, H.; Guo, S.; Hisamitsu, T. Quercetin-induced apoptosis of HT-29 colon cancer cells *via* inhibition of the Akt-CSN6-Myc signaling axis. *Mol. Med. Rep.,* **2016**, *14*(5), 4559-4566.
[http://dx.doi.org/10.3892/mmr.2016.5818] [PMID: 27748879]

[79] Zhang, J.; Onakpoya, I.J.; Posadzki, P.; Eddouks, M. The safety of herbal medicine: from prejudice to evidence. *Evidence-Based Complementary. Altern. Med.,* **2015**, 2015.

[80] Psahoulia, F.H.; Drosopoulos, K.G.; Doubravska, L.; Andera, L.; Pintzas, A. Quercetin enhances TRAIL-mediated apoptosis in colon cancer cells by inducing the accumulation of death receptors in lipid rafts. *Mol. Cancer Ther.,* **2007**, *6*(9), 2591-2599.
[http://dx.doi.org/10.1158/1535-7163.MCT-07-0001] [PMID: 17876056]

[81] Shen, X.; Si, Y.; Wang, Z.; Wang, J.; Guo, Y.; Zhang, X. Quercetin inhibits the growth of human gastric cancer stem cells by inducing mitochondrial-dependent apoptosis through the inhibition of PI3K/Akt signaling. *Int. J. Mol. Med.,* **2016**, *38*(2), 619-626.
[http://dx.doi.org/10.3892/ijmm.2016.2625] [PMID: 27278820]

[82] Li, H.; Chen, C. Quercetin has antimetastatic effects on gastric cancer cells *via* the interruption of uPA/uPAR function by modulating NF-κb, PKC-δ, ERK1/2, and AMPKα. *Integr. Cancer Ther.,* **2018**, *17*(2), 511-523.
[http://dx.doi.org/10.1177/1534735417696702]

[83] Wang, K.; Liu, R.; Li, J.; Mao, J.; Lei, Y.; Wu, J.; Zeng, J.; Zhang, T.; Wu, H.; Chen, L.; Huang, C.; Wei, Y. Quercetin induces protective autophagy in gastric cancer cells: Involvement of Akt-mTOR- and hypoxia-induced factor 1α-mediated signaling. *Autophagy.,* **2011**, *7*(9), 966-978.
[http://dx.doi.org/10.4161/auto.7.9.15863] [PMID: 21610320]

[84] Ward, A.B.; Mir, H.; Kapur, N.; Gales, D.N.; Carriere, P.P.; Singh, S. Quercetin inhibits prostate cancer by attenuating cell survival and inhibiting anti-apoptotic pathways. *World J. Surg. Oncol.,* **2018**, *16*(1), 108-108.
[http://dx.doi.org/10.1186/s12957-018-1400-z] [PMID: 29898731]

[85] Xing, N.; Chen, Y.; Mitchell, S.H.; Young, C.Y.F. Quercetin inhibits the expression and function of the androgen receptor in LNCaP prostate cancer cells. *Carcinogenesis.,* **2001**, *22*(3), 409-414.
[http://dx.doi.org/10.1093/carcin/22.3.409] [PMID: 11238180]

[86]   Xingyu, Z.; Peijie, M.; Dan, P.; Youg, W.; Daojun, W.; Xinzheng, C.; Xijun, Z.; Yangrong, S. Quercetin suppresses lung cancer growth by targeting Aurora B kinase. *Cancer Med.*, **2016**, *5*(11), 3156-3165.
[http://dx.doi.org/10.1002/cam4.891] [PMID: 27704720]

[87]   Yang, J.H.; Hsia, T.C.; Kuo, H.M.; Chao, P.D.L.; Chou, C.C.; Wei, Y.H.; Chung, J.G. Inhibition of lung cancer cell growth by quercetin glucuronides *via* G2/M arrest and induction of apoptosis. *Drug Metab. Dispos.*, **2006**, *34*(2), 296-304.
[http://dx.doi.org/10.1124/dmd.105.005280] [PMID: 16280456]

[88]   Wang, R.; Yang, L.; Li, S.; Ye, D.; Yang, L.; Liu, Q.; Zhao, Z.; Cai, Q.; Tan, J.; Li, X. Quercetin Inhibits Breast Cancer Stem Cells *via* Downregulation of Aldehyde Dehydrogenase 1A1 (ALDH1A1), Chemokine Receptor Type 4 (CXCR4), Mucin 1 (MUC1), and Epithelial Cell Adhesion Molecule (EpCAM). *Med. Sci. Monit.*, **2018**, *24*, 412-420.
[http://dx.doi.org/10.12659/MSM.908022] [PMID: 29353288]

[89]   Chien, S.Y.; Wu, Y.C.; Chung, J.G.; Yang, J.S.; Lu, H.F.; Tsou, M.F.; Wood, W.G.; Kuo, S.J.; Chen, D.R. Quercetin-induced apoptosis acts through mitochondrial- and caspase-3-dependent pathways in human breast cancer MDA-MB-231 cells. *Hum. Exp. Toxicol.*, **2009**, *28*(8), 493-503.
[http://dx.doi.org/10.1177/0960327109107002] [PMID: 19755441]

[90]   Akbas, S.H.; Timur, M.; Ozben, T. The effect of quercetin on topotecan cytotoxicity in MCF-7 and MDA-MB 231 human breast cancer cells. *J. Surg. Res.*, **2005**, *125*(1), 49-55.
[http://dx.doi.org/10.1016/j.jss.2004.11.011] [PMID: 15836850]

[91]   Cao, C. Quercetin Mediates β-Catenin in Pancreatic Cancer Stem-Like Cells (in eng). *Pancreas.*, **2015**, *44*(8), 1334-1339.
[http://dx.doi.org/10.1097/MPA.0000000000000400]

[92]   Nickel, T.; Hanssen, H.; Sisic, Z.; Pfeiler, S.; Summo, C.; Schmauss, D.; Hoster, E.; Weis, M. Immunoregulatory effects of the flavonol quercetin *in vitro* and *in vivo*. *Eur. J. Nutr.*, **2011**, *50*(3), 163-172.
[http://dx.doi.org/10.1007/s00394-010-0125-8] [PMID: 20652710]

[93]   Jin, H.B.; Yang, Y.B.; Song, Y.L.; Zhang, Y.; Li, Y.R. Protective roles of quercetin in acute myocardial ischemia and reperfusion injury in rats. *Mol. Biol. Rep.*, **2012**, *39*(12), 11005-11009.
[http://dx.doi.org/10.1007/s11033-012-2002-4] [PMID: 23053990]

[94]   Li, B.; Yang, M.; Liu, J.W.; Yin, G.T. Protective mechanism of quercetin on acute myocardial infarction in rats. *Genet. Mol. Res.*, **2016**, *15*(1), 15017117.
[http://dx.doi.org/10.4238/gmr.15017117] [PMID: 26985950]

[95]   Zaafan, M. A.; Zaki, H. F.; El-Brairy, A. I.; Kenawy, S. A. Protective effects of atorvastatin and quercetin on isoprenaline-induced myocardial infarction in rats. *Bull. Fac. Pharm. Cairo Univ.*, **2013**, *51*(1), 35-41.
[http://dx.doi.org/10.1016/j.bfopcu.2013.03.001]

[96]   Li, M.; Jiang, Y.; Jing, W.; Sun, B.; Miao, C.; Ren, L. Quercetin provides greater cardioprotective effect than its glycoside derivative rutin on isoproterenol-induced cardiac fibrosis in the rat. *Can. J. Physiol. Pharmacol.*, **2013**, *91*(11), 951-959.
[http://dx.doi.org/10.1139/cjpp-2012-0432] [PMID: 24117263]

[97]   Chen, J.-Y.; Hu, R.-Y.; Chou, H.-C. Quercetin-induced cardioprotection against doxorubicin cytotoxicity. *J. Biomedi. Sci.*, **2013**, *20*(1), 95.
[http://dx.doi.org/10.1186/1423-0127-20-95]

[98]   Davis, J.M.; Murphy, E.A.; Carmichael, M.D. Effects of the dietary flavonoid quercetin upon performance and health. *Curr. Sports Med. Rep.*, **2009**, *8*(4), 206-213.
[http://dx.doi.org/10.1249/JSR.0b013e3181ae8959] [PMID: 19584608]

[99]   Read, M.A. Flavonoids: naturally occurring anti-inflammatory agents. *Am. J. Pathol.*, **1995**, *147*(2),

235-237.
[PMID: 7639322]

[100] Oršolić, N.; Knežević, A.H.; Šver, L.; Terzić, S.; Bašić, I. Immunomodulatory and antimetastatic action of propolis and related polyphenolic compounds. *J. Ethnopharmacol.,* **2004**, *94*(2-3), 307-315.
[http://dx.doi.org/10.1016/j.jep.2004.06.006] [PMID: 15325736]

[101] Batiha, G.E.S.; Beshbishy, A.M.; Ikram, M.; Mulla, Z.S.; El-Hack, M.E.A.; Taha, A.E.; Algammal, A.M.; Elewa, Y.H.A. The pharmacological activity, biochemical properties, and pharmacokinetics of the major natural polyphenolic flavonoid: quercetin. *Foods.,* **2020**, *9*(3), 374.
[http://dx.doi.org/10.3390/foods9030374] [PMID: 32210182]

[102] Bureau, G.; Longpré, F.; Martinoli, M.G. Resveratrol and quercetin, two natural polyphenols, reduce apoptotic neuronal cell death induced by neuroinflammation. *J. Neurosci. Res.,* **2008**, *86*(2), 403-410.
[http://dx.doi.org/10.1002/jnr.21503] [PMID: 17929310]

[103] Kim, H.P.; Mani, I.; Iversen, L.; Ziboh, V.A. Effects of naturally-occurring flavonoids and biflavonoids on epidermal cyclooxygenase and lipoxygenase from guinea-pigs. *Prostaglandins Leukot. Essent. Fatty Acids.,* **1998**, *58*(1), 17-24.
[http://dx.doi.org/10.1016/S0952-3278(98)90125-9] [PMID: 9482162]

[104] Lee, K.M.; Hwang, M.K.; Lee, D.E.; Lee, K.W.; Lee, H.J. Protective effect of quercetin against arsenite-induced COX-2 expression by targeting PI3K in rat liver epithelial cells. *J. Agric. Food Chem.,* **2010**, *58*(9), 5815-5820.
[http://dx.doi.org/10.1021/jf903698s] [PMID: 20377179]

[105] Endale, M.; Park, S.C.; Kim, S.; Kim, S.H.; Yang, Y.; Cho, J.Y.; Rhee, M.H. Quercetin disrupts tyrosine-phosphorylated phosphatidylinositol 3-kinase and myeloid differentiation factor-88 association, and inhibits MAPK/AP-1 and IKK/NF-κB-induced inflammatory mediators production in RAW 264.7 cells. *Immunobiology.,* **2013**, *218*(12), 1452-1467.
[http://dx.doi.org/10.1016/j.imbio.2013.04.019] [PMID: 23735482]

[106] Yang, D.; Liu, X.; Liu, M.; Chi, H.; Liu, J.; Han, H. Protective effects of quercetin and taraxasterol against H_2O_2-induced human umbilical vein endothelial cell injury *in vitro*. *Exp. Ther. Med.,* **2015**, *10*(4), 1253-1260.
[http://dx.doi.org/10.3892/etm.2015.2713] [PMID: 26622474]

[107] Chirumbolo, S. The role of quercetin, flavonols and flavones in modulating inflammatory cell function.," Inflammation & Allergy-Drug Targets (Formerly Current Drug Targets-Inflammation & Allergy)(Discontinued) **2010**, *9*(4), 263-285.
[http://dx.doi.org/10.2174/187152810793358741]

[108] D'Andrea, G. Quercetin: A flavonol with multifaceted therapeutic applications?. *Fitoterapia.,* **2015**, *106*, 256-271.
[http://dx.doi.org/10.1016/j.fitote.2015.09.018] [PMID: 26393898]

[109] Jung, J.H.; Kang, J.I.; Kim, H.S. Effect of quercetin on impaired immune function in mice exposed to irradiation. *Nutr. Res. Pract.,* **2012**, *6*(4), 301-307.
[http://dx.doi.org/10.4162/nrp.2012.6.4.301] [PMID: 22977683]

[110] Dong, Y.; Wang, J.; Feng, D.; Qin, H.; Wen, H.; Yin, Z.; Gao, G.; Li, C. Protective effect of quercetin against oxidative stress and brain edema in an experimental rat model of subarachnoid hemorrhage. *Int. J. Med. Sci.,* **2014**, *11*(3), 282-290.
[http://dx.doi.org/10.7150/ijms.7634] [PMID: 24516353]

[111] Kandere-Grzybowska, K.; Kempuraj, D.; Cao, J.; Cetrulo, C.L.; Theoharides, T.C. Regulation of IL--induced selective IL-6 release from human mast cells and inhibition by quercetin. *Br. J. Pharmacol.,* **2006**, *148*(2), 208-215.
[http://dx.doi.org/10.1038/sj.bjp.0706695] [PMID: 16532021]

[112] Milenković, M.; Arsenović-Ranin, N.; Stojić-Vukanić, Z.; Bufan, B.; Vučićević, D.; Jančić, I. Quercetin ameliorates experimental autoimmune myocarditis in rats. *J. Pharm. Pharm. Sci.,* **2010**,

13(3), 311-319.
[http://dx.doi.org/10.18433/J3VS3S] [PMID: 21092705]

[113]   Kobori, M.; Takahashi, Y.; Sakurai, M.; Akimoto, Y.; Tsushida, T.; Oike, H.; Ippoushi, K. Quercetin suppresses immune cell accumulation and improves mitochondrial gene expression in adipose tissue of diet-induced obese mice. *Mol. Nutr. Food Res.,* **2016**, *60*(2), 300-312.
[http://dx.doi.org/10.1002/mnfr.201500595] [PMID: 26499876]

[114]   Comalada, M.; Camuesco, D.; Sierra, S.; Ballester, I.; Xaus, J.; Gálvez, J.; Zarzuelo, A. *in vivo* quercitrin anti-inflammatory effect involves release of quercetin, which inhibits inflammation through down-regulation of the NF-κB pathway. *Eur. J. Immunol.,* **2005**, *35*(2), 584-592.
[http://dx.doi.org/10.1002/eji.200425778] [PMID: 15668926]

[115]   Nijveldt, R.J.; van Nood, E.; van Hoorn, D.E.C.; Boelens, P.G.; van Norren, K.; van Leeuwen, P.A.M. Flavonoids: a review of probable mechanisms of action and potential applications. *Am. J. Clin. Nutr.,* **2001**, *74*(4), 418-425.
[http://dx.doi.org/10.1093/ajcn/74.4.418] [PMID: 11566638]

[116]   Wang, W.; Sun, C.; Mao, L.; Ma, P.; Liu, F.; Yang, J.; Gao, Y. The biological activities, chemical stability, metabolism and delivery systems of quercetin: A review. *Trends Food Sci. Technol.,* **2016**, *56*, 21-38.
[http://dx.doi.org/10.1016/j.tifs.2016.07.004]

[117]   Xu, H. Anti-malarial agent artesunate inhibits TNF-α-induced production of proinflammatory cytokines *via* inhibition of NF-κB and PI3 kinase/Akt signal pathway in human rheumatoid arthritis fibroblast-like synoviocytes. *Rheumatology (Oxford).,* **2007**, *46*(6), 920-926.

[118]   Haddad, P.; Eid, H. The antidiabetic potential of quercetin: underlying mechanisms. *Curr. Med. Chem.,* **2017**, *24*(4), 355-364.
[http://dx.doi.org/10.2174/0929867323666160909153707] [PMID: 27633685]

[119]   AL-Ishaq, R.K.; Abotaleb, M.; Kubatka, P.; Kajo, K.; Büsselberg, D. Flavonoids and their anti-diabetic effects: cellular mechanisms and effects to improve blood sugar levels. *Biomolecules.,* **2019**, *9*(9), 430.
[http://dx.doi.org/10.3390/biom9090430] [PMID: 31480505]

[120]   Bule, M.; Abdurahman, A.; Nikfar, S.; Abdollahi, M.; Amini, M. Antidiabetic effect of quercetin: A systematic review and meta-analysis of animal studies. *Food Chem. Toxicol.,* **2019**, *125*, 494-502.
[http://dx.doi.org/10.1016/j.fct.2019.01.037] [PMID: 30735748]

[121]   Eid, H.M.; Martineau, L.C.; Saleem, A.; Muhammad, A.; Vallerand, D.; Benhaddou-Andaloussi, A.; Nistor, L.; Afshar, A.; Arnason, J.T.; Haddad, P.S. Stimulation of AMP-activated protein kinase and enhancement of basal glucose uptake in muscle cells by quercetin and quercetin glycosides, active principles of the antidiabetic medicinal plant Vaccinium vitis-idaea. *Mol. Nutr. Food Res.,* **2010**, *54*(7), 991-1003.
[http://dx.doi.org/10.1002/mnfr.200900218] [PMID: 20087853]

[122]   Coskun, O.; Kanter, M.; Korkmaz, A.; Oter, S. Quercetin, a flavonoid antioxidant, prevents and protects streptozotocin-induced oxidative stress and β-cell damage in rat pancreas. *Pharmacol. Res.,* **2005**, *51*(2), 117-123.
[http://dx.doi.org/10.1016/j.phrs.2004.06.002]

[123]   Kobori, M.; Masumoto, S.; Akimoto, Y.; Takahashi, Y. Dietary quercetin alleviates diabetic symptoms and reduces streptozotocin-induced disturbance of hepatic gene expression in mice. *Mol. Nutr. Food Res.,* **2009**, *53*(7), 859-868.
[http://dx.doi.org/10.1002/mnfr.200800310] [PMID: 19496084]

[124]   Vessal, M.; Hemmati, M.; Vasei, M. Antidiabetic effects of quercetin in streptozocin-induced diabetic rats. *Comp. Biochem. Physiol. C Toxicol. Pharmacol.,* **2003**, *135*(3), 357-364.
[http://dx.doi.org/10.1016/S1532-0456(03)00140-6] [PMID: 12927910]

[125]   Haddad, P.S.; Eid, H.M.; Nachar, A.; Thong, F.; Sweeney, G. The molecular basis of the antidiabetic

action of quercetin in cultured skeletal muscle cells and hepatocytes. *Pharmacogn. Mag.,* **2015**, *11*(41), 74-81.
[http://dx.doi.org/10.4103/0973-1296.149708] [PMID: 25709214]

[126] Eitah, H.E.; Maklad, Y.A.; Abdelkader, N.F.; Gamal el Din, A.A.; Badawi, M.A.; Kenawy, S.A. Modulating impacts of quercetin/sitagliptin combination on streptozotocin-induced diabetes mellitus in rats. *Toxicol. Appl. Pharmacol.,* **2019**, *365*, 30-40.
[http://dx.doi.org/10.1016/j.taap.2018.12.011] [PMID: 30576699]

[127] Dai, X.; Ding, Y.; Zhang, Z.; Cai, X.; Li, Y. Quercetin and quercitrin protect against cytokine-induced injuries in RINm5F β-cells *via* the mitochondrial pathway and NF-κB signaling. *Int. J. Mol. Med.,* **2013**, *31*(1), 265-271.
[http://dx.doi.org/10.3892/ijmm.2012.1177] [PMID: 23138875]

[128] Jeong, S.M.; Kang, M.J.; Choi, H.N.; Kim, J.H.; Kim, J.I. Quercetin ameliorates hyperglycemia and dyslipidemia and improves antioxidant status in type 2 diabetic db/db mice. *Nutr. Res. Pract.,* **2012**, *6*(3), 201-207.
[http://dx.doi.org/10.4162/nrp.2012.6.3.201] [PMID: 22808343]

[129] Boots, A.W.; Haenen, G.R.M.M.; Bast, A. Health effects of quercetin: From antioxidant to nutraceutical. *Eur. J. Pharmacol.,* **2008**, *585*(2-3), 325-337.
[http://dx.doi.org/10.1016/j.ejphar.2008.03.008] [PMID: 18417116]

[130] Halliwell, B. Oxidative stress, nutrition and health. Experimental strategies for optimization of nutritional antioxidant intake in humans. *Free Radic. Res.,* **1996**, *25*(1), 57-74.
[http://dx.doi.org/10.3109/10715769609145656] [PMID: 8814444]

[131] Askari, G.; Ghiasvand, R.; Feizi, A.; Ghanadian, S. M.; Karimian, J. The effect of quercetin supplementation on selected markers of inflammation and oxidative stress. *J Res Med Sci: Off. J. Isfahan. Univ. Med. Sci.,* **2012**, *17*(7), 637.

[132] Costa, L.G.; Garrick, J.M.; Roquè, P.J.; Pellacani, C. Mechanisms of neuroprotection by quercetin: counteracting oxidative stress and more Oxidative medicine and cellular longevity. In: *Oxid. Med. Cell. Longev;* , **2016**; p. 2016.
[http://dx.doi.org/10.1155/2016/2986796]

[133] Marunaka, Y. Actions of quercetin, a flavonoid, on ion transporters: its physiological roles. *Ann. N. Y. Acad. Sci.,* **2017**, *1398*(1), 142-151.
[http://dx.doi.org/10.1111/nyas.13361] [PMID: 28574574]

[134] Xiao, L.; Luo, G.; Tang, Y.; Yao, P. Quercetin and iron metabolism: What we know and what we need to know. *Food Chem. Toxicol.,* **2018**, *114*, 190-203.
[http://dx.doi.org/10.1016/j.fct.2018.02.022] [PMID: 29432835]

[135] Huang, H.; Liao, D.; Dong, Y.; Pu, R. Effect of quercetin supplementation on plasma lipid profiles, blood pressure, and glucose levels: a systematic review and meta-analysis. *Nutr. Rev.,* **2020**, *78*(8), 615-626.
[http://dx.doi.org/10.1093/nutrit/nuz071] [PMID: 31940027]

[136] Kuipers, E.; Dam, A.; Held, N.; Mol, I.; Houtkooper, R.; Rensen, P.; Boon, M. Quercetin lowers plasma triglycerides accompanied by white adipose tissue browning in diet-induced obese mice. *Int. J. Mol. Sci.,* **2018**, *19*(6), 1786.
[http://dx.doi.org/10.3390/ijms19061786] [PMID: 29914151]

[137] Dong, F.; Wang, S.; Wang, Y.; Yang, X.; Jiang, J.; Wu, D.; Qu, X.; Fan, H.; Yao, R. Quercetin ameliorates learning and memory *via* the Nrf2-ARE signaling pathway in d-galactose-induced neurotoxicity in mice. *Biochem. Biophys. Res. Commun.,* **2017**, *491*(3), 636-641.
[http://dx.doi.org/10.1016/j.bbrc.2017.07.151] [PMID: 28757412]

[138] Paula, P.C.; Angelica Maria, S.G.; Luis, C.H.; Gloria Patricia, C.G. Preventive effect of quercetin in a triple transgenic Alzheimer's disease mice model. *Molecules.,* **2019**, *24*(12), 2287.
[http://dx.doi.org/10.3390/molecules24122287] [PMID: 31226738]

[139] Samini, M. The neuro-protective effects of quercetin. *Res. J. Pharm.Techn.,* **2019**, *12*(2), 561-568.
[http://dx.doi.org/10.5958/0974-360X.2019.00100.8]

[140] Eftekhari, A.; Ahmadian, E.; Panahi-Azar, V.; Hosseini, H.; Tabibiazar, M.; Maleki Dizaj, S. Hepatoprotective and free radical scavenging actions of quercetin nanoparticles on aflatoxin B1-induced liver damage: *in vitro / in vivo* studies. *Artif. Cells Nanomed. Biotechnol.,* **2018**, *46*(2), 411-420.
[http://dx.doi.org/10.1080/21691401.2017.1315427] [PMID: 28423950]

[141] Muñoz-Reyes, D.; Morales, A.I.; Prieto, M. Transit and Metabolic Pathways of Quercetin in Tubular Cells: Involvement of Its Antioxidant Properties in the Kidney. *Antioxidants.,* **2021**, *10*(6), 909.
[http://dx.doi.org/10.3390/antiox10060909] [PMID: 34205156]

[142] Dong, Y.; Lei, J.; Zhang, B. Effects of dietary quercetin on the antioxidative status and cecal microbiota in broiler chickens fed with oxidized oil. *Poult. Sci.,* **2020**, *99*(10), 4892-4903.
[http://dx.doi.org/10.1016/j.psj.2020.06.028] [PMID: 32988526]

[143] Xu, D.; Hu, M.J.; Wang, Y.Q.; Cui, Y.L. Antioxidant activities of quercetin and its complexes for medicinal application. *Molecules.,* **2019**, *24*(6), 1123.
[http://dx.doi.org/10.3390/molecules24061123] [PMID: 30901869]

[144] van der Woude, H.; Boersma, M.G.; Vervoort, J.; Rietjens, I.M.J.C.t. Identification of 14 quercetin phase II mono-and mixed conjugates and their formation by rat and human phase II *in vitro* model systems. *Chem. Res. Toxicol.,* **2004**, *17*(11), 1520-1530.
[http://dx.doi.org/10.1021/tx049826v]

[145] van der Woude, H. Formation of transient covalent protein and DNA adducts by quercetin in cells with and without oxidative enzyme activity *Chem. Res. Toxicol.,* **2005**, *18*(12), 1907-1916.
[http://dx.doi.org/10.1021/tx050201m]

[146] Marseglia, L.; Manti, S.; D'Angelo, G.; Nicotera, A.; Parisi, E.; Di Rosa, G.; Gitto, E.; Arrigo, T. Oxidative stress in obesity: a critical component in human diseases. *Int. J. Mol. Sci.,* **2014**, *16*(1), 378-400.
[http://dx.doi.org/10.3390/ijms16010378] [PMID: 25548896]

[147] Nabavi, S.F.; Russo, G.L.; Daglia, M.; Nabavi, S.M. Role of quercetin as an alternative for obesity treatment: You are what you eat. *Food Chem.,* **2015**, *179*, 305-310.
[http://dx.doi.org/10.1016/j.foodchem.2015.02.006] [PMID: 25722169]

[148] Ahn, J.; Lee, H.; Kim, S.; Park, J.; Ha, T. The anti-obesity effect of quercetin is mediated by the AMPK and MAPK signaling pathways. *Biochem. Biophys. Res. Commun.,* **2008**, *373*(4), 545-549.
[http://dx.doi.org/10.1016/j.bbrc.2008.06.077] [PMID: 18586010]

[149] Qiu, L.; Luo, Y.; Chen, X. Quercetin attenuates mitochondrial dysfunction and biogenesis *via* upregulated AMPK/SIRT1 signaling pathway in OA rats. *Biomed. Pharmacother.,* **2018**, *103*, 1585-1591.
[http://dx.doi.org/10.1016/j.biopha.2018.05.003] [PMID: 29864946]

[150] Shen, Y.; Croft, K.D.; Hodgson, J.M.; Kyle, R.; Lee, I.L.E.; Wang, Y.; Stocker, R.; Ward, N.C. Quercetin and its metabolites improve vessel function by inducing eNOS activity *via* phosphorylation of AMPK. *Biochem. Pharmacol.,* **2012**, *84*(8), 1036-1044.
[http://dx.doi.org/10.1016/j.bcp.2012.07.016] [PMID: 22846602]

[151] Yang, J.Y.; Della-Fera, M.A.; Rayalam, S.; Ambati, S.; Hartzell, D.L.; Park, H.J.; Baile, C.A. Enhanced inhibition of adipogenesis and induction of apoptosis in 3T3-L1 adipocytes with combinations of resveratrol and quercetin. *Life Sci.,* **2008**, *82*(19-20), 1032-1039.
[http://dx.doi.org/10.1016/j.lfs.2008.03.003] [PMID: 18433793]

[152] Arias, N.; Macarulla, M.T.; Aguirre, L.; Martínez-Castaño, M.G.; Portillo, M.P. Quercetin can reduce insulin resistance without decreasing adipose tissue and skeletal muscle fat accumulation. *Genes Nutr.,* **2014**, *9*(1), 361.

[http://dx.doi.org/10.1007/s12263-013-0361-7] [PMID: 24338341]

[153] Khare, T.; Palakurthi, S.S.; Shah, B.M.; Palakurthi, S.; Khare, S. Natural product-based nanomedicine in treatment of inflammatory bowel disease. *Int. J. Mol. Sci.,* **2020**, *21*(11), 3956.
[http://dx.doi.org/10.3390/ijms21113956] [PMID: 32486445]

[154] Hosseini, A.; Razavi, B.M.; Banach, M.; Hosseinzadeh, H. Quercetin and metabolic syndrome: A review. *Phytother. Res.,* **2021**, *35*(10), 5352-5364.
[http://dx.doi.org/10.1002/ptr.7144] [PMID: 34101925]

[155] Ulusoy, H.G.; Sanlier, N. A minireview of quercetin: from its metabolism to possible mechanisms of its biological activities. *Crit. Rev. Food Sci. Nutr.,* **2020**, *60*(19), 3290-3303.
[http://dx.doi.org/10.1080/10408398.2019.1683810] [PMID: 31680558]

[156] Zhao, L.; Zhang, Q.; Ma, W.; Tian, F.; Shen, H.; Zhou, M. A combination of quercetin and resveratrol reduces obesity in high-fat diet-fed rats by modulation of gut microbiota. *Food Funct.,* **2017**, *8*(12), 4644-4656.
[http://dx.doi.org/10.1039/C7FO01383C] [PMID: 29152632]

[157] Zhao, Y. The beneficial effects of quercetin, curcumin, and resveratrol in obesity Oxidative medicine and cellular longevity. *Oxid. Med. Cell. Long.,* **2017**, *2017*.
[http://dx.doi.org/10.1155/2017/1459497]

[158] Zhao, L.; Zhu, X.; Xia, M.; Li, J.; Guo, A.Y.; Zhu, Y.; Yang, X. Quercetin Ameliorates Gut Microbiota Dysbiosis That Drives Hypothalamic Damage and Hepatic Lipogenesis in Monosodium Glutamate-Induced Abdominal Obesity. *Front. Nutr.,* **2021**, *8*, 671353-671353.
[http://dx.doi.org/10.3389/fnut.2021.671353] [PMID: 33996881]

SUBJECT INDEX

www.ingramcontent.com/pod-product-compliance
Lightning Source LLC
Chambersburg PA
CBHW041707210326
41598CB00007B/557